POCKET
MEDICAL DICTIONARY

Pocket
Medical Dictionary

Rohit Kalra

ANMOL PUBLICATIONS PVT. LTD.
NEW DELHI - 110 002 (INDIA)

ANMOL PUBLICATIONS PVT. LTD.

H.O.: 4374/4B, Ansari Road, Darya Ganj,
New Delhi-110 002 (India)
Ph.: 23278000, 23261597

B.O.: No. 1015, Ist Main Road, BSK IIIrd Stage
IIIrd Phase, IIIrd Block,
Bangalore - 560 085 (India)
Visit us at: www.anmolpublications.com

Pocket Medical Dictionary

© Reserved

First Edition, 1997

Reprint, 2006

PRINTED IN INDIA

Printed at Mehra Offset Press, Delhi.

Preface

This dictionary has been written to provide students of Medical Sciences at all levels with a handy and reliable source for the meanings of terms in the field of Medical Terminology. These terms have been carefully selected and presented in brief analytical or functional phrases, thus avoiding the more comprehensive type of treatment appropriate to larger reference works. An attempt has been made to include new terms which have been introduced and have come into usage with the new invention.

An attempt has been made to write the entries in a clear and lucid style to provide both straightforward definitions and invaluable background information. Line drawings have been included whenever the meaning of a word can be best understood by means of a diagram. The network of cross-references has been kept throughout this book.

The dictionary will of value to students of Medical Sciences and to naturalists, geographers and others studying or working in related fields.

The author is happy to give credit here to all those who had a hand in getting the dictionary into its present form. The care and interest took in clearing up complex points so that they might be put in simple English.

In compiling a dictionary of this kind it becomes necessary to draw upon the work of many authorities and seek the advice of colleagues to all of whom the author is deeply indebted.

Finally the author expresses sincere thanks to the publishers and printer for printing this book promptly.

Constructive comments from users on omissions or short comings will be highly appreciated and shall be incorporated in next edition.

Editor

A

Abdomen. The part of the body cavity below the chest from which it is separated by the diaphragm. The abdomen contains the organs of digestion—stomach, liver, intestines, etc.—and excretion—kidneys, bladder, etc.; in women it also contains the ovaries and womb. The regions of the abdomen are shown in the illustration.

Abortion. The expulsion or removal of an embryo or fetus from the womb at a stage of pregnancy when it is incapable of independent survival (i.e., at any time between conception and the 28th week of pregnancy). In *threatened* abortion there is abdominal pain and bleeding from the womb but the fetus is still alive; once the fetus is dead abortion becomes *inevitable*. It is *incomplete* so long as the womb still contains some of the fetus or its membranes. Abortion may be *spontaneous* (a miscarriage) or it may be *induced* for medical or social reasons (termination of pregnancy). The *abortion rate* (the number of pregnancies lost per 1000 conceptions) is impossible to calculate precisely but is generally reckoned to be between one fifth and one third.

Abortus. A fetus, weighing less than 500 g. that is expelled from the mother's body either dead or incapable of surviving.

Abrasion. Superficial skin wound in which usually only a section of the thickness of the skin is lost, but often covering a large surface area, and showing several small points of haemorrhage; it is also called a graze. Although little or no blood is lost, abrasions are painful because the nerve ends in the skin are damaged.

Abscess (boil). Usually a clearly delineated accumulation of pus forming a cavity within inflamed tissue. On or near the surface of the skin an abscess is usually referred to as a boil. Pus is a fluid consisting of dead tissue, white blood corpuscles and bacteria. Whenever tissue is damaged, for whatever reason, the body reacts with inflammation of the affected area, in order to limit the damage and repair it as soon as possible. Sometimes the inflammation can cause further damage.

Acetanilide. A drug that relieves pain and reduces fever. Since it can cause anaemia and prolonged use may lead to habituation, it has largely been replaced by safer analgesics.

Acetazolamide. A diuretic used in the treatment of glaucoma to reduce the pressure inside the eyeball. Side effects include drowsiness and numbness and tingling of the hands and feet. Trade names: **Acetazide, Diamox**.

Acetohexamide. A drug that reduces the level of blood sugar, used in the treatment of diabetes mellitus. It is administered by mouth; side-effects include headache, dizziness, and nervousness. *See also* talbutamide, chlorpropamide.

Achalasia. Condition of the oesophagus characterized by difficulty in moving food down the lowest part of it, caused by degeneration of the associated parasympathetic nerve cells in the oesophagus. The cardiac sphincter, which connects the oesophagus with the stomach, remains closed, and as a result food is pressed against it, causing widening of the oesophagus (mega-oesophagus). The most important symptom is gradually increasing discomfort when swallowing. Fluids and solid food stick at a point level with the top of the breastbone, causing an oppressive sensation, which is aggravated by large quantities of solid foods or cold drinks. Symptoms may remain fairly constant for years, but usually increase in severity. Later there is persistent pain when swallowing, and food is regurgitated. Such food does not taste sour, because it has not yet reached the stomach.

Achlorhydria. Condition in which the stomach fails to produce hydrochloric acid, even after stimulation (with histamines or gastrins). Hydrochloric acid is important because it destroys bacteria in tissue, plays a part in the digestion of protein and affects the absorption of iron and vitamin B_{12} among other things. Despite this, a shortage does not usually have serious consequences. Only if the stomach wall also fails to produce enzymes for the digestion of food (achylia gastrica) can major digestive problems occur, in which case the missing enzymes have to be taken in tablet form.

Achondroplasia. Uncommon congenital malformation of the skeleton caused by an abnormality of the cartilage. The development of cartilage into bone is disturbed before birth.

Growth of the bones of arms and legs in particular is retarded, causing dwarfism. The affected bones are short and thick; the base of the skull remains small, resulting in enlargement of the cranium to accommodate the brain.

Acid. 1. A chemical compound made up of an electronegative ion and one or more hydrogen ions which may be replaced by another electropositive ion such as sodium. 2. Substances which lower the pH of a solution. 3. The opposite of a base in the sense that an acid forms a compound with a base by accepting electrons from it.

Acidosis. Accumulation of acids in the body. Various chemical substances occur in body tissues, and some of them are acidic. Substances that can neutralize these acids are known as bases. For the body to function properly acids and bases need to be balanced. When excessive acidity threatens, the body loses excess acid via the lungs and kidneys.

Acne. (acne vulgaris). Skin condition common in young people at puberty, which usually clears up between the twentieth and twenty-fifth year, although in some people it can persist until the age of thirty.

Acne results when the sebaceous glands in the skin produce more serum (fat) as a result of stimulation by sex hormones.

Acrocyanosis. Fairly rare condition in which the fingers and toes, and in serious cases the hands and feet, turn blue.

The disease occurs mainly in women and girls aged between 10 and 30 years. Small arterial vessels in the fingers and
toes become narrower, while the veins dilate, causing the bluish colour of the venous blood to predominate. The cause is not
known.

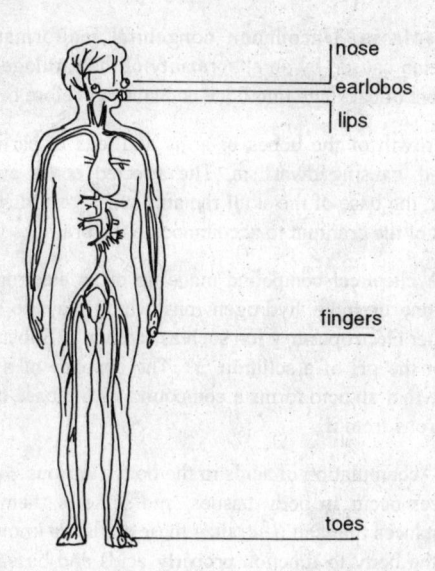

*In acrocyanosis the extremities of the body are coloured
bluish-purple by a disturbance in the arterial blood supply.*

Acromegaly. Growth disturbance in adults, in which overproduction of the growth hormone causes certain parts of the body to
enlarge excessively. Excessive hormone production is usually
caused by a tumour of the pituitary gland.

Actinomycosis. Infection caused by *Actinomyces israeli* bacteria.
It is fairly rare and often occurs in the months of otherwise
healthy people. It can occur in various parts of the body when

gums are inflamed or teeth extracted, and accompanying cases
of persistent inflammation of the lower jaw. A hard, painful,
reddish-blue swelling forms, containing yellow or greyish-white
granular pus. The infection can be transmitted by the pus or
saliva. Other places prone to infection are the lungs and the
abdominal cavity, and from these other organs can be affected
via the bloodstream. It is then a serious condition.

Acupuncture. A traditional Chinese system of healing in which
symptoms are relieved by thin metal needles inserted into selected points beneath the skin. The needles are stimulated
either by rotation or, more recently, by an electric current.

Acute Yellow Atrophy. Rare liver disorder that involves massive
liver cell death (necrosis) as a result of certain liver conditions,
usually hepatitis. The disorder can be very vigorous, in which
case hepatitis develops directly into this life-threatening condition. The condition is characterized by weakness, nausea and
vomiting, pain in the right-hand upper abdomen and jaundice.

Addiction. Psychological and physical dependence on a drug of
stimulant harmful to the user, a self-sustaining process which
the addict is either unable to terminate of his own accord or
can terminate only with great difficulty. The user often needs
more of the substance in order to achieve the same effect (tolerance). As a result of withdrawal symptoms and psychological factors dependence increases and the addict can no longer
do without it.

Addison's Disease. Condition characterized by decreasing production of hormones by the cortex of the adrenal gland (chronic
corticosteroid deficiency). The most important corticosteroid is
hydrocortisone, which maintains blood sugar level and regulates inflammation reactions. Another, aldosterone, plays an
important part in the regulation of water and salt in the body
and of blood pressure. Underproduction of corticosteroids is
usually caused by an autoimmune disease : the body's immune
system produces antibodies which destroy the cells of the ad-
renocortical gland, resulting in tiredness, listlessness and loss
of appetite and weight. Other symptoms are anaemia, abdomi-

nal complaints, thirst, low blood pressure and low blood sugar
level (hypoglycaemia). The skin turns a characteristic brown
colour and in women underarm and public hair disappears.

Adrenal Glands. Adrenals. Two small cones of tissue, one sitting
on top of each kidney. The core or medulla of each gland
produces a hormone, adrenaline. The adrenal cortex or outer
lining of tissue produces a number of different hormones including various sex hormones. The cortical hormones are under control of the pituitary gland by means of a feedback ar-
rangement involving the hormones themselves. Too little hormone in the bloodstream causes the pituitary to release a signal instructing the adrenal cortex to synthesize more. When
the blood level has risen appropriately, the pituitary signal
shuts off. Adrenaline, on the other hand, is produced by medulla cells in response to environmental circumstances either
inside the body or outside.

-AEMIA. Gr: *haem* = blood + ia. Thus, *anaemia* = from
the blood.

Adrenaline (epinephrine) *n.* An important hormone secreted by the
medulla of the adrenal gland. It has the function of preparing
the body for 'fright, flight, or fight' and has widespread effects
on circulation, the muscles, and sugar metabolism. The action
of the heart is increased, the rate and depth of breathing are
increased, and the metabolic rate is raised; the force of muscular cortraction improves and the onset of muscular fatigue is
delayed. At the same time the blood supply to the bladder and
intestines is reduced, their muscular walls relax, and the sphinc-
ters contract. Sympathetic nerves were originally thought to
act by releasing adrenaline at their endings, and were therefore
called *adrenergic* nerves. In fact the main substance released
is the related substance noradrenaline, which also forms a portion of the adrenal secretion.

Adrenaline given by injection is valuable for the relief of
bronchial asthma, because it relaxes constricted airways. It is
also used during surgery to reduce blood loss by constricting
vessels in the skin.

Aflatoxin. A poisonous substance produced in the spores of the fungus *Aspergillus flavus*, which infects peanuts. The toxin is known to produce cancer in certain animals and is suspected of being the causes of liver cancers in human beings living in warm and humid regions of the world, where stored nuts and cereals are contaminated by the fungus.

Agammaglobulinanaemia. Shortage of blood proteins (gamma globulins), antibodies that are a defence against bacteria and infection. To render bacteria harmless the body needs proteins made by white blood cells, the lymphocytes. Agammaglobulinanaemia can be conganitel or occur in later life, in which case the cause is unknown. Sometimes agammaglobulinanaemia is caused by another disease of the white blood cells such as leukemia or Hodgkin's disease, which prevent the cells from making the necessary protein for defence against bacteria. Patients with the complaint run a greater risk of contracting diseases such as pneumonia, meningitis and chronic sinusitis.

Agnosia. Inability to recognize people or things despite intact sensory organs, caused by brain damage, cerebral haemorrhage, cerebral infarction, a tumour or an accident. The patient cannot make sense of anything he sees, hears or feels.

Agranulocytosis. Deficiency of granular leucocytes, a particular kind of white blood cell so called because under the microscope they seem to contain white granules. Their function is to remove harmful bacteria, and agranulocytosis reduces the body's defences against bacteria.

AIDS (acquired immune deficiency syndrome). AIDS is a disease that causes the body's immune system to fail to function against various bacteria, fungi and viruses.

The disease is transmitted by a virus present in the blood and semen of patients suffering from AIDS. The virus is not found universally in the population, but is confined to certain groups. These so-called high-risk groups are promiscuous homosexual males, mainline drug addicts and, until recently, haemophiliacs. Promiscuous sexual contact among homosexual men causes increased risk of infection by blood-blood or blood-semen contact. Drug addicts are at risk through shared use of hypodermic needles.

Infection with the virus need not produce symptoms, but its presence can be established by a special blood test. Only a limited number of those infected become ill, with symptoms such as sore throat, fever, skin eruptions, paid in the joints and muscles and swollen lymph nodes. An even smaller proportion (about 10 per cent) develops AIDS. Roughly six months to a year after infection weight loss, fever, persistent diarrhoea, nocturnal perspiration and skin and mucous membrane infection set in, together with a particular sort of skin tumour (Kaposi's sarcoma).

It has not yet proved possible to detect the virus itself in the blood, although a special test shows whether the patient has been in contact with the virus; this is applied in the case of blood donors, and their blood is not used if the test is positive. For this reason patients with blood diseases are not in the high-risk groups.

An infected patient may remain in normal contact with society. The virus cannot be transmitted by kissing, tears, sweat, sneezing, coughing, or mutual contact with glasses, cutlery etc. More care is required during sexual contact. The use of condoms affords good protection against the AIDS virue. Drug users are advised always to use clean syringes and needles and never to share equipment.

There is no known medicine or vaccine against AIDS. The majority of people contracting the disease die in the course of time from infections against which their bodies are no longer immune.

Alactasia. Absence or deficiency of the enzyme lactase, which is essential for the digestion of milk sugar (lactose). All babies have lactase in their intestines, but the enzyme disappears during childhood in about 10% of northern Europeans, 40% of Greeks and Italians, and 80% of Africans and Asians, Alactasia causes symptoms only if the diet regularly includes raw milk, when the undigested lactose causes diarrhoea and abdominal pain.

Albinism. Rare hereditary deficiency of melanin, the pigment responsible for the colour of the skin, hair and eyes. Albinos have pale skin, very sensitive to the sun because the pigment also normally protects against this. The hair is pale blond to white.

The pigment also performs an important function in the eye by excluding excess light; albinos thus have difficulties in seeing, particularly in bright conditions. The eyes seem red, because the colour of the blood is visible through the iris.

Alcoholic psychosis. Psychosis caused by chronic poisoning of the brain with alcohol and lack of vitamin B, associated with personality changes and delusions: alcoholic paranoia. Long-term vitamin B shortage can lead to Korsakoffs syndrome: amnesia related to recent events, disorientation, confabulation and euphoria.

Alcoholism. Pathological dependence on alcohol, causing mental or physical symptoms. Alcoholism usually develops imperceptibly. At first the patient drinks in the same way as those around him, then an increasing need for relaxation and increasing tolerance to alcohol make him drink larger quantities. The next stage is that alcohol is used as an intoxicant: the patient drinks himself into a stupor. Memory loss sets in and the mind turns more and more to alcohol.

Aldosterone. A steroid hormone that is synthesized and released by the adrenal cortex and acts on the kidney to regulate salt (potassium and sodium) and water balance. It may be given by injection as replacement therapy when the adrenal cortex secretes insufficient amounts of the hormone and also to treat shock.

Algesimeter. A piece of equipment for determining the sensitivity of the skin to various touch stimuli, especially those causing pain.

Alkalosis. Accumulation of bases in the body. The condition is caused by acute hyperventilation : rapid breathing leads to acid loss via the lungs. Prolonged vomiting can also be a cause, because the gastric juices are highly acidic. The condition is identified by blood test, and treated in hospital according to the cause.

Alimentary canal. The long passage through which food passes to be digested and absorbed (see illustration). It extends from the mouth to the anus and each region is specialized for a different stage in the processing of food, from mechanical breakdown in the mouth to chemical digestion and absorption in the stomach and small intestine and finally to faeces formation and storage in the colon and rectum. See also absorption, digestion.

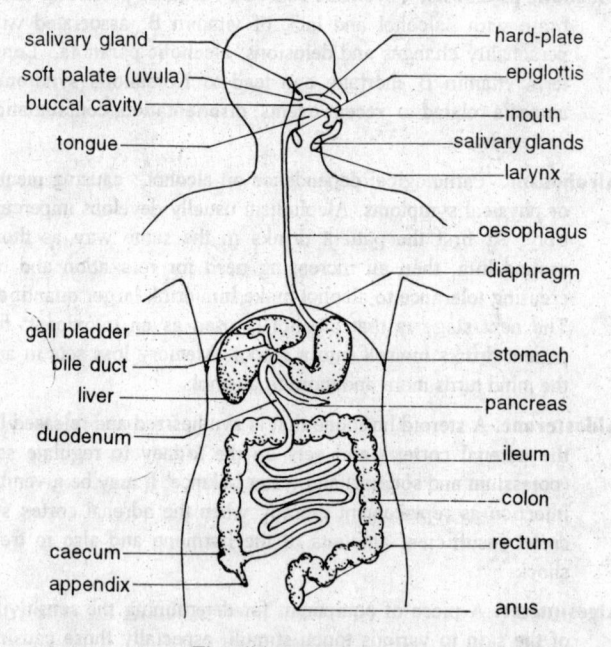

salivary gland — hard-plate
soft palate (uvula) — epiglottis
buccal cavity — mouth
tongue — salivary glands
— larynx
— oesophagus
— diaphragm
gall bladder —
bile duct — stomach
liver — pancreas
duodenum —
— ileum
— colon
caecum — rectum
appendix —
— anus

The alimentary canal

Alkalaemia. Abnormally high blood alkalinity. This may be caused by an increase in the concentration of alkaline substances and/ or a decrease in that of acidic substances in the blood.

Allergy. Variation in the normal immune reaction. Immune reactions normally occur when harmful substances enter the body : antibodies are formed in the blood which render the foreign substances harmless and clear them away. Some people develop the same reaction against harmless substances, against which antibodies are formed on the first contact, without perceptible reaction, but on further contract reaction sets in, usually becoming more violent on each renewed contact. Examples of harmless substances that can cause an allergic reaction are : household dust, grass pollen, fur and feathers, food (strawberries, shellfish), medicines (penicillin) or insect bites.

Altitude Sickness. Condition which occurs when people who live at sea-level suddenly travel to a height of several thousand metres, caused by reduced oxygen pressure : at 5,500 metres the pressure is half that at sea-level. The condition can occur if a patient climbs above 2,000 metres, but not everyone is equally susceptible.

Amblyopia. Irreversible decline in vision, usually in one eye, originating in the brain rather than the eye. The condition can be cogenital: other possible causes of (usually bilateral) amblyopia are poisoning by alcohol, nicotine or quinine. The commonest cause of monolateral (one-sided) amblyopia is a squint, in which sight in the squinting eye is suppressed to prevent double vision (diplopia). Treatment of the squint can prevent amblyopia if it starts when the patient is young enough : it involves correction with spectacles and temporary covering of the good eye to encourage the other to work.

Amnesia. Inability to remember things. There functions are important in memory ; the first is imprinting, the ability to repeat names of sets or numbers; the second is short-term memory; and important events are assigned to the third section, the long-term memory. Memory is seated in the deeper areas of the brain. Sudden temporary loss of memory is a characteristic symptom of concussion caused by a blow to the head. The patient cannot remember what he was doing in the minutes or hours before the injury, the condition known as retrograde amnesia. The contents of the short-term memory seem to have been wiped out; it often also seems that mothing is retained either of what happened immediately after the injury. The patient is clearly conscious, but retains nothing of what is being said. This explains why someone with brain damage so often asks what happened. An epileptic seizure is also often followed by short period of amnesia, as is a blackout from drinking too much alcohol. Presistent memory defects suggest damage to deeper areas of the brain. This occurs in dementia, severe concussion and serve subarachnoid haemorrhage.

Amyloidosis. Refers to condition in which an insoluble protein substance (amyloid) is deposited in the skin and internal organs.

Symptoms are highly dependent on the place in which the amyloid is deposited; the cause, if one can be found, is usually a chronic illness such as rheumatism osteitis, tuberculosis or a cancer. Amyloidosis of the kidneys is particularly common; they are unable to function, and metabolic breakdown products accumulate.

Anaemia. Shortage of red blood cells, the function of which is to transport oxygen (O_2) from the lungs to the tissues and carbon dioxide (CO_2) from the tissues to the lungs. A shortage of red cells thus causes tissue to be starved of oxygen. Such a shortage is first noticed during exertion, when the tissues require more oxygen than when the body is at rest. Symptoms are fatigue, shortness of breath and sometimes headache and dizziness. The body reacts by pumping the remaining red cells around the body as quickly as possible, to optimize the oxygen supply. This can cause palpitations and ringing in the ears. Paleness caused because little blood flows through the skin, is the commonest symptom of anaemia, after tiredness.

Anamia, Aplastic. Form of anaemia that results when the bone marrow produces too few blood cells, as a result of exposure to radioactivity or in rare cases through medication. The condition is often found in cancer patients because on the one hand secondary cancers may develop in the bone marrow and force out the blood-forming cells, and on the other hand cytostatics (medication to check the growth of tumours) also inhibit the growth of blood cells. Usually the cause of aplastic anaemia is unknown.

Anaemia, Haemolytic. Anaemia caused by accelerated breakdown of red blood cells, usually because they are abnormal in form or made up of abnormal components, or because of an autoimmune disease. A particular form of haemolytic anaemia is caused by rhesus incompatibility.

Anaemia, Iron-deficiency. Form of anaemia that arises because of iron deficiency, iron being one of the key constituents of red blood corpuscles. Iron deficiency does not usually result from a lack of iron in the food, because more than enough iron is present in a normal diet. This form of anaemia usually arises as a result of frequent loss of blood. Possible causes are severe menstrual bleeding or haemorrhaging in the gastro-intestinal tract. These can continue for a long time before being noticed. In pregnant women, the growing embryo also absorbs a lot of iron. Since pregnancy and menstruation are major causes of iron-deficiency anaemia, the condition is commoner in women than in men.

Anaemia, Pernicious. Anaemia caused by vitamin B_{12} deficiency, needed for the production of red blood cells.

Vitamin B_{12} can be absorbed from food only with the assistance of a substance found in the gastric juices, and deficiency is usually caused by an inadequate quantity of this substance in the stomach as a result of chronic inflammation or surgical removal of a large part of the stomach.

Anaesthesia. Medically, anaesthesia involves the loss of sensation in the skin, causing an inability to experience touch, temperature changes or pain.

Anal fissure. Longitudinal fissure in the anal mucous membrane, caused among other things by chronic hardness of the faces or by haemorrhoids. Symptoms occur above all during defecation: severe, convulsive pain and loss of blood. The pain can persist for some time. The lost blood is not mixed with the faeces, is bright red, and the loss can be considerable. If the patient was not already prone to hardness of the faeces the condition can cause it, because fear of pain leads to unduly long retention.

Anal fistula. Passage forming a connection between the anal mucous membrane and the skin around the annus, usually caused by an abcen directly above the anus. Rectal fistulas can be caused by other conditions such as ulcerative colitis Conn's syndrome, tuberculosis of the rectum or a tumour.

Anaphylaxis. Particular form of severe allergic reaction. If one comes into contact for the first time with a substance to which one is allergic then antibodies are formed against this substance. In an anaphylactic reaction the antibodies are of a particular kind, If one comes into contact with the substance in question again, the IgE antibodies react with the substance within a few minutes, causing an itchy, red skin eruption with lumps (also called hives or urticaria), constriction of the air passages and lowering of the blood pressure. Serious forms af anaphylactic reaction can result in shock. The most common causes are hypersensitivity to penicillin or similar antibiotics and hypersensitivity to insect stings.

Anaesthetic. 1. An agent that reduces or abolishes sensation, affecting either the whole body (*general anaesthetic*) or a particular region of the body (*local anaesthetic*). General anaesthetics, used for surgical procedures, depress the central nervous system producing loss of consciousness. Anaesthesia is induced by short-acting barbiturates (such as thiopentone) and maintained by inhalation anaesthetics (such as halothane). Local anaesthetics inhibit conduction of impulses in sensory nerves in the region where they are injected or applied; they include cocaine and lignocaine. 2. *adj.* reducing or abolishing sensation.

Analgesic. 1. A drug that relieves pain. Mild analgesics, such as
aspirin and paracetamol, are used for the relief of headache,
toothache and mild rhematic pain. More potent *narcotic analgesics,* such as morphine and pethidine are used only to relieve severe pain since these drugs may produce dependence
and tolerance. Some analgesics, including aspirin, ibuprofen,
ketoprofen, indomethacin, and phenylbutazone, also reduce fever and inflammation and are used in rheumatic conditions.
2. *adj.* relieving pain.

Anencephaly. Congenital abnormality in which a large part of the
top of the skull is missing, and part of the brain has failed to
develop. Under normal circumstances the central nervous system forms an enclosed tube towards the end of the fourth week
of embryonic development. Sometimes however the tube does
not close and nerve tissue is left exposed on the surface. If this
condition occurs in the brain it is known as anencephaly.

Aneurysm. Abnormal dilation of part of an artery. Most aneurysms
occur in the aorta, but they are also found in the femoral and

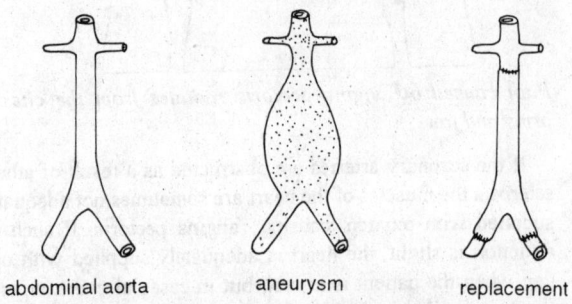

abdominal aorta   aneurysm   replacement

cerebal arteries and the left ventricle of the heart. In most
cases aortal aneurysm is caused by atherosclerosis the calcified arterial wall loses elasticity and stretches through the pressure of the blood, increasing the diameter of the artery. In a
cerebral aneurysm the cause is usually a congenitally weak
spot in the wall of the blood vassel. Cardiac aneurysm develops after cardiac infarction has caused weakness in the wall of
the left ventricle.

Angina Pectoris. Pain in the chest caused by an inadequate supply of oxygen to the heart muscle.

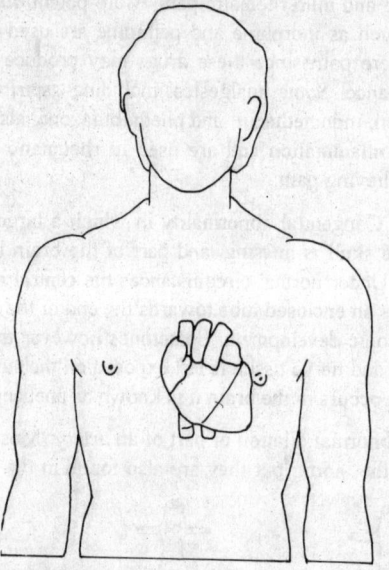

Pain caused by angina pectoris radiates from the chest to arms and jaw.

If the coronary arteries are obstructed as a result of atherosclerosis the muscles of the heart are sometimes not adequately supplied with oxygen, causing angina pectoris. If such obstruction is slight, the heart is adequately supplied with oxygen when the patient is at rest, but in cases of exertion, emotion, or passing from warm to cold surroundings, oxygen supply can be reduced. As obstruction increases, so increasingly less exertion causes discomfort. The pain is oppressive, restricting and cramping, and orginates from directly behind the breastbone. It radiates to the left arm, the neck or the jaw, but sometimes also to the abdomen and back. Shortness of breath may also occur. The attact usually ends when the patient ceases to exert himself. Pain persisting for longer than half an hour may be a sign of a cardiac infarction. If a patient has anginal pains an electrocardiogram (ECG) should be made during exertion; if pain and ECG change are simultaneous, that is evidence of angina pectoris.

Treatment is by giving up smoking, losing weight, regular exercise and medication with nitroglycerin tablets or beta-blockers; if this is unsuccessful a by-pass operation may be performed.

Angioneurotic Oedema. Manifestation closely associated with hives or urticaria. Hives is an itchy red skin eruption with swelling of the skin caused by local dilation of the blood vessels. This can be caused by: anaphylaxis, usually associated with food or medication, infectious diseases (for example glandular fever), low temperature, emotional tension, malignant diseases (e.g. Hodgkin's disease) or diseases of the tissue (e.g., lupus erythematosus).

Ankylosing Spondylitis. Rheumatic disorder involving characteristic chronic inflammation of the joints between the sacrum and the spine, between the vertebrae, and between the vertebrae and the ribs; in 25 per cent of cases the hip, knee and shoulder are also affected.

The condition occurs particularly in men between the ages of 20 and 30, and is often hereditary, and probably caused by a disturbance in the immune system. The first symptoms are pain, worse at night, and stiffness in the back, leading to stiffening and deformation of the spinal column, beginning low and spreading upwards. Stiffening of the joints between vertebrae and ribs reduces mobility of the chest, causing abdominal breathing.

Anopia. Loss of (part of) the normal field of vision, in one or both eyes. The retina is most sensitive at the centre of the field of vision; failure at the centre is thus more serious, because it affects reading and focusing on a particular object. Failure of a small peripheral area is sometimes not even noticed. To a large extent the fields of vision of each eye overlap, so that the healthy eye can sometimes compensate for the defective one.

Loss of vision can be the result of eye disorders, or conditions of the optic nerve or the visual centre in the brain. Haemorrhage or inflammation of the retina cause failure of the central area of the field of vision. In cases of detached retina failure is sudden and normally runs from the edge to the centre. Retrobulbar neuritis causes central failure; a pituitary tumour can cause loss of field of vision in both eyes, with the areas closest to the nose remaining unaffected. Haemorrhage in the cerebral visual centre can cause complete failure, effectively the same as total blindness.

Anorexia Nervosa. ('slimmer's disease') Clinical picture that occurs in young women, and characterized by a particular view of eating and body weight, leading to extreme loss of weight, sometimes associated with freak periods of overeating and self-induced vomiting. The desire of slim can be so great that laxatives are used, causing dehydration. In spite of very poor physical condition bodily activity remains strikingly high; menstruation ceases. The patient does not consider herself slim, and denies abnormality in her eating pattern. If shortage of calories becomes so great that the body starts to break down its own tissue, all sorts of physical abnormalities result and the patient must be admitted to hospital.

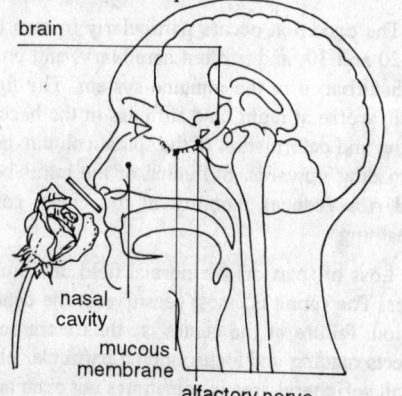

Anosmia, an inability to smell, can be caused by various disorders of the olfactory tract.

Anosmia. Temporary or permanent failure of the ability to smell and taste, because the latter sense is dependent to a large extent upon the former (hence the practice of holding the nose when drinking something unpleasant). The part of the nasal mucous membrane sensitive to smell is high in the nasal cavity on each side of the nasal septum, and contains nerves running from the base of the skull to the olfactory nerves beneath and behind the brain. Anosmia can be caused by cutting or damaging the sensitive nasal mucous membrane, or by temporary or permanent damage to the olfactory nerve sheaths.

Anthracosis. Form of paneumoconiosis caused by long-term inhalation of carbon particles by mine workers. Workers in the mining and ceramics industries can be subjected to a combination of anthracosis and silicosis, causing interstitial fibrosis as a result of exposure to silicosis. Sometimes anthracosis is associated with chronic bronchitis in susceptible patients.

Anthrax. Infection with *Bacillus anthracis*. Anthrax is essentially a disease of large domestic animals such as pigs, cattle and sheep. The animals are infected via skin wounds or through the intestine with bacteria found on the ground or in food.

Antibiotic. Literally, against life. In medicine, a large and growing class of drugs derived from living organisms. The first was of course penicillin, derived from the mould, *penicillium notatum,* by Alexander Fleming (Scottish bacteri—ologist, 1881-1955) in 1928 and introduced into clinical use in 1940. Most of the new antibiotics are synthetic imitations of parts of the molecules of chemicals derived from living organisms. The sulphonamides which were introduced in the 1930s are sometimes incorrectly called antibiotics; they are derivatives of coal-tar dyes.

Antibody. A protein molecule synthesized by cells in the immune defence system in response to challenge by a substance, foreign to the body, called an antigen. Antibodies have several functions. Not only are they designed structurally so that they can attach to and detoxify or destroy the antigen which caused them to be synthesized, but they also play complex and incompletely understood roles in mobilizing other cells and chemicals in the immune defence system.

Antibodies are sometimes called immunoglubulins, especially when they are being considered as constituents of blood in which they are carried around the body as molecules that may actually change their form during the immune process, or as drugs. Broadly speaking, all antibodies consist of four subsections, two of which are heavier and relatively stable in their atomic structure while the two lighter chains vary in accordance with the make-up of the antigen. The fascinating complexity of these vital molecules is further enhanced by the fact that they seem to contradict the fundamental biological principle that every protein produced by an organism is already described in the genes of that organism. Each anbtibody attacks one or a very small group of antigens, but the possible number of antigens in the universe is in practice almost infinite.

Antigen. Any substance foreign to the body which either alone or in combination with some body substance causes the body to produce antibodies against the antigen. Most antigens are proteins, but many large non-protein molecules such as complexes of sugar, (carbodydrates), may be antigenic. Even small molecules may cause the body to produce antibodies, but they must usually combine first with a molecule that is part of the body. Such small molecules are called haptens. They could underlie *autommune disease*.

It follows that antigens have no regular structure. They usually exist in the outer surfaces of invasive substances, like the hard coats of bacteria, where they are intermixed with other structural molecules. However, internal molecules may also be antigenic.

Anticonvulsant *n*. A drug that prevents or reduces the severity of fits (convulsions) in various types of epilepsy. Some anticonvulsants, such as sodium valproate, are used to treat all types of epileptic fits. Others are used only grand mal epilepsy (e.g., ethotioin, phenytoin, and pheneturide) or for petit mal fits (e.g., ethosuximide, phensuximide, and troxidone). Tranquillizers, such as diazepam, are also used to control epileptic fits. Side-effects occur frequently with some anticonvulsants and the dosage must be carefully adjusted.

Antidepressant. A drug that alleviates the symptoms of depression. The most sidely prescribed antidepressants are a group of drugs with a basic chemical structure of three benzene rings, called *tricyclic antidepressants,* which include amitriptyline and imipramine. These drugs are useful in treating a variety of different depressive symptoms. Side-effects commonly include dry mouth, blurred vision, constipation, drowsiness, and difficulty in urination. The other main group of antidepressants are the 'MAO inhibitors, which have more severe side-effects.

Antidote. A drug that counteracts the effects of a poison. For example, dimercaprol is an antidote to arsenic, mercury, and other heavy metals.

Antiemetic. A drug that prevents vomiting. Various drugs have this effect, including some antihistamines (e.g., cyclizine, promethazine) and anticholinergic drugs. They are used for such conditions as motion sickness and vertigo and to counteract nausea and vomiting caused by other drags.

Antihistamine. A drug that inhibits some of the effects of histamine in the body, in particular its role in allergic reactions. Examples include chlorpheniramine, diphenhydramine, and mepyramine. Antihistamines are used mainly for the relief of hay fever, pruritus (itching), rhinitis, urticaria (nettle rash), and other allergic reactions. Many antihistamines, e.g., cyclizine and promethazine, also have strong antiemetic activity and are used to prevent motion sickness. The most common side-effect of antihistamines is drowsiness and because of this they are sometimes used to promote sleep. Other side-effects include dizziness, blurred vision, tremors, digestive upsets, and lack of muscular coordination.

Antiseptic. A chemical that destroys or inhibits the growth of disease-causing bacteria and other microorganisms and is sufficiently nontoxic to be applied to the skin or mucous membranes to cleanse wounds and prevent infections or to be used internally to treat infections of the intestine and bladder. Examples are crystal violet, dequalinium, and hexamine.

Antitoxin. An antibody produced by the body to counteract a toxin formed by invading bacteria or from any other source.

Antrectomy. 1. Surgical removal of the bony walls of an antrum. See antrostomy. 2. A surgical operation in which a part of the stomach (the antrum) is removed. Most secretions of acid, pepsin, and the hormone gastrin occur in the antrum and the operation is used (usually combined with vagotomy) in the treatment of peptic ulcers.

Antrostomy. A surgical operation to produce a permanent or semi-permanent artificial opening to an antrum in a bone, so providing drainage for any fluid. The operation is sometimes carried out to treat infection of the paranasal sinuses.

Anuria. Production of less than 100 ml per day of urine. If urine production is less than 400 ml per day the condition is known as oliguria.

Anuria can be caused by disturbances in the transfer of fluids to the kidneys, by conditions of the kidney tissue and by restrictions in urinary flow, in the latter case only if the flow from both kidneys is blocked. Fluid transfer problems occur if blood supply to the kidneys is reduced, as in shock, blood poisoning, heart failure or closure of the renal valves. Serious fluid shortage through lack of intake or heavy loss (vomiting diarrhoea, perspiration) can also be factors.

Anxiety. Feeling of unease and tension with no apparent cause, sometimes degenerating into panic, and associated with physical manifestations such as hyperventilation.

A patient may be aware of associated physical symptoms, but not of anxiety. If the patient knows the cause, the condition is known as a phobia. Anxiety can be caused by a real problem or danger, in which case no treatment is necessary. Anxiety is also caused by psychotic delusions and hallucinations, in which case it should be treated.

Aortic Valve Disorders. There are two possible abnormalities of the aortic valves of the heart: stenosis and leakage (aortic incompetence). Stenosis usually occurs in later life if the valve becomes calcified or as the result of inflammation (rheumatic fever), and cannot open properly. The condition can be congenital.

Aphasia. Inability to speak normally when the muscles of the tongue, lips and throat are intact, and/or the inability to understand speech. The cause is usually brain damage from a stroke or accident. In most people language is produced in the left cerebral hemisphere, which has two centres important for the use and understanding of speech.

Appendicitis. Inflammation of the vermiform appendix, which is attached to the caecum. The condition can occur at any age, but three-quarters of cases are in young people between the ages of 5 and 35. The cause is not known, but it is possible that a blockage of the appendix by faeces could encourage the growth of bacteria, thus increasing the likelihood of inflammation.

Apraxia. Inability to perform certain acts although the muscles are intact and the patient understands what he should do. The cause is a condition of the cerebral cortex caused by a stocke, dementia with widespread loss of brain cells, or a tumour. In mild cases the patient seems clumsy and absent-minded, in more serious cases simple implements are used wrongly—for example eating with a tooth-brush. Imitation of acts can also be disturbed.

There is no definite treatment; the underlying condition should be identified and treated.

Arteriectomy. The surgical excision of an artery or part of an artery. This may be performed as a diagnostic procedure (for example, to take an arterial biopsy in the diagnosis of arteritis) or during reconstruction of a blocked artery when the blocked segment is replaced by a synthetic graft.

Arteriography. X-ray examination of an artery that has been outlined by the injection of a radio-opaque contrast medium. The major uses of arteriography are to demonstrate the site and extent of atheroma, especially in the coronary arteries (*coronary angiography*) and the leg arteries (*femoral angiography*), and to reveal the site of aneurysms within the skull or cerebral tumours (*carotid* and *vertebral artery angiography*).

Arteritis, Temporal. Inflammation of the wall of the artery which runs over the temple. The cause is unknown, but the condition is often associated with polymyalgia rheumatica; it occurs after the 60th year.

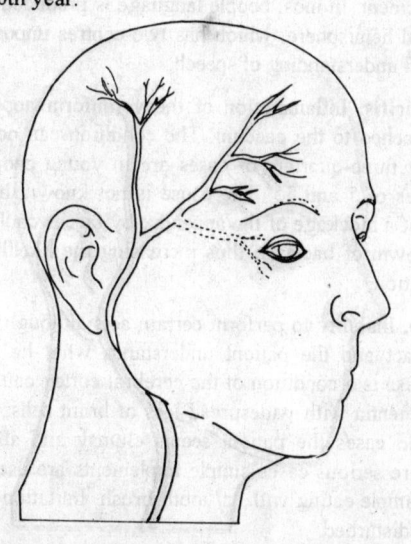

Temporal arteritis causes inflammation and closure of the temporal artery. If the branch leading to the eye is affected, blindness can result.

Arthritis. Inflammation of one more joints (known as polyarthritis in the latter case), which results in pain, swelling and restricted movement of the joint, and warm, red skin. Arthritis can be caused by infection of the joint with germs from the bloodstream, from an open wound or from spreading inflammation of the bone marrow. Infection via the blood occurs in rheumatic fever, tuberculosis and venereal diseases such as gonorrhoea and syphilis.

Arthrography. An X-ray techniques for examining joints. A contrast medium (either air or a liquid opaque to X-rays) is injected into the joint space, allowing its outline and contents to be traced accurately.

Arthroscope. An instrument for insertion into the cavity of a joint in order to inspect the contents, before biopsy or operation on the joint.

Artificial insemination. The instrumental introduction of semen into the vagina in order that the woman may conceive. Insemination is timed to coincide with the day on which the woman is expected to ovulate (see menstrual cycle). The semen specimen may be provided by the husband (*AIH-artificial insemination husband*) in cases of impotence or by an anonymous donor (*AID-artificial insemination donor*) in cases where the husband is sterile.

Asbestosis. Form of pneumoconiosis caused by inhaling asbestos or fibrous silicates over a period of years. It occurs in people who work with insulating materials or in factories in which they are produced.

Ascariasis. Infestation with *Ascaris lumbricoides*, a large worm (15-35 cm long) that occurs throughout the world, and infests about 650 million people. The worms live in the small intestine and feed on its contents; their lifespan is about a year. The female worms can produce large numbers of eggss (up to 200,000 per day) which are excreted in faeces. The larvae develop in the soil. Faeces containing eggs can reach vegetables and fruit as a result of manuring, and man can be infested by eating unwashed produce. The larvae hatch in the small intestine and grow into adult worms, which can cause

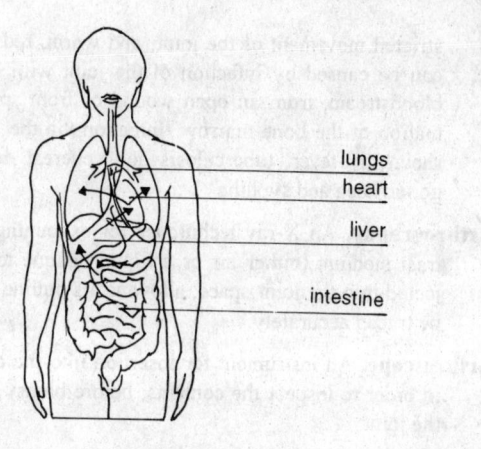

In eel-worm infestation (ascariasis) the larvae reach the lungs because they are discharged into circulating blood by the liver.

discomfort if they crawl through passages such as the junction of the liver and the pancreas. They can also block the intestine, causing obdominal pain, loss of appetite and diarrhoea. Usually infestation causes no discomfort, in which case no treatment is necessary.

Ascites. Accumulation of fluid in the abdomen. Normally there is a very thin film of fluid between individual sections of the intestine, and between the intestine and the abdominal wall. Fluid accumulates in the abdomen for four principal groups of reasons: diseases of or near the peritoneum (tuberculosis, perotonial tumours); restriction of the flow of blood through the liver (usually because of cirrhosis of the liver) causing high pressure in the portal vein and the vessels leading to it, producing fluid; heart failure; low protein content in the blood as a result of severe malnutrition (nephrotic syndrome).

Aspergillosis. Infection with the fungus *Aspergillus fumigatus*.

This fungus occurs throughout nature, usually without causing illness, except under poor hygienic conditions (e.g. in the tropics).

Asphyxia. Threat of suffocation through lack of oxygen. It may occur through failure of respiration in new-born infants in cases of difficult or assisted delivery. The unborn child can suffer from shortage of oxygen as a result of constriction of the umbilical cord, contractions occurring in quick succession, or cerebral haemorrhage. Inhaling meconium or medication from the pregnant mother can also cause the condition. Breathing is affected more quickly than the circulation of the blood from an oxygen shortage. If it persists both heart and circulation will suffer. Thus affected babies very often show symptoms of asphyxia at birth: they are pale and limp, and respiration is absent or occurs only with difficulty. When respiration and circulation are established in the following hours and days there may be symptoms of overexcitability of the brain : tremors, muscular convulsions and fits. The infant is dazed and respiration is laboured and irregular, and there may be cyanosis.

Aspirin (acetylsalicylic acid). A widely used drug that relieves pain and also reduces inflammation and fever. It is taken by mouth-alone or in combination with caffeine, phenacetin, or codeine-for the relief of the less severe types of pain, such as headache, toothache, neuralgias, and the pain of rheumatoid arthritis. It is also taken to reduce fever in influenza and the common cold. Aspirin may irritate the lining of the stomach, causing nausea, vomiting, pain, and bleeding. High doses cause dizziness, disturbed hearing, mental confusion and overbreathing. See also analgesic.

Asthma. Attacks of tightness of the chest, causing difficulty in breathing out. During an attack the patient breathes with a characteristic whistling sound, but suffers little between attacks, except in cases of bronchial asthma, when constriction may occur more persistently. Asthma is one of the group of illnesses affecting the air passages known as CARA.

Astigmatism. Irregular curvature of the cornea or lens of the eye, distorting the image formed on the retina. A dot is seen as a blob or dash.

The most usual condition is regular astigmatism, in which

corneal curvature is asymmetrical. Parallel beams of light entering the eye are normally focussed as a point, but are seen by an astigmatic eye as a stripe. This form of astigmatism is corrected by spectacles with a cylindrical lens.

Atelectasis. Collapse of part of the lung. Normally all the alveoli are filled with air, but this ability can disappear under various circumstances.

In atelectasis the alveoli collapse; a possible cause is blockage of a bronchiole. The affected part no longer functions in breathing.

Atheroma. A deposit on the walls of an artery, usually consisting of fatty materials. The effect is to narrow and roughen the walls of the vessel.

Atherosclerosis. Condition of the arteries characterized by hardening and fatty degeneration of the arterial wall. It is responsible for most deaths in the Western world, and should be considered the number one epidemic.

Athlete's foot (Tinea Pedis). Fungal infection of the skin, but not a form of eczema.

This complaint occurs mainly in people who swim regularly, although other people also suffer from it.

Atopic Eczema. Form of eczema in patients susceptible to allergic reactions. There are two main forms: infantile eczema and adult-type eczema. In infants, atopic eczema can affect the whole face, and the whole face, and there can be patches on arms and legs. The skin is reddened, with small pimples.

Atrial Fibrillation. Heart rhythm disorder characterized by irregular heartbeat. It can occur in all kinds of heart conditions (cardiac valve defects, constriction of the coronary arteries), but also in cases of an overactive thyroid (hyperthyroidism).

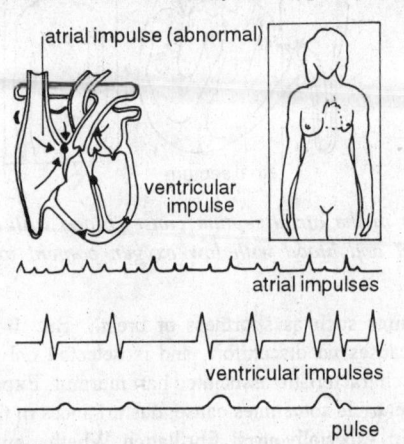

atrial impulse (abnormal)

ventricular impulse

atrial impulses

ventricular impulses

pulse

Atrial fibrillation is caused by unco-ordinated atrial impulses; this often affects the ventricles and the pulse.

Atrial Flutter. Heart condition in which the atria contract irregularly comparable with atrial fibrillation, but characterized by a very rapid but regular rhythm, as opposed to the irregular rhythm of fibrillation.

Atrial Septum Defect (ASD). Congenital heart defect in which there is an opening in the septum between the left and right atria.

The condition has two forms: ASD I, almost always linked with a defective mitral valve, and ASD II, which occurs more

frequently and is not associated with valve defects. Because
the pressure in the left atrium is higher than that in the right
blood flows from one to the other, causing excess blood in
the vessels of the lungs, which can eventually led to lung

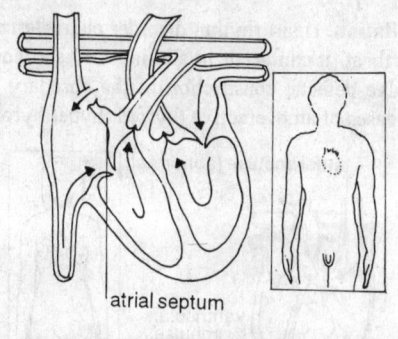

atrial septum

*A hole in the atrial septum causes blood with high oxygen
content and blood with low oxygen content to mix in the
heart.*

complaints such as shortness of breath. But in most cases
ASD causes no discomfort, and is detected only by chance,
from a characteristic associated hart murmur. Expansion of the
right ventricle sometimes cause: dusturbances in the rhythm of
the heart, especially atrial fibrillation. Whether an ASD should
be closed by surgery depends on its type and size. An ASD
with valve defect must be closed when the patient is young. If
the ASD is large lung problems will quickly set in, and action
is certainly required, whereas a small ASD hardly ever causes
complications and therefore no operation is necessary.

Auriscope (otoscope). An apparatus for examining the eardrum
and the passage leading to it from the ear (external meatus). It
consists of a funnel (speculum), a light, and lenses (see
illustration).

Auscultation. The process of listening, usually with the aid of a
stethoscope, to sounds produced by movement of gas or liquid

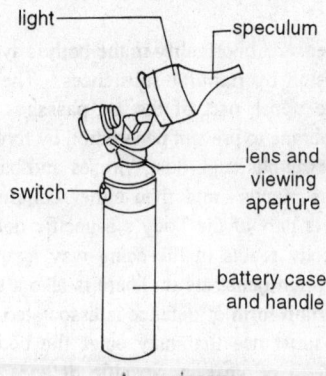

light — speculum

lens and viewing aperture

switch —

battery case and handle

An auriscope

within the body. Auscultation is an aid to diagnosis of abnor- malities of the heart, lungs intestines, and other organs according to the changes in sound pattern caused by different disease processes.

Autism. Severe disturbance in emotional development in which a child becomes withdrawn and incapable of social communication.

All the symptoms of autism are present at birth but often are not recognized until later. An autistic child does not allow itself to be cuddled, does not laugh at its parents, and it is difficult to make eye contact with the child. It can be captivated by moving objects. Speech develops slowly, or not at all. Sometimes there will be parroting. As well as avoiding or even being afraid of human contact, the autistic child shows characteristic stereotyped behaviour patterns such as rocking or endlessly repeating a certain movement. He or she is also afraid of change, which can cause panic.

Autograft. A tissue graft taken from one part of the body and transferred to another part of the same individual. The repair of burns is often done by grafting on strips of skin taken from elsewhere on the body, usually the upper arm or thigh. Unlike homografts, autografts are not rejected by the body's immunity defences. See also skin graft.

Autoimmune disease. Abnormality in the body's system of defence
against invasion by harmful substances. The interior of the
nose and the upper part of the air passages are lined with
mucous membrane to prevent penetration by foreign substances,
such as for example sand, dust, viruses and bacteria; they are
caught in the mucus and then either coughed up or swallowed. This is part of the body's aspecific defence system in
which the body reacts in the same way against all sorts of
substances which penetrate it. There is also a specific defence
system: a certain form of defence is associated with a particular harmful substance that may enter the body, in this case
usually bacteria or viruses. Specific defence is provided by
white blood cells and antibodies present in blood plasma. The
first time a bacterium or virus penetrates the body, resistant
antibodies are formed; they react with no other bacteria or
viruses, but render the specific bacterium or virus harmless.

Autoimmunity. A disorder of the body's defence mechanisms in
which antibodies (*autoantibodies*) are produced against certain components or products of its own tissues, treating them
as foreign material and attacking them. See autoimmune disease, immunity.

Autovaccine (autogenous vaccine). A vaccine prepared by isolat-
ing specimens of bacteria from an infected patient, culturing
them, and killing them. By injecting this vaccine back into the
patient, it was hoped that the body's resistance to the infection
would be stimulated. Although such vaccines were once much
favoured for the treatment of boils, there is no good evidence
that the dead bacteria are any more likely to stimulate immunity than the living and dead bacteria already present in the
body.

B

Baby, Overdue. Child that has remained in the womb for more than 42 weeks, also termed a post-mature baby. If labour has not started by this time it is often induced because placental function then begins to decline, reducing the child's supply of food and oxygen. Most of these babies seem thin and desiccated at birth; the skin is dry, and sometimes scaly, and there is no skin lubricant. Nails are long, and the child has a lot of hair. Such children are usually overexcited and restless, sleep little and feed badly. There are often respiratory difficulties. Their lack of nutrition can cause other complications such as blood-sugar deficiency (hypoglycaemia), resulting in convulsions. A post-mature baby needs extra attention, and admission to hospital may be necessary.

Baby, Premature. Child born between the 28th and 38th weeks of pregnancy. The earlier the child is born, the more striking the outward signs of premature birth will be. The skin is thin and red, and there is little subcutaneous fat, but skin lubricant and hair are present in large quantities. This skull is large in relation to the body, the fontanels are large, and there is a tendency to swelling (oedema) of hands and feet. Boy's testicles have not usually descended, and girls' labia minora have not yet been covered by the labia majora. The child cries feebly and complainingly. All organs are immature, and not completely ready for independent function. There may be respiratory disorders (hyaline membrane disease), waste products are not excreted properly by the kidneys, jaundice and haemorrhage are caused by the immature liver, and convulsions resulting from cerebral haemorrhage or blood-sugar deficiency (hypoglycaemia) can endanger life. Complication can result from brain damage caused by jaundice, anaemia and infections.

Baby, underdeveloped. Infant whose birth weight is lower than the length of pregnancy would suggest. There are various possible causes: general backwardness in growth through underfeeding, genetic tendencies, congenital abnormalities, excessive smoking or alcohol consumption by the mother during pregnancy. The condition affects weight above all.

Backache. Extremely common symptom that can be caused by a bumber of disorders. The source of the pain can be in the spine, in nerves entering or leaving the spinal cord, or in the back muscles. Disorders of the abdominal organs such as the kidneys, gall bladder and womb are also often responsible for back pain. The commonest cause, however, is overloading of the spine or back muscles.

Balance, disorders of. Difficulties in keeping one's balance are the consequences of disturbances to one or more of three systems: the organ of balance, the eyes and certain receptors in muscles and joints which perceive the position of various parts of the body in relation to themselves. Wnen information from these three systems is in phase, we are hardly aware that we know the position in which we stand, but if the information is out of phase, problems arise, particularly in the form of vertigo. The cause of balance disturbances is on three different levels: firstly in the organ of balance and its connection with the brain, for example labyrinthitis, Meniere's disease concussion or inflammation of the nerve controlling balance. A second group of causes includes disorders that affect the organ of balance in one way or another: anaemia, high or even low blood pressure, infectious diseases, and some medicines and alcohol. The third group are abnormalities of the other systems that affect balance (eyes, joints), such as double vision or wear on the vertebrae of the neck.

Balanitis. Inflammation of the glans penis, usually associated with inflammation of lthe foreskin. It is most often caused by inadequate hygiene, which allows bacteria and smegma to accumulate in the groove behind the glans, leading to inflammation involving redness and swelling of the glans, and usually also the foreskin. The patient complains of pain, itching and an odorous discharge.

Baldness (alopecia). Condition caused by various skin disorders of the head which bring about abnormalities of the hair roots. Examples are deep infections, burns or the effect of chemicals, lichen planus and other skin diseases. Baldness can be normal in men, as an effect of male sex hormones, beginning about the age of twenty and spreading more or less rapidly across the entire head. There is no medical treatment. In women the administration of a drug to block male sex hormones can improve a similar condition, but this treatment cannot be used for men. Sometimes baldness occurs in patches (alopecia areata).

Ballottement. The technique of examining a fluid-filled part of the body to detect a floating object. During pregnancy, a sharp tap with the fingers, applied to the womb through the abdominal wall or the vagina, causes the fetus to move away and then return to impart an answering tap to the examiner's hand as it floats back to its original position. This confirms that swelling of the uterus is due to a fetus rather than a tumour or other abnormality.

Bandage. A piece of material, in the form of a pad or strip, applied to a wound or used to bind around an injured or diseased part of the body.

Barber's Rash (sycosis barbae). Chronic skin condition in the beard area of the face, caused by *staphylococci* or a fungus, leading to suppurating pimples which often leave scars; beard hairs fall out.

Barbiturate. Any of a group of drugs, derived from barbituric acid, that depress activity of the central nervous system. Most barbiturates, including amylobarbitone and pentobarbitone, are taken as sleeping pills. Very slow-acting barbiturates (such as phenobarbitone are used as sedatives and to control epilepsy; those with a rapid and short-lived effect (such as thiopentone) are injected as anaesthetics. Because they produce tolerance and psychological and physical dependence, have serious toxic side-effects (see barbiturism), and can be fatal following large overdosage, barbiturates have been largely replaced in clinical use by safer drugs.

Barotrauma. Damage to the middle ear and the eardrum resulting from a sudden change in atmosphere pressure, a condition prevalent in pilots and divers. The Eustachian tube connects the middle ear (tympanic cavity) with the nasal cavity, and maintains equal pressure between them. Normally the tube is closed, but it opens to equalize pressure during swallowing or yawning, for example. In barotrauma the function of the Eustachian tube is disturbed.

Bartholinitis. Inflammation of the Bartholin glands, which are located in the vagina at the rear of the labia majora, with a duct 1 to 2 cm long leading to the inner side of the labia minora. The glands produce a fluid which keeps the vagina supple. Usually they are the size of a bean. In gonorrhoea the ducts are often inflamed. Sometimes bacteria can cause an infection of the glands themselves, which swell and become very painful, and the ducts are often blocked. A round, hard swelling can be felt on the labia majora.

Battered Baby syndrome. Injuries inflicted on babies or young children by their parents, who are often emotionally disturbed or have themselves suffered from physical abuse in infancy or early childhood. The highest incidence of battering occurs in the first six months of life; it commonly takes the form of facial bruises cigarette burns, bites, head injuries (often with brain damage), and fractured bones. Child abuse may be triggered by such crises as an unwanted pregnancy, unemployment, and debts; frequently, signs of older bruises, fractures, etc., are revealed when the child is brought for treatment. 60% of battered children suffer from further injury if discharged from hospital without the intensive support of a social worker and surveillance of family doctor health visitor; a care order is often necessary to safeguard a child from further abuse.

Bazin's disease. A disease of young women in which tender nodules develop under the skin in the calves. The nodules may break down and ulcerate though they may clear up spontaneously. The cause is unknown but the disease may be associated with tuberculosis or, more commonly, perniosis. Medical name: erythema induratum.

BCG (bacille Calmette-Guerin). A strain of tubercle bacillus that has lost the power to cause tuberculosis but retains its antigenic activity; it is therefore used to prepare a vaccine against the disease.

Beclamide. An anticonvulsant drug used in the treatment of epilepsy. It is administered by mouth and often given together with phenobarbitone. Side-effects may include stomach upsets, dizziness, and nervousness. Trade name: Nydrane.

Beclomethasone. A corticosteroid drug that reduces inflammation and is applied externally in the treatment of various skin disorders. High dosage may cause retention of sodium and water and delayed wound healing. Trade name: **Propaderm.**

Bedbug (Cimex lectularius). A blood-sucking pest 5-8 mm long, which can drink quite large quantities of blood in one meal, enabling it to live for months without feeding again. Bedbugs occur in temperate zones and have a characteristic smell. They like warmth but not light and are thus often found in old houses behind wallpaper or in beds.

Bedsore (decubitus ulcer). Skin condition that occurs as a result of protracted pressure on an area of skin, often immediately next to part of a bone, such as the lower part of the back (sacrum), heel, hip, etc. The sores are caused because the blood vessels in the skin are closed by pressure between the bone and the surface on which the patient is lying. If this persists for a long time without interruption, the skin cells do not receive enough oxygen and die.

Bed-wetting (nocturnal enuresis). Involuntary nocturnal urination after the age of four years. Bed-wetting occurs frequently, particularly in boys, usually with no clear cause, but a thor-

ough check should be lmade to exclude   underlying disorders
before starting treatment. Physical disorders can include congenital conditions such as spina bifida and abnormalities of the
urinary tract, infection of the urinary tract, diabetes mellitus
constipation, mental retardation and nocturnal epilepsy. The
most common causes, however, are emotional.

Behaviour Therapy. The treatment based on the belief that psychological problems are the products of faulty learning and not
the symptoms of an underlying disease. Treatment is directed
at the problem or target behaviour and is designed for the
particular patient, not for the particular diagnostic label that
has been attached to him. See also aversion therapy, conditioning, desensitization.

Bell's palsy. Paralysis of one side of the face, caused by swelling
and trapping of the facial nerve (nervus facialis). The cause is
unknown, although cooling (by a draught) is often a factor; it
is possibly a viral infection.

Benethamine Penicillin. An antibiotic effective against most
Grampositive bacteria (streptococci, staphylococci and pneu-
mococci). A derivative of benzylpenicillin, it can be administered by mouth but is usually given as an intramuscular injection, from which it liberates benzylpenicillin slowly. Patients
hypersensitive to penicillins may suffer allergic reactions. See
also penicillin.

Benzathine Penicillin. A long-acting antibiotic, given by mouth or
intramuscular injection, that is slowly absorbed and effective
against most Gram-positive bacteria (streptococci, staphylococci, and peneumococci). Patients hypersensitive to the penicillins suffer allergic reactions. Trade names: **Bicillin,
Penidural.** See also penicillin.

Benzhexol. A drug that has actions and side-effects similar to those
of atropine. Taken by mouth, it is used mainly to reduce
muscle spasm in parkinsonism. Trade names: **Artane, Pipanol.**

Benzocaine. A local anaesthetic used in the form of an ointment, suppository, or aerosol to relieve painful conditions of the skin and mucous membranes. Virtually non-toxic, it can also be given by mouth to treat such conditions as lacerations of the mouth or tongue and gastric ulcers.

Benzodiazepines. A group of pharmacologically active compounds used as minor tranquillizers and hypnotics. The group includes chlordiazepoxide, diazepam, and oxazepam.

Benzoic acid. An antiseptic, active against fungi and bacteria, used as a preservative in foods and pharmaceutical preparations, as well as for the treatment of fungal infections of the skin.

Benzphetamine. A drug with actions and side-effects similar to those of amphetamine. It is given by mouth in the treatment of obesity. Trade name: **Didrex.**

Benzthiazide. A diuretic used in the treatment of conditions involving fluid retention such as congestive heart failure, oedema, hypertension, and obesity. Trade name: **Exna.**

Benztropine. A drug similar to atropine, but that also acts as an antihistamine, local anaesthetic, and sedative. Given by mouth it is used mainly in the treatment of parkinsonism to reduce rigidity and muscle cramps. It is well tolerated, but produces drowsiness and confusion.

Beriberi. Condition caused by shortage of vitamin B^1 (thiamine hydrochloride) in the food. Symptoms occur gradually, starting with loss of appetite, muscular cramps, tingling, and pain in the calves, followed by more severe symptoms, at which point the illness may properly be described as beriberi: general inflammation of the nerves (polyneuritis), paralysis, weakness of the heart and fluid retention (oedema). Heart conditions are particularly frequent and can endanger life.

Bile. An oily, viscous fluid secreted by the liver, normally yellowish-brown in colour, but it may become green. It looks and feels a little like fresh motor oil. The liver secretes about a litre a day, but it becomes concentrated in the gall bladder where it is stored. It is required for normal digestion of fats.

When fat from a meal appears in the upper small intestine, a sequence of events causes the gall bladder to contract and discharge bile into the intestine. Fats are insoluble in water, and therefore not easily absorbed into the cells lining the intestines. Bile consists of molecules so constructed that while one end can be dissolved in water, the other is water-repellant. In water, all of the bile molecules try to turn so as to maximize these molecular preferences; the lowest energy state for doing so is a tiny ball of molecules each aligned with the water-soluble moiety turned out and the water-repellant moiety in toward the centre. Within the pocket formed by this micelle a single molecule of fat can be transported through the cells of the intestinal walls into the lymph. Such molecules may be cholesterol or any of the fat soluble vitamins, A, D, E or K. If the bile is inadequate, any of these vitamins may be deficient.

Bile aids excretion largely by helping to carry waste out of the body, for example the non-reusable breakdown products of haemoglobin, the oxygen-carrying pigment inside red blood cells. Bile derivatives also add the colour and smell to faeces.

Bilharziasis (schistosomiasis). Infection caused by the *Schistosoma* worm, roughly 1 cm long, which has a fresh-water snail as intermediate host.

The worms lie twisted in the blood vessels of the intestine or bladder, where they live on blood. The female lays her eggs in the blood vessel; they are excreted into water in urine or faeces, develop into larvae, enter a snail and multiply; they then leave the snail and are able to infest man (e.g. swimmers) by penetrating the skin. The larvae develop into full-grown worms in the liver and then enter the blood vessels.

Biopsy. Surgical removal of living tissue from some part of the body for examination, usually microscopic, in order to diagnose a disorder affecting that part of the body. The technique is most familiar in the diagnosis *of cancer* but may be used for any other condition that caused characteristic changes in the cells affected.

Biperiden. A drug with effects similar to those of atropine, used in the treatment of parkinsonism, certain forms of spasticity, and to control the muscular incoordination that may result from the use of some tranquillizers. It is given by mouth; side-effects are those of atropine. Trade name: *Akineton*

Birth injuries. Usually caused by difficult labour or an assisted delivery, the injuries can take various forms. Excessively rapid delivery, breech delivery, forceps delivery or other operations can all place the child slightly at risk. The least serious complication is deformation of the skull by a cephalic haematoma or caput succedaneum, which disappear without treatment. More serious is damage to brain tissue through shortage of oxygen during labour (asphyxia), as is haemorrhage and tearing of the cerebral mucous membrane. In both cases the child will be delivered in a very poor condition: limp, pale and hardly breathing. These symptoms may take one or two days to disappear. They can cause spasticity or mental retardation.

Birthmark. Conganital abnormality of the skin, usually not serious. The commonest is a mole, caused by an abnormal accumulation of skin pigment. The dark spots are sometimes large and hairy, and can be a cosmetic problem.

New-born infants sometimes have small white spots on their nose and cheeks (milia), or light red colouring of the nose, eyelids and neck as a result of swollen blood vessels; these disappear of their own accord.

Bisacodyl. A laxative that acts on the large intestine to cause reflex movement and bowel evacuation. It is administered by mouth or in a suppository. The commonest side-effect is the development of abdominal cramps. Trade name: **Dulcolax.**

Black eye. Swelling and blue discoloration around the eye as a result of haemorrhage under the skin. The cause can be a blow to the eye, or a fracture in the facial region of the skull. The skin tissue around the eye is loose-textured, which can cause severe swelling, to the extent that the upper eyelid cannot be opened. If the skull is fractured, both eyes may be blackened.

Fracture of the cheek-bone or severe haemorrhage can cause double vision (diplopia), because the eye cannot be directed properly.

Blackwater fever. A rare and serious complication of malignant tertian (falciparum) malaria in which there is massive destruction of the red blood cells, leading to the presence of the blood pigment haemoglobin in the urine. The condition is probably brought on by inadequate treatment with quinine; it is marked by fever, bloody urine, jaundice, vomiting, enlarged liver and spleen, anaemia, exhaustion, and-in fatal cases—a reduced flow of urine resulting from a blockage of the kidney tubules. Treatment involves rest, administration of alkaline fluids and intravenous glucose, and blood transfusions.

Bladder, Disorders of. The most important bladder conditions are concerned with urination. Difficulty in urination can be the result of sclerosis of the neck of the bladder, stricture of the urethra or pressure of a tumour on the urethra, a pregnant uterus or prolapse of the floor of the bladder, common in women. Failure of part of the nerve supply to the bladder associated with some conditions of the spinal grey matter can also cause difficulty in urination. Often such difficulties cause urinary retention, urine retained in the bladder after urination which, by increasing the pressure in the bladder, can cause diverticulitis of the bladder as well as increasing the likelihood of bladder stones and cystitis (inflammation of the bladder), the latter associated with pain when urinating, and an increased need to do so. Tumours of the bladder are often benign polyps, which may develop into cancers of the bladder. A fairly common condition in women is urinary incontinence, involuntary urination when the pelvic muscles are used or when coughing or laughing.

Bladder, Diverticulitis of. Inflammation of sac-like dilation of the wall of the bladder. The dilations can be small, but are sometimes larger than the bladder itself, and several may appear at the same time.

Bladder, Sclerosis of neck of. Usually congenital stricture of the neck of the bladder, caused by excessive muscle and connective tissue in the ring muscles (sphincter) slowing down urination. Children with this condition take longer to urinate than their contemporaries; the condition is often hardly noticed between the ages of 10 and 30.

Bladder, tumour of. Various tumours occur in the bladder, 95 per cent of them originating in the inner lining.

Bladder polyps are benign tumours which sometimes occur in large numbers, usually causing no discomfort, although blood may appear in the urine. They can be burnt off (cautery), but tend to recur and can sometimes become malignant.

Malignant tumours of the bladder occur particularly in men over the age of 50. Bladder cancer can be caused by lengthy exposure to aniline (an intermediate product in the manufacture of dyestuffs), and by infection with bilharziasis. Cigarette smoking also increases the likelihood of cancer of the bladder.

Bladder stone (calculus). Bladder stones may be formed in the bladder or deposited there via the ureters from the pelvis of the

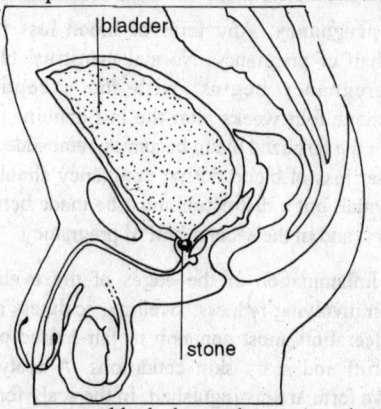

A bladder stone can block the urethra, preventing the discharge of urine and causing the bladder to become overfull.

kidneys. Stones are usually formed in the bladder if urine is contaminated with bacteria responsible for the breakdown of urine, particularly in cases of urinary retention. A stone some- times forms around a foreign body in the bladder, for example hairpin. Other stones 'grow' on much smaller ones that have originated in the kidney. Bladder stones usually produce the symptoms of cystitis; also the stone can abruptly close the junction of bladder and urethra during urination, caus-ing acute retention. Stones or foreign bodies are often visible on X-rays, and diagnosis may be confirmed by examination with an instrument inserted through the urethra (cystoscope).

Bleeding (haemorrhage). Escape of blood from the vascular system.

Haemorrhage can occur in various forms and to various extents. External haemorrhage is loss of blood from the sur-face of the body, and usually not dangerous; it stops of its own accord or can be staunched by firmly applying a dressing. Internal haemorrhage cannot be seen from outside, is thus not usually discovered until late, by which time a great deal of blood can be lost. The danger of heavy blood loss is that shock may set in.

Bleeding in pregnancy. Any form of blood loss in the first or second half of pregnancy. Normal menstrual bleeding ceases when pregnancy begins, with the exception of slight haemorrhage four weeks after the last genuine period, associ-ated with the fertilized ovum becoming embedded in the womb. Any other loss of blood during pregnancy should be regarded as abnormal, but a distinction must be made between bleeding in the first and in the second-half of pregnancy.

Blepharitis. Inflammation of the edges of the eyelids, a chronic condition involving redness, swelling, scaliness and sometimes slight ulceration, most common in fair-haired people inclined to dandruff and scaly skin conditions. A scaly form and an ulcerative form are distinguished. In the scaly form small white scales occur between the eyelashes, which may also fall out to some extent. The condition is aggravated by chemicals, smoke, fatigue or other irritation of the eyelid. In the ulcerative form, bacterial infection causes inflammation of the sebaceous glands at the base of the eyelashes, and a yellow crust and scales form on the inflamed, thickened edges of the lids. The roots are affected, and eyelashes fall out. The scaly form is the more common.

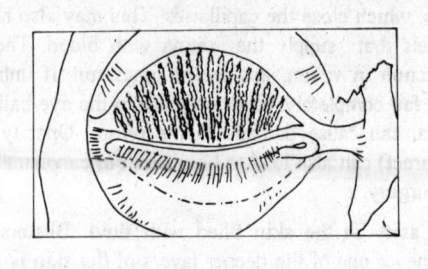

Blepharitis is inflammation of the edge of the eyelid, often aggravated by blockage of the sebaceous glands.

Blindness (amaurosis). Complete absence of vision in one or both eyes, the condition can be congenital, or develop during the

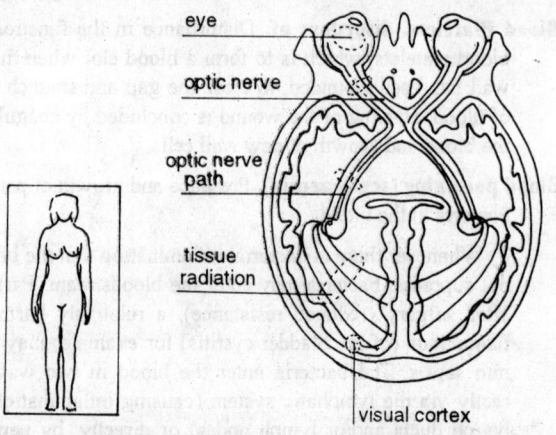

eye

optic nerve

optic nerve path

tissue radiation

visual cortex

Blindness or partial blindness can be caused by a disorder of one of the named structures.

patient's lifetime; the latter is uaually the case. The cause of
blindness can be in the eye itself, in the nerve that carries
information to the brain, or in the part of the brain that processes the information (occipital cortex).

High blood pressure and diabetes can damage blood capillaries and cause thickening of their walls and the formation of
clots, which close the capillaries. This may also happen to the
vessels that supply the retina with blood. The result is a
reduction in vision, and in the long, run, if untreated, sight
may fail completely. High pressure in the eye ball, as in glaucoma, can cause damage to the retina. Opacity of the lens
(cataract) can also lead to blindness but can usually be treated
by surgery.

Blister. Cavity in the skin filled with fluid. Blisters are caused
whenever one of the deeper layers of the skin is damaged, so
that fluid can accumulate underneath it. There are various
ways in which such damage may be caused, the commonest
being pressure or friction from badly fitting shoes. Burn blisters are caused by second-degree burns. There are also various skin diseases linked with blistering, including pemphigus.

Blood Platelets, disorders of. Disturbance in the function of the
blood platelets, which is to form a blood clot when the vessel
wall has been wounded, to close the gap and staunch the loss
of blood. Healing of the wound is concluded by coagulation of
the blood and growth of new wall cells.

Blood poisoning (septicaemia). Presence and growth of pathogenic
bacteria in the blood.

Whenever there is bacterial inflammation that the body cannot suppress, bacteria may enter the bloodstream. Particularly
after surgery (reduced resistance), a relatively harmless inflammation (of the bladder cystitis) for example) may develop
into sepsis. The bacteria enter the blood in two ways, indirectly via the lymphatic system (causing inflammation of the
lymph ducts and/or lymph nodes) or directly, by penetrating
capillary walls. The presence of bacteria in the blood is known
as bacteriaemia, and is often associated with high fever and

cold shivers. If the bacteria are rendered harmless before they can multiply, recovery soon takes place; sepsis sets in if they are allowed to multiply. The patient becomes seriously ill within a few hours, with high fever, often over 40°C. The bacteria in the blood can reach any part of the body and cause inflammation. In serious cases a condition like paralysis occurs in the walls of all blood vessels, causing them to dilate, leading to shock (known as septic shock).

Blood pressure. The pressure of blood against the walls of the main arteries. Pressure is highest during systole, when the ventricles are contracting (*systolic pressure*), and lowest during diastole, when the ventricles are relaxing and refilling (*diastolic pressure*). Blood pressure is measured—in millimetres of mercury-by means of a sphygmomanometer at the brachial artery of the arm, where the pressure is most similar to that of blood leaving the heart. The normal range varies with age, but a young adult would be expected to have a systolic pressure of around 120 mm and a diastolic pressure of 80 mm. These are recorded as 120/80.

Individual variations are common. Muscular exertion and emotional factors, such as fear, stress, and excitement, all raise systolic blood pressure (see hypertension). Systolic blood pressure is normally at its lowest during sleep. Severe shock may lead to an abnormally low blood pressure and possible circulatory failure (see hypotension). Blood pressure is adjusted to its normal level by the sympathetic nervous system and hormonal controls.

Blue baby. An infant suffering from congenital malformation of the heart as a result of which some or all of the blue (deoxygenated) blood is pumped around the body instead of passing through the lungs to be oxygenated. The skin and lips have a purple colour. Advances in cardiac surgery have enabled remedial operations or even total correction to be performed, usually in the first few days or weeks of life. Those that cannot be corrected or improved may survive for months or years with persistent cyanosis.

Boils. Suppurating inflammation of a hair follicle and the surrounding area; the condition is now less common, as hygiene has improved. The cause is the bacterium *Staphylococcus aureus*, which penetrates the follicle and causes folliculitis, which can then spread and form a boil; a cluster of boils is known as a carbuncle. A boil develops from a normal pimple; a slight subcutaneous swelling develops around it, and a rigid disc can be felt under the skin. The skin is locally red and painful. At a later stage the rigid disc becomes liquid, forming an abscess. The boil ripens to a head, which shows white through the skin; the boil then bursts, or can be opened by a doctor. When the pus has been released the abscess cavity cleans itself and heals in a few days.

Bone, tumour of. Accumulation of tissue caused by excessive cell division in the bone. Tumours can originate in bone, cartilage, periosteum (the layer of connective tissue that sheathes a bone) or bone marrow, although the latter are usually secondary tumours, which are always malignant. Bone tumours are painful, usually limit the movement of the affected part of the body, and can affect normal bone tissue to the extent of causing fracture. There are benign and malignant forms.

Bone disorders. Disorders may affect one or more bones, or possibly the whole skeleton. Age is an important factor in the origin and consequence of bone conditions. In children, for example, they can affect growth.

The most frequent disorders are fractures, as the result of an accident or weakening of the bone.

Bone inflammation is usually associated with bone-marrow inflammation. Bone tumours can originate in bone tissue, cartilage, the connective tissue in an around bone and bone marrow. Usually, however, they occur by metastasis from tumours elsewhere in the body.

Bornholm disease (Pleurodynia). Inflammation of the muscles of the chest, named after the Danish island which suffered an epidemic of the disease in 1930. The infection is caused by coxsackievirus.

The symptoms of Bornholm disease are sudden spasms of muscular pain, especially between the ribs. Breathing is extremely painful. Fever can occur. The clinical picture looks very serious—the chest pain can sometimes seem like a heart attack—but recovery is generally complete. Treatment is by controlling the pain; there is no medication effective against the virus.

Botulism. Serious form of food poisoning caused by eating foodstuffs containing *Clostridium botulinum* bacteria, which multiply and form neurotoxins in sausage, meat or in tinned vegetables under certain circumstances (including temperatures above 17°C). The toxins are quickly destroyed by raising the temperature above boiling point for several minutes. Botulism hardly ever occurs in Britain because of good hygienic practice and improved techniques in handling foodstuffs.

Bradycardia. Heart rate of fewer than 60 beats per minute. Well-trained sportsmen often have a slow pulse, because their heart contracts so powerfully that it can maintain adequate blood pressure with fewer beats per minute, and in such cases the condition is harmless. But it can be caused by a disorder elsewhere in the body. A rise in brain pressure, hepatitis and hypothyroidism are associated with slowing of the heartbeat; also damage to the system of impulse and transmission caused by cardiac infarction.

Bradyphrenia. Marked slowing-down in thinking and the ability to react.

The condition is often associated with psychological fatigue, and consists of reduced ability to concentrate, apathy and lack of initiative. The cause can be organic, as in dementia, but the condition can also be a symptom of depression. It can also be caused by alcohol and tranquillizer overdose or poisoning, or extreme fatigue.

Brain disorders. Brain disorders can be classified by cause, a useful division because it also indicates something about their amenability to treatment and the treatment required.

Circulatory problems of the brain (stroke) include cerebral infarction and cerebral haemorrhage, in which blood is discharged into brain tissue. Haemorrhage outside the brain but inside the skull (between the meninges) are subarachnoid, subdural and epidural haemorrhage. The last two in particular can occur after an injury involving brain damage. Various tumours, benign and malignant, can occur in and around the brain. The brain can also be affected by infection-encephalitis or meningitis according to the site.

Brain infarct. Circulatory disturbance in the brain (stroke resulting in brain tissue death through oxygen deficiency, occurring particularly in later life. An important cause is narrowing of the blood vessels and possible clot formation as a result of atherosclerosis.

Brain tumour. May be benign or malignant, but because the skull is an enclosed space even a benign tumour can endanger life. Brain tumours can originate in the cerebral support tissue (glioma), meninges (meningioma) connective tissue surrounding the cerebral nerves (neurinoma), or in the pituitary gland. Cancer originating in the lung, prostate or breast can metastasize to the brain. Symptoms occur according to the speed of growth of the tumour, taking weeks or months. As soon as a tumour reaches a certain size, pressure rises in the skull. The patient complains of a headache and vomiting (particularly in the morning) with no associated nausea, possibly followed after some time by epilepsy, character changes and memory problems. There may be associated faculty failure caused by pressure of the tumour as a result of local pressure on brain tissue. A tumour in the frontal lobes causes character changes and memory problems; a tumour in the motor cortex, unilateral paralysis. If such a tumour is in the left-hand side of the brain the paralysis is often associated with speech defects (aphasia), and sometimes an inability to perform everyday tasks (apraxia). A tumour in the rearmost section of the brain can affect the ability to process visual information (hemianopia). Stimuli can also lead to hallucinations. Finally consciousness is lowered. If pressure in the brain increases too much, part of the brain can be trapped, a life-endangering condition.

Breast cancer. The commonest potentially fatal cancer in women. The peak age for breast cancer is between 40 and 50, but it can occur in much younger women. It seems that an abnormal reaction to oestrogen is a factor in its origin; use of the contraceptive pill on the other hand does not seem to have an effect. Research has also established a number of the other risk factors: early first menstruation, child-bearing at a late age, and breast cancer in other members of the immediate family. The role of breast-feeding is not clear.

Treatment of breast cancer can be by surgery, associated with radiation therapy and the use of anti-hormones, hormones and medication to inhibit cell division. Treatment depends on the extent of the cancer and the type of cancer cell.

Breast disorders. The breast is a sensitive organ in which a number of abnormalities may occur, usually after puberty, but generally not after the menopause, because no more sex hormones are produced, although breast cancer occurs more frequently at this age. There are actually only three abnormalities found in the breast. Mastitis (inflammation of the breast) results from small cracks or wounds in the breast caused by suckling a child. Sore breasts and benign tumours (fibroadenoma) occur frequently in young women of childbearing age. Although the condition requires no treatment the woman must establish with certainty that the tumour or cyst is benign. Finally, there is the possibility of breast cancer.

Breast tumour. Thickened tissue in the brest which feels abnormal to the touch. Nowadays almost everyone is aware of the of the necessity of paying careful attention to possible tumours breast, and more and more women are undertaking self-examination. Tumours of all kinds occur after the age of sexual maturity, and after the menopause they are even more suspect.

If a woman discovers a lump in a breast she should check the following points: does it alter under influence of the menstrual cycle; does it get bigger; if so, how quickly; how long has it been there, and has anything that could have caused it (such as haemorrhage after a fall). In many cases the tumour will turn out to be benign, but this has to be proved.

Breath, shortness of (dyspnoea). The feeling of not getting enough air, often connected with a low level of oxygen and high level of carbon dioxide in the blood. The later condition stimulates the respiratory centre in the brain (causing a feeling of shortness of breath), which then causes the lungs to make respiratory movements. If one deliberately holds one's breath, it is this mechanism that makes it impossible to avoid taking a breath in due course. One form of shortness of breath is familiar to everybody: being 'out of breath' as a result of physical exertion, but this should not occur as a result of light activity. Shortness of breath in such cases can occur in lung conditions such as CARA, serious anaemia, and heart diseases. Heart failure in particular can cause construction through occasional accumulation of fluid in the lungs. Acute shortness of breath causes anxiety-in an attack of asthma, for example, in which the air passages are narrowed and exhalation is restricted. An entirely different type of shortness of breath is hyperventilation in which the victim is anxious, fears that he is not getting enough air, and breathes too much. In this case blood-oxygen levels are normal.

Breath-holding attack. Attack in which a baby or small child holds his breath in a fit of temper. He cannot cry or shout, and turns blue. It is sometimes although rarely associated with loss of consciousness and convulsions, sometimes reminiscent of epilepsy, but different from these in that there is always an identifiable cause pain, temper or another emotion, in that the child sees no other way of working out his frustration. Although the condition is often alarming, it is not dangerous, and no treatment is necessary, certainly not by medication. The best therapy is to provide the child with an alternative means of expressing his frustration. Respiration always returns spontaneously, and the attacks do not occur after the age of five or six.

Breech presentation. Abnormal presentation of a baby in which the buttocks are born before the head. This is not without danger for the child. The stimulus of cold may start the baby breathing before the head is born, and amniotic fluid may be inhaled into the lungs; also the umbilical cord may be crushed between the head and the exit from the womb. Both situations cause serious constriction. The head must be born a few minutes after the feet and buttocks, or the baby may die. Breech presentation is caused by a narrow pelvis, uterine tumour or hydramnios.

Bromodiphenhydramine. An antihistamine given by mouth to relieve the symptoms of allergic reactions, especially hay fever and rhinitis. It is also used to prevent travel sickness. Common side-effects include drowsiness, dizziness, dryness of the throat, and digestive upsets. Trade name: **Ambodryl.**

Bronchiectasis. Severe dilation of the bronchi, the larger branches of the air passages to the lungs. Repeated inflammation or a congenital flaw can weaken the bronchial wall, so that it blows up like a balloon on each intake of breath. In the past this occurred frequently in tuberculosis patients, today only in patients with a lung abnormality or children with mucoviscidosis. Frequently there are few symptoms pointing clearly to the condition. The most important is repeated pneumonia. A lung X-ray shows a picture typical of bronchiectasis. Round or tubular cavities are visible in the lungs, sometimes containing a layer of mucus. Coughing up blood can also be a sign of this condition.

Bronchiolitis. Inflammation of the smallest branches of the lung's air passage, the bronchioles. Acute bronchiolitis occurs predominantly in babies and young children under the age of two, caused by a kind of influenza virus. The child usually has a cold, but then suddenly becomes really ill, coughs, becomes constricted, and blue around the mouth. Narrowing of the air passages causes a whistling. difficult exhalation. The disorder often disappears spontaneously within a few days, but sometimes leads to bacterial inflammation, and can also cause pneumonia.

Bronchitis. There are two forms of bronchitis: acute bronchitis and chronic bronchitis. Acute bronchitis is a sudden inflammation of the bronchi, a larger air passages of the lungs. The illness can occur once or a number of times in a lifetime. Chronic bronchitis is a persistent, often debilitating, form of the disorder.

During respiration air is carried to the lungs via the air passages. Inflammation of the bronchi can impair the air supply to the tissue of the lung. Acute bronchitis is largely caused by viruses, and is usually preceded by common cold.

Brucellosis. Infectious disease caused by *Brucella* bacteria, which occur in animals (goats, pigs, cattle and sheep). The disease cannot be passed from one human being to another. Cattle infected with brucellosis are probably the principal cause of the spread of the disease in Europe. The varieties of bacteria produce various clinical pictures. Bang's disease, caused by *Brucella abortus*, comes from cows and can occur in abbatoir workers, veterinary surgeons and farmers throughout Europe. Pig brucellosis, from *Brucella suis,* occurs in some Eastern European countries and in the United States. Malta fever, caused in goats by *Brucella melitensis,* mainly occurs in the Mediterranean region.

Buerger's disease. An inflammatory condition affecting the arteries, especially in the legs of young male Jews who smoke cigarettes, intermittent claudication (pain due to reduced blood supply) and gangrene of the limbs may develop. Coronary thrombosis may occur and venous thrombosis is common. The treatment is similar to that of atheroma but cessation of smoking is essential to prevent progression of the disease. Medical name: **thromboangiitis obliterans.**

Bulimia. Exaggerated increase in appetite, with characteristic sessions of eating to excess followed by self-induced vomiting, Bulimia is usually associated with, or follows, anorexia nervosa, but can occur independently. Certain heart conditions can also lead to bulimia. The characteristics of typical bulimia are that eating bouts often take place when the patient is alone, in the evening or at night. It is preceded by a period of excited anticipation, followed by an irrepressible urge to eat without stopping. There is a preference for high calory, ready-to-eat foods, and the session ends with an action aimed at forgetting or showing that the bout is over (going to sleep or to work, taking laxatives or inducing vomiting). Bulimia must not be confused with over-eating.

Bupivacaine. A Potent local anaesthetic, used mainly for regional nerve block. It is significantly longer-acting than many other local anaesthetics. It has been used in childbirth, but may cause slowing of the baby's heart, with a risk of death. Trade name: **Marcain.**

Burns. Very painful sterile inflammation of the skin caused by heat or chemicals. There are three degrees of burn. In a first-degree burn the skin looks red, is very painful and may be slightly swollen. Only the uppermost part of the skin is affected. In a second-degree burn, the skin is also blistered. Infection can occur, and scars may form when the burn heals. A third-degree burn extends into connective or even muscular tissue. This is no longer painful, bacause the pain nerves are also burned. A third-degree burn is generally surrounded by a border of second-degree burn, in its turn surrounded by an area of first-degree burn.

Bursa. A sac or pocket lined with a slippery membrane like that lining a joint and filled with a viscid fluid. They are situated where friction might otherwise develop, for example the places where ligaments or tendons move over bones. Thus, although some bursae are normal adjuncts of anatomical development, like the hollow, moving joints which they resemble, others may develop in response to unusual pressure. *Inflammation* of a bursa is called *bursitis*.

Bursitis. Inflammation of a bursa, a sac-like cavity lined with connective tissue and containing mucous fluid. Bursitis is usually the result of chronic irritation; tenosynovitis can spread to a neighbouring bursa. The condition causes pain, particularly when the patient moves, and the bursa swells as a result of excess moisture production. The skin above the bursa becomes red and warm. Bursitis occurs particularly in the knee, especially in patients whose work involves kneeling, hence the name housemaid's knee.

Butacaine. A local anaesthetic used to produce surface anaesthesia, mainly in eye, ear, nose, and throat surgery. Trade name: **Butyn.**

Butobarbitone. (Butobarbital) An intermediate-acting barbiturate, used for the treatment of insomnia and for sedation. It produces sleep within 30 minutes when given by mouth and its sedative effect lasts for about six hours. Prolonged administration may lead to dependence and its use with alcohol should be avoided; overdosage has serious effects (see barbiturism). Trade name: **Soneryl.**

C

Caisson disease. (Decompression sickness; the bends) Formation of gas bubbles in blood and body fluids as a result of a sudden drop in pressure. The condition occurs particularly in divers who have been breathing air under pressure and are then brought to the surface too quickly.

Callus. Local thickening of the horn layer of the skin in areas exposed to pressure or friction, such as the feet, or workmen's hands, with the original function of protecting the skin from damage. This protective layer cannot form unless pressure is eased occasionally; if it is not, bedsores form. Cuts and cracks in calloused skin can be very painful. Corns are a troublesome form of callus. Cracks and corns may need treatment by a chiropodist; corns may even need surgical attention.

Candidiasis. (moniliasis) Infection caused by the fungus *Candida albicans*. In healthy human beings the fungus occurs on the skin and in the intestines, and often causes no infection or difficulties. Infection can occur in patients with reduced resistance caused by long illness, blood abnormalities, certain medicines (such as anti-cancer drugs, corticosteroids or antibiotics) or radiation. If a bacterial infection is treated with antibiotics, harmless bacteria are also destroyed, the fungus grows more vigorously and candidiasis can occur. In some illnesses, diabetes for example, the condition of the tissue is so altered that the fungus can cause infection.

Caput Succedancum. Swelling on the head of a new-born child which can occur in the course of labour, the result of oedema under the scalp of the most deeply recessed part of the skull; the oedema is caused by pressure and obstruction to the removal of venous blood. The swelling is doughy in consistency and, because it is subcutaneous, extends beyond the joints of the skull, thus differing from a cephalic haemotoma.

CARA. (Chronic aspecific respiratory ailments) Combination of disorders of the air passages and lungs, sometimes grouped together for diagnostic convenience. The group includes chronic bronchitis asthma and emphysema. None of these has a specific cause, but some patients are highly susceptible to them. They often run in families and are associated with allergies and hypersensitivity of the mucous membrane of the air passages. CARA occurs more in men than women.

Carbon Monoxide Poisoning. Caused by breathing carbon monoxide (CO), which is formed during the incomplete combustion of many fuels. CO combines (in preference to oxygen) with haemoglobin in the red blood cells, making the transport of oxygen impossible. The symptoms of sudden poisoning are headache, dizziness, nausea, vomiting and lowered consciousness. The skin turns red. Severe cases can lead to heart damage, unconsciousness (coma), and cessation of respiration often leading to death. Gradual poisoning is associated with headaches and other symptoms include sweating and constriction of the chest.

Treatment is by administration of oxygen, possibly with artificial respiration in a high-pressure chamber, thus driving out CO from the haemoglobin. The patient gradually brightens up with treatment; there may be residual symptoms such as muscular quivering (tremor), and symptoms similar to paralysis or Parkinson's disease; serious cases may lead to permanent dementia.

Diagnosis is by the symptoms and the presence of excess CO-haemoglobin in the blood.

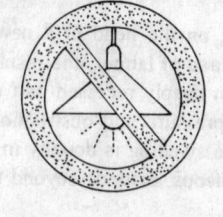 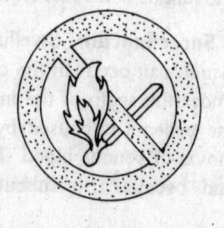

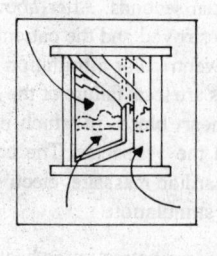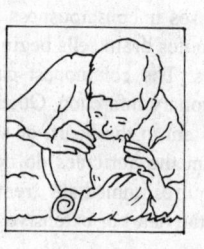

If someone has been overcome by poisonous gas, the following points should be borne in mind: extinguish lights and naked flames (risk of explosion), open windows and administer mouth-to-mouth resuscitation.

Carbuncle. Accumulation of interconnected boils occurring almost exclusively in conditions of poor hygiene or when a patient's resistance is reduced. The disorder is associated with fever and a general feeling of malaise, largely caused by the size of the area affected.

There is a strong likelihood that bacteria from the carbuncle will enter the bloodstream and cause inflammation elsewhere; for this reason antibiotics are usually prescribed. They do not help to cure the carbuncle itself, which should be treated like a boil.

Carcinoid Syndrome. Combination of symptoms caused by hormone-producing intestinal tumour. These rare tumours are malignant, but behave in a relatively benign fashion, growing slowly and metastasizing late.

They can occur throughout the alimentary tract, but are usually found in the appendix or the end of the small intestine.

The characeristic symptoms of the carcinoid syndrome are caused by the production of serotin, histamine and related hormones.

Cardiac arrest. Circulatory failure caused by non-contraction of the heart. This cuts off the oxygen supply to the brain and causes unconsciousness within ten seconds. After about three minutes brain cells begin to be destroyed and the patient finally dies. The commonest cause is ventricular fibrillation after a coronary infarction. Other causes are total failure of the impulse system in the heart, or serious heart block, in which impulses from the auricules do not reach the ventricles. The condition requires immediate treatment: cardiac massage, electric shock to the heart or extensive cardiac stimulation.

Cardiac Asthma. Breathing difficulty originating in the heart rather than the lungs or air passages, characteristically occurring at night. It is caused by failure of the left side of the heart because of abnormalities of the aortic or mitral valve, or after a coronary inflarction. The heart cannot pump blood away from the lungs rapidly enough and it accumulates there. By day this causes little or no discomfort, but at night the sleeping posture brings more blood into circulation from the legs, and even a small increase in the quantity of blood in the lungs can cause an attack. Because not enough oxygen can be taken from the lungs, cyanosis sets in. A cardiac asthma attack can endanger life and must be treated promptly by the administration of oxygen and medication: rapidly effective diuretics, digitalis and morphine.

Cardiac Infarction. Death of part of the heart muscle caused by sudden interruption in the arterial blood supply to that section of the heart. It is caused by blockage of a coronary artery, almost always as a result of a coronary artery already constricted by atherosclerosis, in which even a small blood clot can then block the artery completely. Many patients who suffer cardiac infarction have angina pectoris, but it can occur without warning. Symptoms are the same as those of angina but more severe, and they persist for longer : severe, convulsive pain behind the breastbone, often radiating to left arm neck and jaw, associated with nausea vomiting, shortness of breath, sweating and acute feelings of anxiety.

Cardiomyopathy. Any condition of the heart muscles associated with cumulative damage to heart muscle cells, but not including cardiac muscles degeneration caused by disorders of the coronary arteries or of the cardiac valves.

Symptoms of cardiomyopathie are always the same, regardless of the cause. Because the heart is no longer able to pump adequately, heart rhythm disorders occur, causing problems such as shortness of breath on exertion, fatigue, and oedema of the ankles. Symptoms increase in severity as the muscle deteriorates.

Cataract. Clouding of the lens of the eye, causing a decline in vision and sometimes blindness. In advanced stages of the disorder the clouded lens can be seen as a grey mass in the eye. The condition is painless. Cataract may be congenital, occur as a result of hereditary factors or through German measles in the mother in the 5th to 8th week of pregnancy. Cataract can also occur as a result of irradiation of the eye or injury to the lens. Diabetes mellitus can also cause cataract, especially if blood-sugar content is not carefully controlled. The commonest form, however, is senile cataract, after the age of 60. In the early stages the edge of the lens becomes opaque, and the condition proceeds gradually to the middle of the lens. At the same time vision is increasingly impaired, until the eye is blind when the lens becomes completely opaque. Cataract usually occurs in both eyes, but not necessarily to the same extent. Treatment is by surgery, but not usually until vision is affected. The opaque lens is removed, and after healing vision is restored with spectacles or contact lenses, or sometimes an artificial lens is implanted surgically. If the eye was otherwise healthy vision can be restored completely, but because the lens is missing the eye cannot accommodate to different distances, thus the patient needs different spectacles for close and distant work.

Catarrh. Clear fluid dribbling from-nose, usually caused by inflammation of the nasal mucous membrane. A typical symptom of a cold, troublesome catarrh can also be a side-effect of hay fever. The nasal mucous membrane contains many mucus-producing cells. When the membrane is stimulated by a virus or by pollen in the case of hay fever, the cells produce mucus of a watery consistency, and when this happens in quantity it causes a runny nose. When the cause is a virus, such as a cold, the nose will dry up again in a few days to a week, but in the case of hay fever the runniness may persist for as long as there is pollen in the air in large quantities.

Catatonia. Bizarre movement disorder not based on delusions or hallucinations, but a rare symptom of conditions such as schozophrenia. Strange postures and movements may persist for hours. The condition is extremely rare nowadays because of modern medication and the positive attitude of psychotherapy.

Cellulitis. Acute inflammation of the skin and sub-cutaneous connective tissue. Cellulitis is caused by bacteria penetrating the skin through a small wound, often not visible to the eye. The disorder is associated with fever and general malaise, with localized skin swelling; subcutaneous infiltration may develop, tissue feels stiffer than normal, and there seems to be a hard layer under the skin.

Central Nervous System (CNS). The brain and spinal cord. All other neurons form the peripheral nervous system.

Cerebral Haemorrhage (apoplexy) Caused by rupture of a blood vessel in the brain, possibly made vulnerable through atherosclerosis a congenital condition (aneurysm) or an abnormality or inflammation of the vein, and usually occurring in old age or as a result of arteriosclerosis. The risk is increased by high blood pressure and the use of anticoagulant drugs. Haemorrhage deprives the brain cells of oxygen and puts pressure on the cerebral tissue, causing cell death. In serious cases the symptoms are sudden severe headache and vomiting; the patient may go into coma, the increasing pressure on the brain can be life-threatening. Smaller haemorrhages also cause headache and possibly slight lowering of the level of consciousness. Faculties fail according to the site of the haemorrhage. Usually one side of the body is affected by paralysis; haemorrhage in the cortex of the dominant (left) half of the brain can cause aphasia and apraxia; haemorrhage in the area of the nearmost cortex can cause hemianopia (loss of half the field of vision). Recovery is often not complete. and can take several months; repeated haemorrhage is a dangerous complication.

Cerebral Palsy. Abnormalities of muscles and nerves in new-born babies, resulting from brain damage. The following symptoms can occur: paralysis, muscular weakness, stiffness, spasticity, involuntary movements, tremors and problems of muscular co-ordination possibly together with convulsions, mental defi-ciency, defects of vision and hearing, and emotional problems. The cause is not always clear. Damage can occur before or shortly after birth. Causes in pregnancy can be hereditary fac-tors, exposure to X-ray, haemorrhage or infection in the mother (such as German measles), and during or shortly after birth, lack of oxygen, blood group antagonism, haemorrhage or in-fection.

Cervical Cancer. The commonest form of gynaecological cancer. It seems that women who were sexually active at an early age and who have had a lot of partners are at risk. Jewish women are rarely affected, possibly through hereditary immunity or male circumcision. Cervical cancer is practically never found in women who live a life of strict celibacy, such as nuns. The disease can be detected at an early stage by a smear test. If the cancer is restricted to the surface of the cervix the chance of recovery is almost 100 per cent. The spread of cervical cancer is divided into stages; in the later stages the cancer is larger and/or metastasized. Symptoms occur only in the later stages: irregular menstruation, loss of blood during sexual intercourse, pain and vaginal discharge.

Treatment depends on the stage of development of the can-cer. If it is restricted to the cervix an operation is possible; if it has advanced further, treatment is radiotherapy.

Cervical Incompetence. Inability of the cervix of the womb to remain closed during pregnancy, causing miscarriage or pre-mature birth. Normally the cervix does not open until the onset of labour.

Cervical incompetence is usually caused by damage in previous labour, forceps delivery, induced abortion or cervical surgery. Cervical function can usually be restored by stitching, permitting a pregnancy to proceed normally.

Cervical Myelopathy. Damage to the spinal grey matter in the neck by narrowing of the vertebral canal caused by arthrosis (wear) of the vertebrae, leading to thickening and protrusions. Neck movement continually damages the spinal grey matter. This condition occurs particularly in older people, who suffer from slight loss of feeling and strength in the fingers, with pain radiating to the arms, caused by pressure on the local nerves in the spine. Damage to other areas of the spinal grey matter affects different parts of the body: there may be diminished feeling in the legs, with resultant stiffness and uncertainty in walking, or impotency and urinary problems. The severity of the disorder can vary greatly. Narrowing can be established by spinal X-ray and contrast medium pictures, showing that cerebral fluid cannot pass freely. This examination also eliminates other possible causes such as a tumour or slipped disc. Treatment is by surgery to widen the vertebral canal.

Cervical smear. Test to seek abnormalities, visible under the microscope, in cells coming from the area around the cervix. A smear using the Papanicolaou method (the Pap smear) is used as a test to detect cervical cancer at an early stage. Cells and mucus are scraped from the cervix with a spatula, smeared on to a microscope slide and then fixed with fluid. The slide is then sent for examination. No smears can be taken during menstruation.

Cervicitis. Inflammation of the cervix, one of the most frequently occurring gynaecological conditions, roughly 50 per cent of women suffer from it at some time, and it almost always occurs in childbirth. Use of the contraceptive pill, pessaries or intra-uterine devices (coils) slightly increases the probability of the disorder.

It can be caused by fungi (candidiasis), bacteria or viruses, and the most usual symptoms are vaginal discharge and itching. When the cervical mucus is affected the white blood cells contain a factor which make it impenetrable for sperm, thus causing temporary infertility.

Chagas' disease. An infectious disease transmitted by insects and caused by a protozoan parasite (*Trypanosoma cruzi*). It occurs principally in South and Central America, where about 10 million people are infected. The trypanosomes are very small and move by means of a flagellum through the human circulatory system. Blood-sucking insects suck up blood containing trypanosomes and deposit them on the skin of other human beings in their excrement while sucking blood. The insects are intermediate hosts (vectors).

Chalazion. Small, firm, painless swelling in the upper or lower eyelid. the skin moves freely over the swelling. A small blob is visible on the inside of the eyelid some distance from the edge, without signs of inflammation such as redness or accumulation of fluid. Chalazion results from blockage of a sebaceous gland; the sebaceous glands have large number of exits in the upper and lower eyelids just below the roots of the eyelashes. If a chalazion causes discomfort-to contact lens wearers for example—it can be removed by an ophthalmic surgeon making a small incision inside the eyelid. If no discomfort is caused no treatment is necessary.

Character disturbances. Character traits which are problematical to the extent that life is seriously disturbed by them.

Character disturbances in the psychiatric sense are those that originate in the earlier stage of development, the first two years of life.

They can come to light later as disturbances which trouble only the patient himself, such as a neurosis (e.g. a compulsive neurosis), or it can be that only those around the patient suffer (e.g. psychopathy). Most character disturbances fall between these two extremes.

Cheilosis. Condition of the lips, usually beginning with a pale area at the corner of the mouth which later becomes calloused and possibly cracked, and then inflamed as bacteria enter the cracks.

Cheilosis is usually caused by deficiency of riboflavin (one of the B vitamins) in which case there are associated abnormalities of the tongue and eyes; but it can also be 'normal' in older people. Treatment is with vitamin B; inflammation subsides spontaneously.

Chickenpox (varicella) Virus disease of children. The incubation period is two to three weeks, and the disease is contagious from one day before the skin rash appears until all the vesicles have dried up. Chickenpox begins with a high temperature, listlessness, poor apetite and headache. After a few days small red lumps develop and these becomes itchy vesicles containing a clear fluid. The visicles dry out to form scabs which drop off after a few days. The chickenpox rash mainly occurs on the trunk, head and oral mucous membrane. The younger the child is when he or she is infected, the fewer the symptoms.

Chilblains. Skin condition characterized by red and intensely itchy hands and feet. It occurs mainly in cold weather. Chilblains develop rapidly during damp cold conditions, such as fog. The skin can swell up, and in severe cases blisters or ulcers can form. It is most common among young people.

The cause is an abnormal reaction of the capillaries to cold. Instead of closing, these vessels open. The blood flows too slowly as a result, and this leads to the development of the symptoms.

Childhood Disorders. Infectious diseases that affect children almost exclusively, because they are so infectious that anyone who comes into contact with them for the first time catches the disease but then normally acquires immunity for life. These illnesses do not usually occur until the child is at least three months old, because he or she receives some immunity from the mother, and this period of passive immunity is lengthened by breast feeding. Later the child has to establish his own immunity, either by contracting the disease or through vaccination. The most important infectious diseases with which a child can be confronted are measles, German measles, scarlet fever poliomyelitis, whooping cough (pertussis), mumps, chickenpox and diphtheria. A number of these have been stamped out for all practical purposes by preventive immunization, originally developed to counteract the consequences of the more dangerous diseases, such as paralysis from polio, suffocation from diphtheria, and so on. Modern vaccines have been developed to give protection against a number of the diseases in a single injection, such as the DPT (diphtheria, pertussus, tetanus) vaccine.

Chlamydia. Pathogens which can cause various diseases. In Europe and North America one of them causes a common venereal disease, a certain form of urethritis more common than gonorrhoea. Ten to twenty days after infection in men the penis discharges a slimy fluid containing pus, caused by inflammation of the urethra, and associated with frequent urination and pain when doing so. The inflammation can spread to the prostate and the epididymis. Chlamydia can also cause urethritis in women, but more often results in cervical inflammation and grey vaginal discharge. The infection can spread to the womb and the Fallopian tubes, resulting in fever, stomachache and nausea. Infection of the Fallopian tubes can lead to infertility. Babies born of mothers with this disease can themselves be infected during birth. Between the fifth and fourteenth days of life a slight inflammation of the eyes occurs, and sometimes inflammation of the ears and lungs. The infection usually clears up without residual symptoms.

Chloasma. Disturbance in the normal distribution of pigment during pregnancy. A patchy brown discoloration develops on the face. The alternation in the distribution of pigment is less striking elsewhere in the body.

If a woman suffers from chloasma during her first pregnancy, she will suffer from it again in a subsequent one.

Choking. Chocking occurs when a morsel of food lodges in the larynx or windpipe instead of passing down the oesophagus, causing immediate closure of the glottis and a violent fit of coughing which dislodges the food from the larynx. Someone who is choking can be helped by patting on the back between the shoulder blades. If a morsel of food or other object remains in the windpipe, acute and severe chest constriction occurs. It is then necessary to act quickly. The object can sometimes be expelled from the windpipe by grasping the victim from behind below the ribs and pulling him backwards.

Cholangitis. Inflammation of the bile ducts, which carry bile from the liver to the gall bladder and thence to the duodenum. Such inflammation is always the result of a temporary and partial blockage of the bile duct, by a gallstone, a (tissue) stricture or a tumour, and results in attacks of pain (colic) and fever with cold shivers. Restriction of bile flow causes jaundice, through accumulation of bilirubin in the body; excess acid gall salts cause itching.

Cholecystitis. Inflammation of the gall bladder, which collects bile from the liver and releases it into the duodenum. Almost always a complication of a gallstone, it can be acute, with severe pain, or chronic, with nagging pain.

The acute form is caused by a gallstone blocking the exit from the gall bladder, leading to increased pressure, swelling and colicky pain. Sometimes the stone returns into the bladder, in which case the symptoms disappear.

Cholera. Acute, contagious intestinal dosorder caused by the *Vibrio cholerae* bacillus. Infection is from man to man, or from contaminated food; the bacillus can survive only with difficulty except in man. After a short incubation period (2 to 5 days) the disease begins suddenly with violent diarrhoea and vomiting, faces are watery, and may be discharged upto twenty times a day, but without pain or spasms. As much as 15 litres of fluid and 30 grams of salt can be lost in 24 hours, causing serious dehydration, resulting in severe thirst, sunken eyes, low blood pressure and very low urine production; it can cause death within hours or days, Diagnosis can be difficult because the disease is rare and the symptoms are similar to gastroenteritis. Blood tests show acidity and accumulation of toxins through poor kidney function.

Treatment is by infusion of fluid and salt and antibiotics to remove the bacteria; recovery is usually within a few days.

Cholesteatoma. Benign tumour of the middle ear, consisting of a slowly accumulating mass of layers of dead cells from the lining, containing cholesterol crystals. The cause is not yet fully established, although the condition is always associated with chronic otitis media and / or a perforated eardrum. Growth of the cholesteatoma and release of enzymes graduelly destroy the auditory ossicles (the bones of the middle ear), and the condition can spread to the inner ear. Symptoms are slight at first: an odorous discharge of pus and sometimes blood from the ear. Hearing gradually deteriorates with destruction of the auditory ossicles; earache is rare, but can be caused by inflammation of the auditor canal.

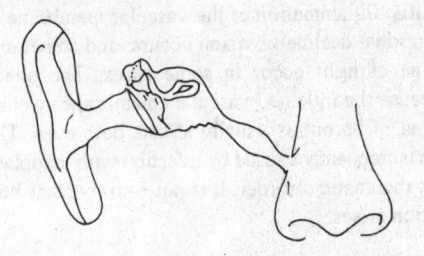

Cholesteatoma is an inflamed accumulation of sebum and skin cells in the middle ear.

Cholesterol. A fatty chemical obtained from food but also synthesized in the liver. It is a steriod and necessary in the biosynthesis of several hormones bile and the white sheaths, surrounding many nerves, called myelin. Adults have about 140 gms or 5 ozs of cholesterol in their bodies of which 4 to 6 gms is being transported in the blood. The blood cholesterol tends to rise in older people. It can be reduced temporarily by reducing the dietary intake of fatty foods, but the liver tends to maintain a steady amount of cholesterol in the blood. Cholesterol is undoubtedly a major constituent of atheromas, but the evidence that it causes *atheroscalerosis* or *hypertension* is still circumstantial and inconclusive. Most authorities would now accept no more than that it may be a contributing factor.

Choriocarcinoma. Malignant tumour of the trophoblast, usually after a previous hydatidiform pregnancy; the cause is unknown, and this cancer is rare in the West (1 in 20,000 pregnancies). The cancer can metastasize to brain, lungs and liver. Symptoms are loss of blood after a hydatidiform pregnancy, and sometimes pregnancy symptoms, because a great deal of the hormone HCG is produced; its presence is important in diagnosis and checks. Women who have had a hydatidiform pregnancy must undergo careful checks and not become pregnant for a year. Treatment is by drugs to inhibit cell division; recovery rate is about 80 per cent.

Choroiditis. Inflammation of the vascular membrane of the eyeball. A gradual decline in vision occurs, and sometimes parts of the retina of light occur in some cases. The phenomena arises because the inflamed vascular membrane swells, affecting the retina. Choroiditis usually affects both eyes. This rare condition is frequently caused by infection with toxoplasmosis, syphlis or a rheumatic disorder. It is not entirely clear how this inflammation arises.

Chromosome. A very large molecule containing genes and thus governing part of the inheritance of the individual. Normal humans have 46 chromosomes, 44 of them called autosomal because they seem to govern characteristics of the body, like eye colour, and 2 sex chromosomes which contain, among other genes, those determining biological sex.

Chromosomes are long assemblages of similar segments called nucleic acids. During most of the life of a cell, they seem to be arranged more or less at random in the nucleus of the cell. However, just before cell division is to occur, the chromosomes form a line across the centre of the nucleus organized so that their long axis is parallel to the line of division.

Before division begins, the two mirror-image strands of each chromosome separate, one strand entering each daughter cell. Once the two new cells are organized, each chromosome strand immediately governs the synthesis of its mirror image. The normal condition of a chromosome consists of these two strands tightly coiled together. However, in order to perform their genetic functions, the two strands must unwind and separate partially in the region of the gene required. The chemical regulation of these complex events is not yet fully understood.

Cirrhosis of the liver. The final stage of a number of liver conditions. The characteristic features of cirrhosis are widespread cell death, the formation of inflexible connective tissue (fibrosis), regeneration of liver cells and formation of connecting blood vessels. Various forms are distinguished according to the size of the knobs of liver tissue between the connective tissue; the forms overlap to a large extent.

Important causes cirrhosis are: excess alcohol consumption over a long period, viral hepatitis which does not clear up properly, long-term bile blockage (as a result of gallstones, etc.), blockage of blood flow in the liver by heart function failure and chronic (protein) malnutrition.

Cleft palate. Congenial condition arising very early in pregnancy from defective fusion of the two halves of the palate. Although it often occurs in conjunction with a hare lip, there is no genetic connection between the two, although a hereditary factor is present in both. Cleft palate is less common than hare lip; it occurs as 1 in every 2,500 births, more commonly in girls than boys.

The disorder is often not noticed immediately at birth, particularly if the gap is small and there is no associated abnormality of the lip, and may be discovered because the child cannot take milk properly, or because food is returned down the nose. The danger here is that food can enter the air passages, causing chocking or pneumonia. It is thus important that new-born children are examined for the condition.

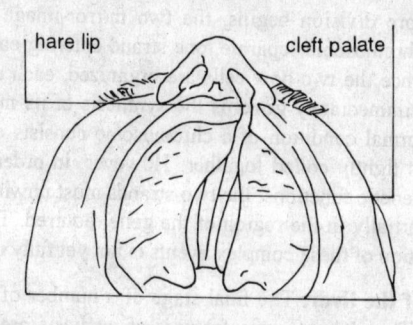

Cleft palate and hare lip often occur together. These conditions cause feeding problems at first, and speech defects at a later stage

Coarctation. Congenital abnormality of the aorta involving obstruction at the point at which it leaves the heart, just beyond the point at which the arteries leading to the head and the arms branch off. The rest of the body can be supplied adequately with blood only if it is pumped vigorously past the obstructed

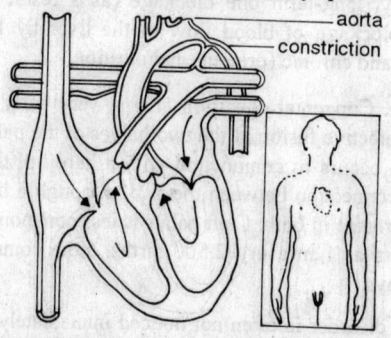

Constriction of the aorta raises the blood pressure in the head and arms and lowers it in the rest of the body.

part of the aorta, and in order to do this blood pressure in the part of the aorta in front of the obstruction and in the arteries of the head and arms has to be kept high; thus the left ventricle has to work very hard and signs of overload can show over the course of years (heart failure).

Coccidioidomycosis. Fungus disease caused by *Coccidioides immities*. The infection occurs through inhaling spores or through skin wounds which come into contact with the soil. The fungus lodges in the lungs. The clinical picture is very similar to tuberculosis with fever, coughing, chest pain and constriction as the most common symptoms. The fungus can live in the lungs for a long time and cause recurring sumptoms over the years. In rare cases it can spread in the bloodstream throughout the entire body.

Cold (coryza) Viral infection of the mucous membrane of the nose. There are many viruses that can cause a cold, which explains why someone can have several colds a year, each being caused by a different virus. The first symptoms are a runny nose, sneezing fits, red eyes and a tired, listless feeling. Breathing is impaired by the red, swollen mucous membrane, and the patient tends to breathe through the mouth, causing throat complaints such as hoarseness a dry feeling in the throat, slight pain and coughing, and the lymph nodes in the neck are often tender. The nasal mucous membrane is readily susceptible to bacterial attack in this condition, and when they are involved in the infection the nasal mucus bedomes a thick, yellowish - green secretion. After this the swollen membrane subsides, and breathing through the nose is easier again. The mucous is 'nice and loose'. Usually a cold does not last for longer than seven days. If it persists for longer, the sinuses, throat and middle ear are often inflamed as well, and a doctor should be consulted. The early symptoms of a cold can also be the first signs of various children's illnesses such as measles, chickenpox and scarlet fever. Influenza is also a possibility.

Cold sore (herpes labialis) Eruption on the face caused by the herpes simplex virus (HSV type I). Herpes simplex infections are very common, and by later life almost everyone will have experienced one, usually without discomfort. One of the characteristics of the virus is that after infection it remains in the body during the patient's lifetime, usually without causing any other manifestations of disease. However, it is also possible for the virus to produce recurrent infection, of which cold sores are an example. The venereal disease Herper genetalis is another example of a herpes simplex infection, although it is produced by a different, HSV type I generally occurs in the second to fourth year of life, usually without symptoms at that time. The virus then established itself in the nerves, from which it can later cause cold sores.

Colic. Attack of severe, stabbing pain caused by convulsive movement of smooth muscular tissue in the alimentary canal or the ureters, caused by irritants (laxatives etc.) in the stomach or intestine, or by restriction of the intestines, (intestinal obstruction), the bile ducts (gallstones) or the ureters (kidney stones). Colic is thus not a disorder in its own right, but a symptom. Pain occurs in fits, and because it is reduced by movement the patient is unlikely to lie still in bed. The site of the pain or radiation can give an indication of its cause: in gallstones the pain is at the topmost right-hand point of the abdomen and radiates to the back; in kidney stones it is most severe in the side and radiates to the groin.

Colour Blindness. Cogenital inability of the retinal cones to distinguish colours usually reduced ability to perceive shades of green. About 50 per cent of colour-blind people have reduced green vision; 25 per cent cannot see the colour at all. Total colour blindness, in which the person sees only black, white and grey, is very rare. Sometimes colour vision is disturbed by inflammation in the centre on the retina, where the most cones are. Normal vision usually returns on recovery.

There are various tests for colour blindness consisting of figures made up of spots in various colours, which have to be recognized.

Coma. Condition of unconsciousness from which the patient cannot be roused, with various causes and varying degrees of depth. Normally consciousness is maintained by an activating centre in the brain stem which stimulates the rest of the brain. If this centre or a large part of the cerebral cortex fails, consciousness can no longer be maintained. Coma can occur in brain conditions such as stroke, encephalitis, meningitis brain injury, brain tumour and serious attacks of epilepsy. Non-cerebral causeds are a severe drop in blood pressure (through cardiac infraction or serious haemorrhage), metabolic disturbances (including inadequate blood sugar content or hypoglycaemia in diabetics) or serious liver and kidney disorders.

Concussion. Usually short disturbance of brain function caused by a head injury. A distinction is made between 'normal' concussion and cerebral contusion, according to the seriousness of the injury. In the case of concussion the patient loses consciousness for a few minutes after the incident, and cannot remember the period immediately before it (retrograde amnesia). Nausea and vomiting often occur as a result of short-term lack of control of the central nervous system, possibly associated with headache. In contrast with cerebral contusion there are no faculty failures (such as paralysis or reflex disorders), because the brain is probably undamaged. Headache and dizziness may persist for days or weeks.

Condylomata Acuminata. Small warts caused by a viral infection at the conjunction of mucous membrane and skin around the anus, vulva and penis. They can spread to the vagina, and they grow rapidly in a warm, moist environment. The infection can be transmitted by sexual intercourse and is thus a venereal disease to a certain extent.

Confabulation. Invented story told to make an impression or to conceal amnesia.

Young children often try to make an impression with invented stories and at their age this is a normal fantasy outlet, but if it occurs too often, or if older children or adults do it, it can be abnormal, and is a symptom of some neuroses; it is as though the patient is addicted to his fantasy.

Congential abnormalities. Abnormalities present at birth; they are not necessarily hereditary and not always immediately apparent. They occur in 5 per cent of babies. New congenital abnormalities are still being discovered, but their nature is less important to parents and medical science than their cause. An important discovery was that the cause of certain abnormalities is already present in the fertilized ovum (hereditary). Such hereditary qualities are transmitted through the chromosomes in the nucleus of every cell. Some are sex-linked determined, such as haemophilia: others, like Down's syndrome (mongolism), are caused by an abnormal number of chromosomes. Abnormalities in the chromosome pattern are almost always linked with backwardness in mental development. External influences on the developing embryo as well as hereditary factors can cause congenital abnormalities, although usually only in the first three months of pregnancy, when the organs are formed.

Congenital heart disorders. Deformities of the heart and adjacent blood vessels which are present at birth. They are usually discovered shortly after birth if they cause serious symptoms, but problems may not occur for years, and sometimes not at all. Congenital heart conditions occur through constructional faults in the first months of pregenncy; they can be caused by some infectious diseases such as German measles in the mother, but in most cases no cause can be found. Cyanosis can point to a congenital heart disorder, as can poor growth, shortness of breath and heart murmurs. Specialist examination is necessary to determine the nature of the condition and whether or not surgery is necessary and possible. Holes in the heart (atrial and ventricular septal defect) are the commonest congenital heart abnormalities (40 per cent).

Conjunctivitis. Inflammation of the mucous membrane that covers the surface of the eye and the underside of the eyelids. The condition can be caused by bacteria, viruses or irritation of the eye by an allergy or harmful substances. The commonest cause is a viral infection, usually during influenza or a cold, often first on one side only, then spreading to both. The eye becomes red, and weeps. The membrane swells, and small bubbles can form inside the eyelid. The eye smarts, the patient becomes hyper-sensitive to light, and the whole eye can swell. Conjunctivitis occurs about two weeks after the eye is infected with the virus. A viral infection heals spontaneously, and medication is unnecessary. Viral conjunctivitis can sometimes develop into the bacterial form. Symptoms are the same, but more severe. Discharge from the eyes contains pus, and the patient's eyelashes are stuck together on waking in the morning. Bacterial inflammation starts about two days after the eye is infected with bacteria. A possible complication is ulceration of the cornea. Treatment is by antibiotics in the form of eye drops of ointment.

Conn's syndrome. Uncommon condition in which the adrenal cortex produces too much aldosterone, which inhibits the excretion of sodium and stimulates that of potassium, thus disturbing their balance in the blood. The condition is associated with high blood pressure, headache, and copious urination, particularly at night.

Constipation. Lack of bowel movement for several days, usually associated with hard, dry faeces, which can be excreted only with difficulty. There are many possible causes. In the colon, rectum or anus a tumour of the colon, diverticulosis, haemorrhoids, an anal fistula or anal fissure may be responsible. In these cases bowel movement is painful, visits to the toilet are postponed (thus making the faeces harder still) and their passage more painful. Spastic colon is also often associated with constipation. Diet as well as conditions of the intestine may have an influence; too little fibre (eating too much whitebread, little fruit, and only easily digested food) and lack of fluid intake have a constipating effect: the intestine becomes lazy. This is also the case if the patient takes too little exercixe (a sedentary lifestyle or confinement to bed). Metabolic disturbances such as hypothyroidism or disturbed function of the adrenal glands can also cause constipation. Medicines that can cause constipation include opiates (codeine, morphine, etc.) and diuretics, Strangely enough laxative abuse can also cause constipation: the intestine becomes dependent on the laxative, and cannot function unless they are used. Usually however there

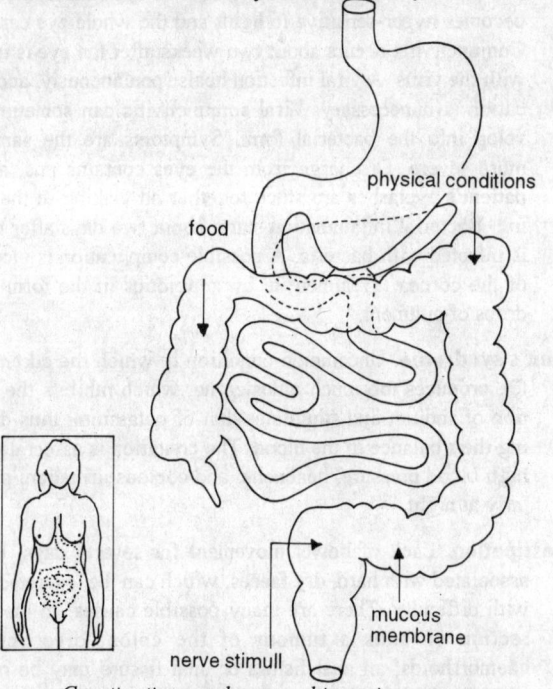

Constipation can be caused in variaous ways.

is no clear cause. Also there is a tendency to assume the existence of constipation even if there is no bowel movement for one or two days, and patients who immediately reach for laxatives in such a case should be aware of what they might bring upon themselves. Characteristic symptoms of chronic constipation are hard, dry faeces once or twice per week, associated with a full feeling in the abdomen and an increasing sense of pressure which decreases after defecation.

Contracture. Constraint of a joint or part of the body caused by shrivelled tissue, usually scar tissue. Intense scarring which can cause contracture occurs after severe burns or inflammation. Scars in muscle are caused by tissue decline during inflammation or by a blood supply disturbance after wounds. Ligaments and capsules can shrivel after injury of inflammation of the joint. Contracture commonly results from a long-term inability to move a joint: muscles and the tissue of the joint shrink. This can occur in paralysis, after long spells in bed, through temporary immobilization of joints after injury, or if a joint is kept immobile to avoid pain.

Contusion (bruise) Tearing of internal tissue and blood vessels, causing haemorrhage, by a blow from a blunt instrument whereby the skin remains intact. Because all that is visible from the surface is discoloration of the skin, there is a danger that the seriousness of the internal injuries might not be recognized. The symptoms are pain and swelling caused by the haemorrhage, and accumulation of fluid in the damaged tissue (oedema). In bone contusion there can be haemorrhage between the bone and the periosteum, which can cause local bone death, because the periosteum is normally a source of bone nutrition. Contusion of a joint often causes extra production of synovial fluid, and thus severe swelling. Muscle is rich in blood vessels, so muscular contusion can cause severe haemorrhage within the muscle. Because it is surrounded by fibrous connective tissue (the fascia) pressure in the muscle is increased, reducing the blood supply and possibly leading to muscle death; dead muscular tissue is replaced by connective tissue, which can shrivel to cause contracture.

Conversion. Unconscious conversion of tension or psychological conflict into physical discomfort or symptoms. The least serious form of conversion is well known: headache intestinal disorders and fatigue as a result of tension. If a patient responds to psychological problems physically, refusing to accept a cause of mental origin, the condition is known as emotional hyperaesthesia or neurosis.

Convulsions. Suddents involuntary movement associated with low-
    ered consciousness, lasting for a few minutes, usually a symp-
    tom of a disorder; they are caused by abnormal stimulation of
    the brain. This can, in turn, be caused by an abnormality or
    disease of the brain itself (encephalitis, meningitis, brain tumours
    or epilepsy). Other causes are possible, such as lack of sugar
    or calcium in the blood. The commonest cause in children,
    however, is high fever. Convulsions then occur when the tem-
    perature rises rapidly, and can recur with each bout of fever.
    Fever convulsions do not affect children over the age of six.

Corn. Highly localized callus formation. Persistent pressure on a
    particular small patch of skin causes a small callus which grows
    inwards, forming a horn-like piece of tissue which in some
    cases can penetrate to the bone; it exerts pressure on nerves,
    causing pain and making walking painful. Corns are most usu-
    ally caused by ill-fitting shoes or foot abnormalities that press
    the toes against the shoes. Treatment in the first place is by
    removing the cause, either by buying new shoes or having an
    operation on the foot. If the corn is very painful it can be
    removed by a surgeon, or in some cases a chiropodist. It is
    important to remove the whole of the corn because even a
    small remaining fragment can be painful. If the cause is not
    removed, the corn soon returns.

Coronary Heart Disease. Disorder of the coronary arteries that
    leads to malfunction of the heart. Atheroscalerosis is the most
    important of these, involving thickening of the walls of the
    arteries by deposits of calcium and fat, reducing the internal
    diameter and finally closing the vessel completely and starving
    the heart muscle of oxygen. Narrowing of the coronary arter-
    ies causes angina pectoris, and closure of these arteries causes
    coronary infarction.

Coronary Thrombosis. Process by which a coronary artery is
    blocked, causing cardiac infarction (death of part of the heart
    muscle). When a coronary artery is affected by atherosclerosis
    its internal diameter decreases and the interior surface is rough-

ened; blood cells and platelets can then stick to the surface, causing thrombosis. As soon as the clot is large enough to block the artery completely part of the heart muscle receives no more oxygen and dies off (infarct). The precise reason for a clot to start to form is not known; it is possible that the size of the calcified patch, exertion and stress are factors.

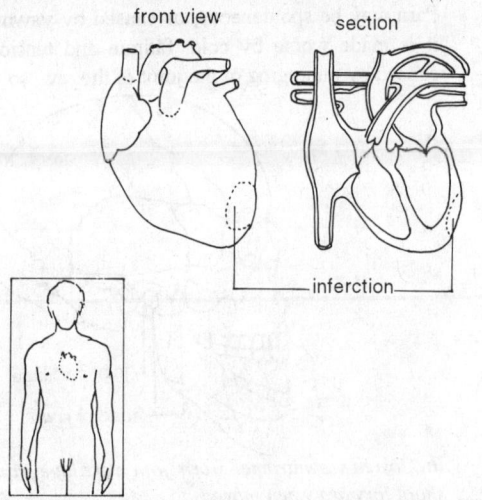

front view   section

inferction

Coronary thrombosis involves closure of a blood vessel in the heart muscle, causing the death of a piece of heart tissue (infarction).

It is sometimes possible to disperse a clot by injecting anticoagulants, but only if this is done within a few hours of the occurrence of the clot and the infarction. This procedure can reduce the number of heart muscle cells affected, but cannot restore tissue which has died.

Corticosteroid. A steroid hormone produced by cells in the cortex of the adrenal glands. Hydrocortisone is the most prolific corticosteroid, but the sex hormones, oestrogen and progesterone, may also be produced by cells in the adrenal cortex as well as in the ovaries and placenta.

Costen's syndrome. Painful spasm of the jaw muscles as a reaction
to pain or irritation in the joint of the jaw, equally common in
men and women.

    The pain, localized in the cheek around the eye, in the
lower jaw and/or in front of the ear, varies in kind can be dull,
searing or nagging; when the pain abates, the face feels tense.
Ringing in the ears (tinnitus) and dizziness may also occur.
Pain may be spontaneous, or caused by yawning or chewing;
it is made worse by cold, fatigue and tension. It is usually
caused by unhinging of the joint of the jaw, so that the end of

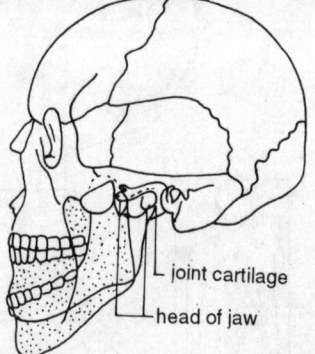

    joint cartilage

    head of jaw

*In Costen's syndrome, worn join cartilage causes the jaw to
shoot forward when moved.*

the lower jaw is not properly seated in the joint, or by abnormalities in the cartilage disc in the joint. Grinding the teeth at
night or ill-fitting dentures can also be the cause. Treatment is
by exercises to relax the jaw muscles and alteration of eating
and chewing habits; dentures may need replacing.

Cough. Reflex movement by means of which the air passages keep
themselves clear; dirt, mucous and bacteria are forcibly expelled. The air passages are also supplied with hairs which
keep up a continuous waving movement to sweep out dirt.
Coughing can be a symptom of almost any condition of the air
passages and lungs. A distinction should be made between
normal coughing, in which mucus (sputum) is coughed up, and
a dry, irritable cough. The colour of the mucus is important:

white mucus suggests irritation of the air passages by a cold, for example; yellow-green mucus points to a bacterial infection such as bronchitis and blood in the mucus can be a sign of a serious condition such as bronchiectasis, tuberculosis or lung cancer, but this is by no means always the case. Coughing can be acute, in a cold, bronchitis or pneumonia, or chronic, as in chronic bronchitis. Smoker's cough is also chronic, caused by continual irritation of the air passages by the smoke, but is often not even noticed because it has persisted for so long.

Coughing blood (haemoptysis) Appearance of blood in the mouth after coughing. This can be the consequence of various disorders, and can vary in severity from a streak of blood in phlegm which is coughed up to the coughing up of large quantities of blood. It is important to establish for certain that the blood was definitely coughed up, and did not come from the mouth (haemorrhage of the mucous membrane), the nose (nosebleed), or the throat. Vomiting blood (haematemesis) is also easily confused with this condition.

The countless causes include many harmless ones; it may be simple bronchitis, bronchiectasis, tuberculosis, a lung embolism or a deficiency in the clotting of the blood. Another cause can be reduced effectiveness of the left-hand side of the heart, causing increased pressure in the blood vessels in the lungs. In the case of cigarette smokers aged over forty lung cancer should not be ruled out. If blood is coughed up a doctor should be consulted; he will produce a diagnosis by means of associated symptoms, physical examination, and possibly an X-ray of the lungs and examination of phlegm which has been coughed up.

Cramp. Involuntary powerful contraction of one or more muscles, generally very painful. Cramp is often caused by poor blood supply to the muscle, with the result that the products of metabolism cannot be removed rapidly enough. This occurs particularly in sports training, and especially in cold weather, massage can decrease the risk. Cramp can also occur as a reaction to muscular tearing, inflammation or dislocation. Lum-

bago is a reaction cramp caused by overloaded or cold back
muscles Circulatory difficulties can also be caused by keeping
muscles tense for too long, as in writer's cramp, for example.
Cramp in various muscles can occur in epilepsy tetanus or
abnormalities of blood calcium level, as in hyperventilation.

Cretinism. Disturbed mental and physical development caused by
thyroid deficiency (hypothyroidism).

Thyroid hormones are important from birth for both physical
and mental development, and if a baby's thyroid gland is missing
or malfunctions, or if food received from the mother does not
contain sufficient iodine, normal development is disturbed.

Crohn's Disease (regional ileitis) Chronic inflammation of the intestine without a specific bacterial or viral origin. Usually the
last section of the small intestine (terminal ileum) is affected,
but other parts may be involved. The disorder occurs particularly in young adults, and hereditary factors may be significant. Discomfort arises from inflammation of the intestinal wall,
sometimes a single section or sometimes several sections, associated with thickening of the wall, inflammation and thickening of the lymph ducts, and ulceration of the mucous membrane. Symptoms vary in severity, consisting principally of
persistent or colicky abdominal pain, with attacks of diarhoea
alternating with periods of normal defecation. There is also
loss of weight and (slight) fever. A possible complication is
fistula formation between the infected area of the intestine and
the anus, another part of the intestine, or even the bladder, skin
or vagina. The condition can lead to peritonitis or disorders of
the joints.

Crush Syndrome. Serious, potentially fatal deficiency in urine production resulting from extensive tissue damage caused by serious injury or severe burns. Another possible cause is excessively long interruption of blood supply to one or both legs,
particularly if a tourniquet is applied to stop arterial bleeding,
a procedure that can cause tissue death. Serious crushing or
death of part of the body causes massive internal bleeding and

circulatory failure, which can be fatal. The damaged tissue produces large quantities of protein, especially muscle protein, which is transported by the blood to the kidneys, damaging them and reducing urine production. Finally production of urine can stop completely, and breakdown products accumulate in the blood, which can lead to death.

Cushing's syndrome. Condition characterized by an excess of corticosteroids in the bloodstream. The most important corticosteroid is cortisol, which regulates carbohydrate metabolism among other things, raising the blood sugar level and controlling inflammation reactions, the adrenal cortex also produces hormones which regulate water and salts in the body, and male sex hormones.

Excess corticosteroid production can result from stimulation by a tumour on the adrenal cortex, or by a pituitary tumour, but Cushing's syndrome usually follows treatment with artificial corticosteroids, much used because of their effectiveness in controlling inflammation in asthma and rheumatoid arthritis sufferers.

Cyanosis. Blue colouring of the skin and mucous membranes. The condition is the result of oxygen shortage in the tissue, and occurs whenever capillary oxygen content falls below a certain level. There are two kinds of cyanosis, central and peripheral. The central type is caused by too little oxygen reaching the blood from the lungs, leading to oxygen shortage in all tissues and often originating in a lung condition such as ephysema, severe pneumonia or interstitial fibrosis. It is also caused whenever too little blood reaches the lungs, e.g. in congenital heart abnormalities (e.g. Fallot's tetralogy). Central cyanosis can also occur as a result of heart failure, when too little blood reaches the heart, or when there is a shortage of oxygen in the air, in the mountains, for example, or in an unventilated room.

Cystic fibrosis. Congenital disorder with secretion of viscous mucus in the air passages and the gastro-intestinal tract. This disease occurs only in children who have inherited the géne for this congenital abnormality from both their parents. The parents are healthy and do not know that they are carriers. The disorder occurs in 1 in 3,000 to 4,000 births, It is caused by an abnormality in the body's exocrine glands: the sweat glands exude sweat with an unusually high salt content, the pancreas does not function well, and there is thick, viscous mucus in bronchi, clogging the air passages.

Cystitis. Inflammation of the urinary bladder by contamination of urine with micro-organisms, usually intestinal bacteria which arrive in the bladder via the urethra. The condition occurs more frequently in women than men, because a woman's urethra is shorter and its opening nearer the anus.

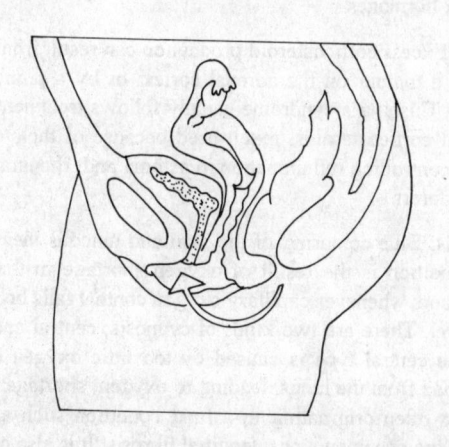

The end of the urethre is nearer the anus in women than men, which means that women are more susceptible to inflammation of the bladder (cystitis).

Cytomegalovirus. Virus of the herpes group, which can remain in the host for a lifetime after first infection. The name refers to the fact that the virus enters a cell and causes it to swell considerably (cysto = cell, megalo = large).

D

Dacryocystitis. Inflammation of the tear discharge system in the corner of the eye next to the nose, usually caused by a blockage of the tear duct (as in new-born babies). In older people, inflammation of the tear duct usually leads to chronic inflammation. The symptoms are continual watering of one eye, and pus in the eye. Pus is released when there is pressure in the corner of the eye next to the nose. Chronic inflammation of the lachrymal can develop into acute inflammation, with a painful red swelling occurring in the corner of the eye. The eyelids also swell up as a result of the inflammation, and the patient may have a fever.

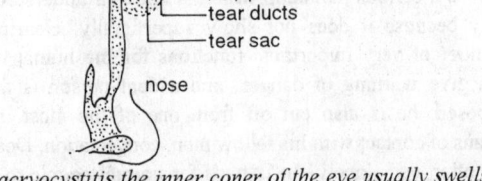

In dacryocystitis the inner coner of the eye usually swells up.

Dacryostenosis. Blockage of the tear duct between the inner corner of the eye and the nasal cavity.

The eye waters continuously because the discharge of lachrymal fluid is blocked. Tear-duct blockage can be congenital; in this case the tear duct often becomes inflamed (dacryocystitis).

Dandruff. Irksome scaliness of the skin of the head; the scales show
as small white flecks in the hair and on the shoulders. Some
scaliness is normal, but not to the extent that it occurs in
dandruff. A number of skin disorders can cause dandruff. Infection with fungoid micro-organisms can usually be controlled
with anti-dandruff shampoo, but if this does not give a satisfactory result, the condition could be an eczema of the head or
psoriasis. A doctor can determine cause and treatment by examining the patient's head.

Deaf-Mutism. Hearing deficiency combined with impaired speech.
If a child is born completely deaf it will not learn to speak of
fits own accord. Shortly after birth a child begins to imitate
the sounds its parents make; hearing other people speak is
essential for speech development.

Cogenital deafness often occurs within the same family.
Hearing can also be damaged during pregnancy, by an illness
such as German measles in the mother, or by the use of certain
medicines. Sometimes damage is perinatal, caused by oxygen
deficiency or severe jaundice in the infant, leading to brain
damage (kernicterus). Some cases of congenital deaffness are
inexplicable.

Deafness. Complete or partial absence of hearing. Genuine deafness is a serious handicap which is not well understood, probably because it does not show superficially. Hearing has a
number of very important functions for the human being. It
can give warning of danger, and a deaf person is thus very
exposed; he is also cut off from one of the most important
means of contact with his fellow men, conversation. Deaf people
are often very lonely—it is hard for normal people to imagine
what it is like to live one's life in complete silence.

Hardness of hearing is of two kinds: conductive deafness
and perceptual deaffness. Conductive deafness is caused by
impaired conduction of sound from the outside world to the
cochlea. Thus the cause may be in the auditory canal (blockage
with ear-wax, ruptured eardrum) or in the middle ear (otitis
media, otosclerosis, low pressure caused by closure of the

Eustachian tube or a cholesteatoma). These conditions can often be treated by medication or surgery to restore conduction of sound.

Perceptual deafness is caused by damage to the cochlea, the auditory nerve or parts of the brain. The most common form is deafness in old age, and another important cause is noise damage.

Death in utero. The pre-natal death of the foetus after the 16th week of pregnancy. The older the foetus, the greater the chance of the death of the foetus being followed by spontaneous abortion (stillbirth). Death in utero occurs much less frequently (in about eleven per thousand pregnancies) than miscarriage (before the 16th week). The suspicion that the child is dead develops in the pregnant woman when, over a period of time, she can no longer feel the child moving. This may be normal in the fourth to sixth months. However, the question of whether the child is still alive must be decided by an examination.

Dehydration. Fluid deficiency in the body caused by the loss of much liquid. This loss of fluid can arise as a result of severe vomiting and/or diarrhoea, but also through the excessive production of urine and/or too low a fluid intake. Children are especially susceptible to dehydration. Acute vomiting and diarrhoea with considerable loss of liquid are often the result of infection caused either by a virus (gastric flu) or a bacterium. Bacterial infections, in particular, can give rise to dehydration, and some examples are tropical forms such as cholera and dysentery. Other forms of diarrhoea are not usually serious enough to lead to dehydration. Dehydration caused by increased urine production is a complication of diabetes mellitus.

Delirium. Condition of lowered consciousness, associated with disorientation, confusion, hallucinations, compulsive movement and often great fear. The cause is always physical: infectious diseases (such as typhoid), pneumonia, heart conditions and oxygen deficiency in the brain. Delirium also occurs in poisoning, as in alcoholic delirium tremens and uraemia. Children may respond to fever with delirium. Treatment is according to symptoms and the underlying illness.

Delusions. A false idea of reality which does not agree with what other people in the same environment believe. The idea cannot be corrected and is not shared by a group of like-thinking people. It is not always possible to draw a clear dividing-line distinguishing delusion from bigotry, prejudice, idealism and other very firm and consistently maintained opinions. A person suffering from delusions usually displays enough other sychotic symptoms, such as lowered consciousness and hallucinations to confirm that the patient has a delusion.

Dementia. General deterioration of mental faculties caused by gradual decay of brain cells. The condition is sometimes temporary, particularly if it results from conditions such as epilepsy, brain tumours or an increase in brain pressure caused by disorders such as hydrocephalus. In such cases dementia is the result of treatable disorder, but senile and presenile dementia are untreatable. The most important form of persistent dementia is senile dementia, caused by atherosclerosis (fatty degeneration of the blood vessels of the brain, which can lead to a stroke). It usually occurs between the ages 60 and 70 with amnesia, reduced emotional control and character changes.

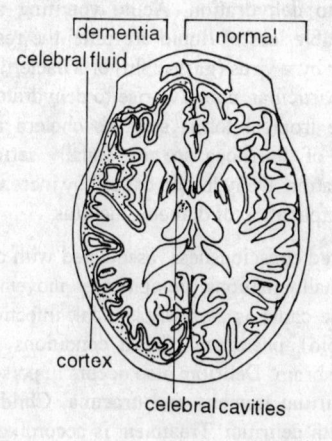

dementia | normal
celebral fluid

cortex

celebral cavities

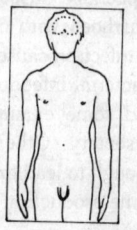

In dementia the cerebral cortex shrinks as a result of cell decay; this causes enlargement of the cavities in and around the brain.

Dental caries (tooth decay) The process by which teeth are broken down by the action of bacteria in the mouth. Three factors must coincide if dental decay is to occur: the presence of bacteria, the presence of food (sugar) for the bacteria, and a set of teeth which is susceptible to the effects of bacterial products. Bacteria which are always in the mouth, such as certain streptococci, convert sugars into acids which attack tooth enamel.

Dental decay or caries is characterized by sudden discoloration, softness, and, subsequently, loss of tooth tissue, with the appearance of the characteristic small cavities. If not treated these cavities progressively increase in size, and intense pain and complications, such as inflammation at the tip of the root can arise.

Caries is treated by the usual dental procedures.

Depersonalization. Feeling of alienation from self, body and surroundings. The patient may feel that he is not in the room, but looking at it through glass: not talking to people, but watching a film; senses that his arm is not his arm. The sense of judgment is not impaired, as in delusion. Depersonalization is unplesant because it is often associated with loss of emotional reactions. The patient sees himself as cold and empty. Despite

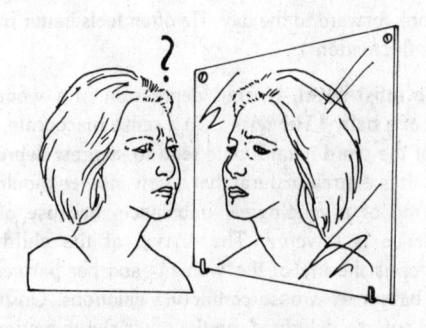

Sufferers from depersonalization do not always recognize their own face.

this, the condition often occurs without serious abnormality in cases of fatigue, poor physical condition or stress. Chronic depersonalization occurs at certain stages in life (puberty, menopause, shortly after childbirth) and in association with neuroses such as hysteria. Depersonalization can also be associated with more serious disorders (such as schizophrenia).

Depression. Mood of extreme gloom not associated with any particular cause or stimulus, or blackness of mood out of proportion to its cause. It can be a phase of manic-depressive psychosis, but is also a clinical picture in its own right. It can be a reaction to a shocking event ('reaction' depression), or the result of neurotic problems ('psychogenic ' or 'neurotic' depression).

The cause can be brain disorder (atherosclerosis, Parkinson's disease), a general physical illness (hypothyroidism, Addison's disease, myasthenia gravis) or poisoning (corticosteroids, some drugs to lower blood pressure). Sometimes there is no demonstrable cause ('endogenous' depression). The latter case is often hereditary. Any form of depression, but particularly endogenous depression, can be associated with physical symptoms, such as marked slowness of thinking, inhibition of movement, and mimicry. The patient may complain of loss of appetite and constipation, wake earlier without being rested, and not look forward to the day. He often feels better in the evening ('day fluctuation').

Depression, post-natal. Serious depression in a woman after the birth of a baby. The term is in a sense inaccurate, because the use of the word natal would tend to suggest depression in the baby. It is entirely natural that a new mother should go through a period of psychological imbalance, because often psychic resilience is lowered. The arrival of the child completely transforms the life of the woman and her partner. The newborn baby may arouse conflicting emotions. On the one hand she is entirely delighted, on the other she in anxious about the future and motherhood; this anxiety may become directed at the child, arousing guilt feelings. The mother is often moved

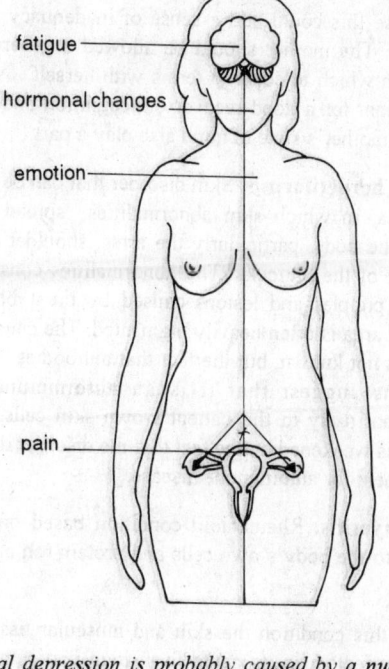

fatigue

hormonal changes

emotion

pain

Post-natal depression is probably caused by a number of factors.

to tears by trifles, and is quickly irritated by those around her; she may herself find these feelings and emotions difficult to understand. In serious cases, when the mother is without all spirit as well as in a state of physical and mental hypersensitivity, the depression can be so severe that there is danger of violence towards the child, or suicide. The cause lies in interlinked factors. Physically speaking, pregnancy and labour are considerable exertions; hormonal changes at the end of pregnancy occur from one moment to the next; and aswell as these physical matters the mother's character and environment also affect the situation. If her feelings are misunderstood by those around her, she may feel acutely lonely and deserted. It is counterproductive to appeal to her to resist these emotions, because this could add a sense of inadequacy to her general gloom. The mother should be allowed a generous amount of time in which to come to terms with herself. Not only rest is important for a good recovery, recognition and understanding of the mother's state of mind also play a part.

Dermatitis herpetiformis. Skin disorder that can be very similar to eczema, in which skin abnormalities spread symmetrically over the body, particularly the arms, shoulder blades and the crease of the buttocks. The abnormalities consist of blisters, small pimples and lesions caused by burst blisters. The affected area is often heavily pigmented. The cause of the condition is not known, but the fact that antibodies are found in the lesions suggest that it is an autoimmune disease, an oversensitivity to the patient's own skin cells, but the argument is weakened by the fact that the disorder does not react to treatment for autoimmune disease.

Dermatomyositis. Rheumatoid condition based on defence reactions to the body's own cells and protein (an autoimmune disease).

In this condition the skin and muscular tissue are particularly affected; in-its acute form it is particularly common in children. The symptoms are accumulation of fluid (oedema), and pain in the muscles associated with loss of energy and swelling of the eyelids, and possible eruptions on the face and neck. General symptoms are fever, loss of weight and fatigue. All the muscles in the body can be affected, but usually the flexors of the limbs and neck are involved. If the respiratory muscles become affected there can be shortage of breath, and contracture can occur in the tissue concerned. Chronic dermatomyositis occurs in adults, beginning gradually, then increasing in severity. If the condition affects only the muscles and not the skin it is known as polymyositis. Malignant tumours, particularly of the stomach and intestine, occur in 20 per cent of sufferers.

Deviated septum. Common condition in which displacement of the septum causes unequal width of the two inner parts of the nose. It is in fact rare for them to be equal in width, and the condition usually causes no complications, even if the deviation is large, although it can lead to slight breathing difficulties and inadequate warming and moistening of the air. Also bacteria and other foreign bodies are not properly filtered out of inhaled air. Deviated septum can be caused in two ways. The nasal septum develops in the embryo from a price of cartilage and a piece of bone, and thickening of the bone and projection can occur at the joint. The deviation can also result from damage (such as a blow) to the nose. The condition can cause nasal blockage; most people are aware that they can breathe better through one nostril than the other. A dry throat can also result, because air passing through the nose is insufficiently moistened; sinusitis also occurs more frequently because the nose is not so effective in removing pollen and viruses from the air, causing headache or a congested feeling in the head. The patient usually suffers discomfort from a combination of deviated septum and some other factor that impairs breathing, e.g. swollen mucous membranes if the patient has a cold. When the membrane returns to normal, discomfort will be reduced or disappear.

Diabetes insipidus. Disorder in the regulation of the body's salt and water content, caused by antiduiretic hormone deficiency as a result of a disturbance in the pituitary gland.

In order to keep a constant balance of salt and water in the body the kidneys produce large or small quantities of urine, containing salts and waste products in solution. The quantity of water which leaves the body in this way is regulated by a hormone produced by the pituitary gland, which inhibits the secretion of water-hence its name antiduiretic hormone (ADH). In diabetes insipidus the production of this hormone is disturbed.

The most important cause of the deficiency is an injury to the skull. A tumour of the pancreas can also result in lowered hormone production. Sometimes no cause at all can be found. Up to 20 litres of water can be lost in the urine within

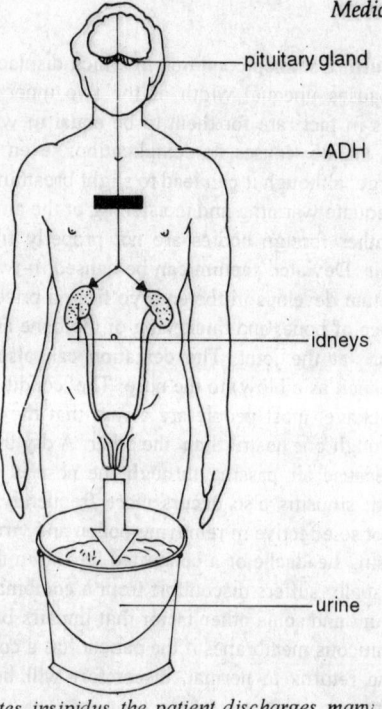

pituitary gland

ADH

kidneys

urine

*In diabetes insipidus the patient discharges many litres of urine
per day because the pituitary gland is not producing enough antidiuretic hormone to allow the kidneys to balance the body's fluids.*

24 hours, causing unquenchable thirst. Other symptoms are
associated with constant loss of fluid, such as a dry throat and
constipation. There is a danger of dehydration, particularly if a
patient is bedridden and not enough fluid can be provided. A
thirst test is sometimes used to confirm diagnosis; the patient
is not allowed to drink, and urine production is measured over
a period of hours. Under normal circumstances ADH ensures
that no more urine is produced, but in patients with diabetes
insipidus too much urine continues to be produced; if after an
ADH injection urine production is lowered, the ieagnosis is
certain. Treatment is by removal of any tumour and administration of an artificial ADH preparation. This can be by injection, but there are also preparations that can be placed on the

nasal mucous membrane and inhaled. This treatment usually
has to be maintained throughout the patient's lifetime. If brain
damage is the cause the condition may be temporary, and the
pancreas will later produce sufficient ADH, when treatment
can stop.

Diabetes mellitus. Metabolic disorder in which the body is unable
to control the levels of blood sugar (glucose). Diabetes is a
common complaint, particularly in older people; it affects
roughly 2 per cent of the population. It is not hereditary, but
heredity seems to play a part: if both parents are diabetic,
there is a high probability that their child will be diabetic. This
is particularly true in the case of maturity-onset diabetes. There
are several types of diabetes mellitus. The first form begins in
childhood or at puberty. The onest is sudden; usually no insulin
is formed at all, so that insulin injections are necessary. The
cause is probably that the body produces antibodies which
affect the cells of the pancreas. Maturity-onset diabetes
sometimes occurs in youth, but usually not until the age of 40.
This form develops very gradually. The patient is often
overweight; the pancreas is not able to make enough insulin
to deal with this excess tissue, and a deficiency develops. In
the case of maturity-onset diabetes it is important to lose weight:
when the weight is reduced, it is often possible for the pancreas
to produce adequate insulin. Pregnancy of certain medicines
(the contraceptive pill, corticosteroids or diuretics) can cause
the onset of diabetes in patients prone to it. After the birth of
the baby or ceasing to use the drugs in question symptoms
disappear, but sometimes only temporarily. In the early stage
the symptoms of both forms of diabetes mellitus are the same.
Excess urine formation is the most marked; sugar 'syphons'
water away with it. A great deal has to be drunk to combat
this fluid loss, but if sweetened drinks are consumed the
condition is exacerbated. In the youthful type of diabetes in
particular loss of sugar via the kidney is so great that the body
has to produce energy by burning fat and protein, causing
tiredness, loss of weight and also a serious disturbance of blood
acidity. In severe cases this can lead to unconsciousness.

Resistance to infection is greatly reduced. Boils, infections of the urethra, inflammation and itching of the vagina or penis are also common: the sugar-drenched tissue is a good breeding-ground for infection. Other possible symptoms are muzziness, impotence and menstrual difficulties.

Diarrhoea. Frequent passing of faeces with a high water content, causing increased volume. Because the normal pattern of bowel evacuation varies considerably this should be taken into account before diarrhoea is diagnosed (three times per day can be normal; the important factor is whether it is exceptional). Sometimes diarrhoea contains blood, mucus or pus, which may help to identify the cause. The condition can be acute, severe or even chronic; there are many causes, discussed below in groups, but it must be pointed out that despite the variety of possible causes, most cases of diarrhoea result from eating the wrong or too much food or from a slight infection of the stomach and intestines, and clear up of their own accord without medical assistance.

The following are the important groups of causes: infections (including food poisoning, typhoid, dysentery salmonella), malabsorption (digestive troubles occurring in galactosaemia, thrush, after operations etc.), pancreatic disorders (e.g. chronic inflammation), restricted bile discharge (for example as a result of gallstones), metabolic disturbances (e.g. hyperthyroidism), food allergies, use of certain antibiotics, misuse of laxatives, aspecific inflammation such as Crohn's disease or ulcerative colitis, and psychological causes (nervousness). Severe diarrhoea (possibly with vomiting) can lead to complications such as mineral deficiency, dehydration (particularly in the young and the elderly) and acidification of the blood (acidosis). Chronic forms cause malnutrition, weight loss and vitamin deficiency.

Diptheria. Infectious disease of the throat which can be serious in children. It is caused by the diphtheria bacillus, which established itself in the mucous membrane of nose and throat, producing a greyish-white false membrane on the tonsils. The disease is dangerous because this false membrane can cause suffocation, and the toxins produced by the bacillus can lead to serious complications elsewhere in the body. The infection is contracted via the air (droplets) and the incubation period lasts for a few days.

Diplopia. Double vision, a condition in which vision in one eye is no longer co-ordinated with vision in the other, so the patient sees the same object in two different places, displaced in any direction or partly overlapping. Double vision can have various causes, some of them relatively innocent—for example through excessive alcohol consumption, overtiredness or slight concussion, in which cases it disappears with the cause. Presistent double vision can be caused by injury to an eye muscle, or detachment of the muscle from the eye socket; the eye cannot then move in all directions, and thus sees double in certain fields. Sometimes the head has to be held in a certain position to avoid double vision. Such failure can be caused by a tumour, inflammation, and accident or haemorrhage. In a few cases a certain nerve is absent at birth, and the condition is congenital. In myasthenia gravis double vision arises in the course of the day because the muscles function improperly. Treatment of double vision depends on the underlying cause. A paralysed eye muscle sometimes heals of its own accord, but surgery may be advisable. Covering the abnormal eye gives temporary relief.

Dislocation. Pushing apart of bone ends in a joint by an injury, often associated with tearing of the joint capsule and ligaments which normally hold the joint together. Damage to blood vessels can cause haemorrhage in the joint. Further characteristics of dislocation are abnormal position of the joint, abnormal shape, and inability to move the ends of the bones in relation to each other. The last effect is increased by muscle cramps as a reaction to the dislocation. There are also congenital dislocations such as congenital hip displacement, caused by imperfect alignment of the ball and socket of the joint.

Disorientation. Condition in which the patient no longer knows what time or place he is living in.

   Disorientation can occur if a person loses his way, has been concentrating hard or busy with something, or simply wakes from a deep sleep. In such cases new information or a simple correction are enough to change the thought pattern.

Dissimulation. Refusal to recognize or making light of something of which the patient is perfectly well aware, especially in the realm of health. Physical complaints (pain) may be ignored, as may feelings (fear or anger) or illness (acting as if nothing were wrong). Alcoholics do it with respect to their memory difficulties (confabulation), and sufferers from anorexia nervosa with respect to their poor physical condition.

Diverticulitis. Diverticulosis of the large intestine, complicated by inflammation; it is estimated that 20 to 25 per cent of patients with diverticulosis develop diverticulitis. The condition is caused by infection from contents of the large intestine which have accumulated in the diverticula. Symptoms are pain on the left of the abdomen (the descending section of the large intestine), associated with fever and malaise in acute cases, and with constipation, a bloated feeling and sometimes diarrhoea in the chronic form.

Diverticulosis. Protrusion of mucous membrane through the intestinal wall, usually in the colon, but in rare cases in the small intestine. Diverticula are usually found in the descending section of the intestine in the lower left-hand side of the abdomen, where pressure is highest. They do not usually cause discomfort until after the 40th year. One of the causes of the condition is the low-fibre Western diet, leading to hard faeces and strain on evacuation, and thus herniation in weak spots. Spastic colon is another source of the condition.

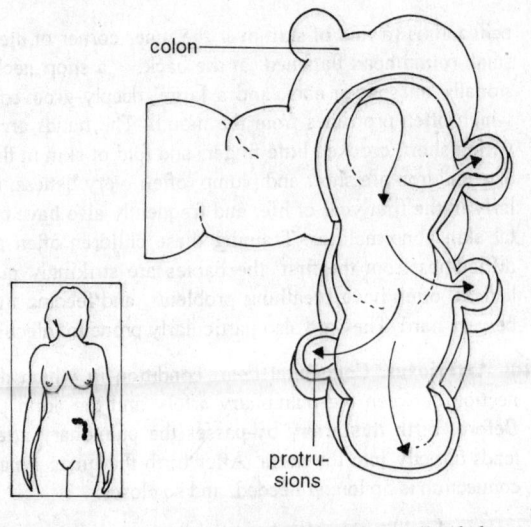

Diverticulosis involves protrusions in the wall of the colon, often caused by eating food with too little fibre.

Down's Syndrome. Best-known and commonest congenital disorder, sometimes called mongolism because of its effect on the set of the eyes. The condition is associated with mental deficiency and occurs in 1 in 600 live births. The percentage is higher in babies born to older mothers. Many congenital disorders occurs as the result of an error of cell division in the fertilized ovum; in Down's syndrome the ovum has received two many chromosomes, 47 instead of the normal 46; chromosome 21 is represented three times instead of twice (trisomy 21), although other deviations are possible. Heredity affects only 1 to 2 per cent of cases.

The outward signs of Down's syndorome are usually clear at birth, but not always recognized, because the baby's behaviour is not significantly different from the norm. After a few weeks or months the baby's backwardness shows clearly. The most important characteristics are a slight slant in the eyes running from underneath on the inside to above on the outside;

pelicanthus (a fold of skin over the inner corner of the eye); a small round head flattened at the back; a short neck; occasionally misshapen ears; and a large, deeply-grooved tongue which often protrudes from the mouth. The hands are plump, with a short, crooked little finger, and fold of skin in the palm. The children are short and plump, often very listless, particularly in the first year of life, and frequently also have congenital skin abnormalities. Training these children often presents difficulties from the first; the babies are strikingly quiet and listless, often have breathing problems, and feeding them can be very hard. They are also particularly prone to infection.

Ductus Arteriosus. Congenital heart condition in which the connection between the pulmonary artery and the aorta persists. Before birth this artery by-passes the pulmonary artery and leads directly into the aorta. After birth the lungs expand, the connection is no longer needed, and so closes.

Inexplicably, this closure does not occur in some children, and because pressure in the aorta is higher than that in the pulmonary artery, pressure in the pulmonary blood vessels rises, causing shortness of breath and pneumonia and also bringing about a mixture of blood with high and low oxygen content. The heart functions less effectively. Babies with this condition sometimes grow slowly. Treatment is by surgery to close the ductus: it is tied and cut, ideally a few months after birth.

ductus arteriosus

Ductus arteriosus allows extra blood to be pumped through the blood vessels of the lungs, thus overloading them.

Dumping syndrome. Symptoms caused when excessive quantities of food enter the intestine shortly after a meal. The stomach's reservoir function is lost, particularly after the removal of (part of) the stomach (stomach resection), in cases of stomach ulcer or cancer of the stomach. The excess food attracts too much blood to the intestine before gastric juices are produced and nutrients can be removed, thus causing a feeling of slackness, lassitude, yawning, drowsiness, sweating etc. Symptoms can also occur in the intestine itself, such as nausea, a full feeling and rumbling always half an hour to an hour after a meal. They are more acute immediately after a stomach operation, and decrease in the course of time. Symptoms may be alleviated by a change of diet. Full dairy produce is best avoided; dry food and small, frequent meals often have a favourable effect.

Dupuytren's contracture. Hand condition in which the fingers are forced into a claw shape and cannot be used. The first symptoms are small lumps on the fibrous sheet under the palm of the hand. The tendons of the fingers adhere to the fibrous sheet, or fascia, which shrinks at a later stage, pulling the tendons and bending the fingers; they cannot be straightened even if the patient uses his other hand. The condition usually starts with the little or ring finger, and in severe cases the little, ring and middle fingers can be pulled against the palm of the hand, but it is usually treated by surgery before it reaches this stage.

Treatment is by removal of the lumps on the fascia to release the fingers. The hand can be used normally again, although the fingers may be stiff for some time, and there is a risk that the contracture may recur.

Dwarfism. Growth disturbance in children in which annual growth is slow, and the final height attained abnormally small. Growth to a normal height required optimal nutrition, the absence of metabolic or other chronic deficiencies, correct growth hormone levels, normal puberty-and parents of more or less normal height.

Deviations from the norm are of two kinds. Usually the growth disturbance is proportional, but in the case of some metabolic disorders (including some hereditary metabolic disorders) bodily proportions are also altered; growth of the limbs is much more restructed than that of head and body.

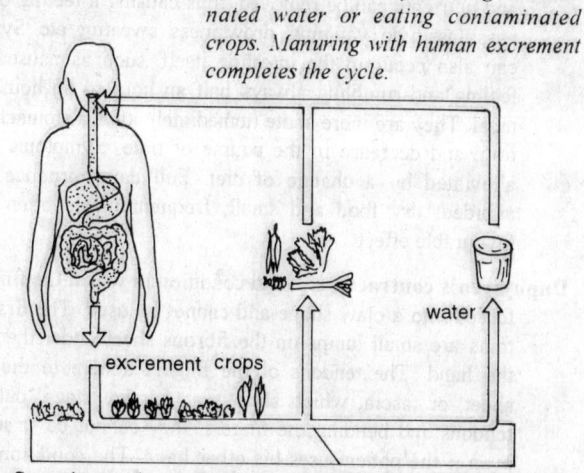

Dysentery is caused by drinking contaminated water or eating contaminated crops. Manuring with human excrement completes the cycle.

Sometimes slow growth is perceptible from birth, in others the growth spurt is delayed (delayed puberty); in the latter case normal height will probably be reached after puberty.

Dysentery. Infection of the large intestine caused by *Shigella* bacteria (bacillary dysentery) or-only rarely in Europe-amoeba (amoebic dysentery). Infection is through food or by contact. The disorder is always epidemic in character occurring most often in the late summer. After 1 to 4 days a serious clinical picture emerges consisting of high fever (39 to 40°C), abdominal convulsions and diarrhoea. Faeces contain mucus and often blood, and are passed 10 to 20 times a day. Dehydration occurs very quickly, and for this reason the disease is dangerous for children in particular, and can be fatal. Possible complications are cerebral oedema, and painful joints and eyes. The illness lasts approximately 3 to 7 days. Diagnosis is by culture from the faeces (directly after it is passed), to establish the source of the infection from the bacteria which have damaged the intestinal mucous membrane. Dysentery must be distinguished from other forms of gastroenteritis such as paratyphoid and similar disorders, and other colonic conditions. Treatment is by antibacterial medication; dehydration should also be prevented, for which purpose an intravenous drip may be needed.

Dyslexia (word-blindness) Inability to assemble letters into a word-picture. It is nevertheless usually possible to read, but there are always particular words that are bit recognized or reading is slower than normal. Dyslexic children fall behind their classmates even if they are normal intelligence. They make 'stupid' errors in writing and appear not to understand written text. Vexation, and mistakes which are not understood, cause tension which worsens the dyslexia. If the problem is not recognized, The child may be thought to be suffering from mental deficiency. However, most sufferers are well able to follow normal teaching. The cause is a disorder in the brain's co-ordination. Treatment consists of well-directed assistance in the form of teaching from a speech-trainer working in the field of listening to language and reading and writing it.

Dysphagia. Pain during and after swallowing, and difficulty in moving food. Conditions that can cause such problems are stricture of the oesophagus (as in achalasia Plummer-Vinson's syndrome or as a result of tumour of the oesophagus). Damage to the oesophagal mucous membrane by gastric acid reflux causes pain when swallowing irritants such as coffee or alcoholic drinks. Pain is sometimes caused by a foreign body, such as a fish bone in or at the entrance to the oesophagus.

E

Earache. Pain which may originate in the ear itself, or elsewhere in the head and body. In children earache with fever is usually caused by inflammation of the middle ear (otitis media). Pus in the middle ear causes a slight decline in hearing. Another common source of earache is inflammation of the ear canal (otitis externa); this may involve the whole canal, or may be local (a boil, for example). The condition is often caused by poking with sharp objects; a characteristic symptom is pain caused by pressure on the ear canal or pulling the ear. The eardrum can also become inflamed, often associated with a cold, and also causing severe pain, but without impairment of hearing. Finally earache can result from reduced pressure in the middle ear. If the Eustachian tube is closed by swollen mucous membrane when the patient has a cold, or by abrupt pressure changes when flying, pressure drops sharply, causing pain (barotrauma).

Eardrum, ruptured. A condition that can result from an accidental direct blow with a sharp object or by indirect means such as very loud bang or an explosion, or by sudden greatly increased pressure resulting from a slap on the ear. Children can perforate their eardrum by accidentally sticking an object in their ear. The fact that the eardrum has been ruptured is usually apparent from a diminished sense of hearing. It is essential to examine the ear in order to establish whether the auditory ossicles, or even the inner ear itself, is damaged. A small tear in the eardrum generally heals of its own accord. If this does not occur within a few weeks, it may be necessary to close it by means of an operation.

Ears, protruding. Condition caused because the fold in the carti-lage where the ear meets the head fails to form during embryonic development. Contrary to popular opinion it is not useful to secure the ears to the head with plaster at night, although plastic surgery is possible after the age of 4 to 5, when the ears are more or less fully grown. The missing fold is made in the cartilage, and the ear placed closer to the head.

Ear-wax blockage. Accumulation of wax in the ear canal, sometimes causing hearing loss. A wax plug can be caused by inexpert cleaning of the outer ear canal. Ear-wax is produced by small glands in the skin of the ear canal, and has a protective function. Normally it is self-clearing, presumably by chewing movements: the head of the lower jaw is just below the ear canal. If the canal is malformed, outward movement does not occur, and plugs of wax may accumulate. But usually the cause is cleaning the ear with unsuitable instruments, which is not only superfluous, but damaging, because it pushes the wax farther into the canal, gradually causing a blockage. A wax plug usually causes no problems until the canal is completely blocked, which can happen suddenly if water gets into the canal and the plug swells causing poor hearing, buzzing in the ears, a sensation of pressure and sometimes dizziness.

Echolalia. Automatic repetition of everything which is said to the patient. Many people are inclined to repeat questions or the last words of a sentence; echolalia is an exaggerated form of this, and a fairly rare symptom of schizophrenia. Echopraxia, imitation of others' actions by the patient, is related to echolalia; both conditions are primitive forms of behaviour adopted to replace answers and deliberate, appropriate activity.

Eclampsia. Convulsions that accompany advanced stages of toxaemia during pregnancy (pre-eclampsia).

Convulsions can occur in the last three months of pregnancy, during labour, and even in the first 48 hours after delivery. Characteristic features are unconsciousness and spasms in all the body muscles. Breathing fails and the woman turns blue. Such a fit can last for a few minutes and the immediately followed by another one. It is a very serious condition.

Ectopic beats. Extra heart beats which disturb the normal cardiac rhythm, caused when a stimulus somewhere in the cardiac the heart to contract. The most important symptom is the sensation that the heart is missing a beat, because the pause between the extra beat and the next normal one is longer than the pause between two normal beats. The condition occurs without a clear cause, and is usually harmless; it is encouraged by large quantities of coffee, alcohol or nicotine.

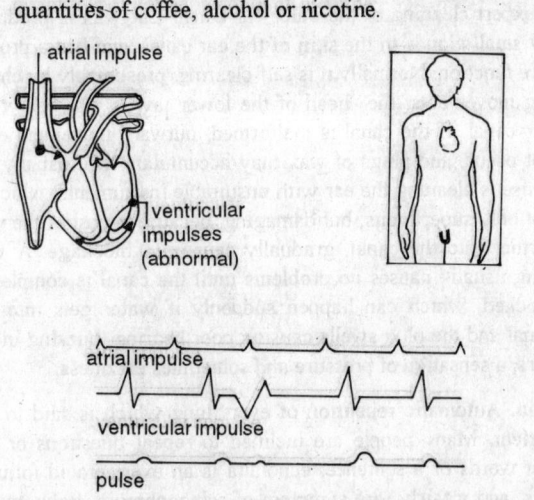

In extrasytole an extra impulse occurs from time to time in the ventricle as well as the normal impulses. The resultant irregularity in the flow of blood can be felt in the pulse.

Ectropion. Condition in which the lower eyelid has sagged downwards, away from the eyeball. It is caused by loss of muscle tone and elasticity, usually in older people. The entrance to the tear duct in the inner corner of the lower eyelid loses contact with lachrymal fluid in the eye and can no longer remove it, causing weeping; the patient has to wipe away tears constantly from cheeks and eyes, and this dabbing again causes irritation of the mucous membrane. The eyelid thickens. Treatment is by surgery to shorten the muscle in the lower eyelid.

Eczema (dermatitis) Non-infectious inflammation of the skin, characterized in its acute phase by one or more of the following symptoms; redness, pimples, blisters and/or scales, and scab formation. The affected patches itch or cause searing pain. There are a number of forms of eczema, which can be subdivided according to cause and clinical picture.

Contact eczema is caused by contact with a particular substance, either an irritant, which would cause eczema in anybody (orthoergic contact eczema), or with an ordinary substance to which the patient is hypersensitive (allergic contact eczema). Contact eczema occurs only at the point of contact, and clears up of its own accord when the substance is avoided.

Ejaculation, premature. Ejaculation of semen before the penis has entered the vagina, or the inability of the man to recognize and delay the moment of orgasm.

There are two forms of premature ejaculation. The first is hypotonic, in which ejaculation takes place without any powerful pulses and is more continuous, with a much reduced orgasm. This form is usually caused by conscious or unconscious psychological problems. The second form of premature ejaculation hypertonic, in which haste and greatly increased tension are the cause of rapid ejaculation. It may occur in men who have had no sexual intercourse for a long time, in inexperienced men who are sexually very stimulated, and in men having too tight a foreskin (phimosis), in whom rapid ejaculation is a means of preventing pain. Situations where there is a danger of discovery or interruption during the sex act sometimes also lead to premature ejaculation.

Electroencephalogram (EEG). The graphic recorder obtained by measuring the electrical activity in the brain. The record may be observed on an oscilloscope or recorded on a continuous roll of paper. By placing electrodes at various places on the scalp, readings can be obtained from the region of the brain beneath the electrodes. The electrodes are usually attached regardless of the hair, using a water-based jelly to make good contact.

The interpretation of electroencephalograms is difficult because the nature of the electrical signals is not easily explained. They almost certainly originate in nerves cells, but what causes them to maintain normal or to develop abnormal rhythms is not understood. The experienced operator can distinguish states of consciousness, for example, waking, sleeping, and unconsciousness. The electroencephalogram is used to diagnose *epilepsy*, and to distinguish amongst forms of that disease. It may also help to locate a brain tumour.

Embolism. Blockage of a blood vessel by a lump of material formed elsewhere in the body and transported by the bloodstream. It is usually a blood clot, but may consist of calcareous matter from a blood vessel affected by atheroscalerosis, clumps of cancer cells, fatty tissue and even small air bubbles.

Embolism, Pulmonary. Blockage of a branch of the pulmonary artery by a blood clot. The clot does not originate in the pulmonary artery itself, but comes from one of the large veins.

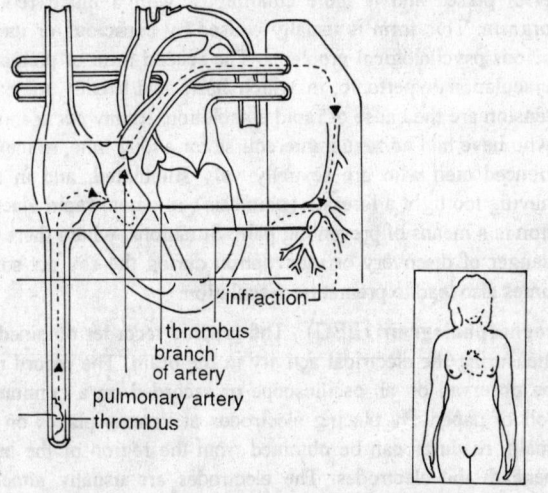

infraction
thrombus
branch
of artery
pulmonary artery
thrombus

A pulmonary embolism is an infarction of lung tissue caused by a thrombus which has worked loose.

Whenever a clot is loosened in a vein it is carried by the bloodstream to the right atrium and right ventricle of the heart, and from there to the pulmonary artery. There it may may stick in one of the large or small branches, according to its size, blocking the branch.

Symptoms include constriction, chest pain and sometimes the coughing up of blood.

Pulmonary embolism caused by a small clot usually causes little or no discomfort, but a large clot can block the pulmonary artery itself, and cut off the blood supply to the lungs, causing immediate death.

Emotional Hyperaesthesia. Disturbance of mood with characteristic anxiety, gloom, bad temper and lack of equilibrium. The patient cannot concentrate, and loses the facility to suppress irrelevant environmental stimuli. He sleeps poorly, and loses his appetite. In general thoughts and emotions are dominated by a feeling of powerlessness and inadequacy. Some people are like this throughout their lives, in which case congenital factors are involved; in others the condition is caused by physical illness, or being run down. Viral infections such as glandular fever are often associated with emotional hyperaesthesia, and it is also common in sufferers from an inferiority complex. Such people are perfectionists, and excessively concerned with tidiness and neatness. In this form of neurosis, stamina decreases as workload increases, or increasing old age means that demands can no longer be met.

Emotional instability. Inability to control the emotions or their expression, with the result that they fluctuate enormously. It is not good always to keep emotion under control, but under normal social conditions some restraint is necessary. In cases of severe fatigue, reduction of resistance by viral diseases, and glandular fever, hypertension, and dementia the patient can burst into tears or a fit of rage over trivia, and then be laughing with others a little later. Associated phenomena are blushing, dizziness, nausea and bouts of heavy perspiration.

Treatment depends on the actual cause.

Emphysema. Destruction of the smallest branches of the air passages of the lungs, the broncheoli and the alveoli, caused by

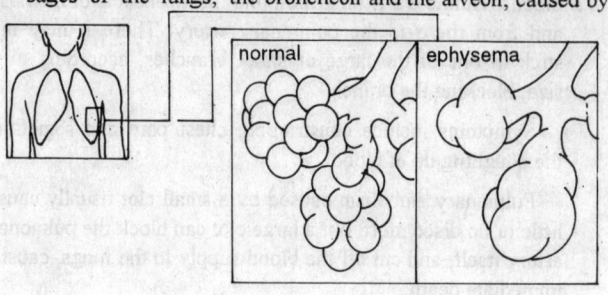

Emphysema involves stretching of the alveoli, reducing the ventilating surface area of the lung tissue.

abnormal dilation and loss of elasticity, and associated with destruction of the wall of the alveoli. The condition is common in later life, although it is usually not severe.

Empyema. Accumulation of pus on a body cavity, as opposed to an abscess, which develops within tissue. It can occur in the nasal sinuses, gall bladder, pulmonary cavity, abdominal cavity, marrow cavity of bones, lachrymal glands and so on. Pus consists

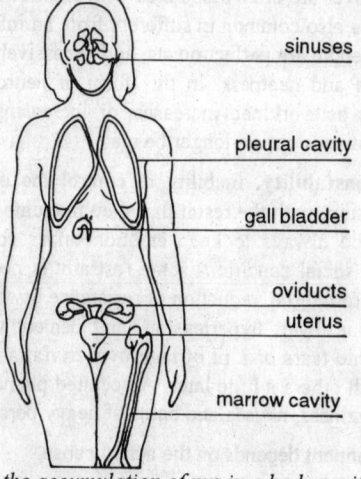

Empyema is the accumulation of pus in a body cavity.

of dead tissue, dead and living bacteria and white blood cells attempting to destroy the bacteria. There is thus always infection, caused by the closure of the cavity and spreading of infection within it. The commonest form is sinus empyema or sinusitis, ofter following a cold in the nose. Infection spreads to the sinuses, which close as a result of swelling of the mucous membrane. Symptoms depend on the place affected, but almost always include redness, pain disturbed function and swelling if the infection is deep in the cavity.

Encephalitis. Inflammation of brain tissue, usually associated with meningitis. Various viruses (including mumps and cold viruses) can cause mild encephalitis, but herpes and rabies viruses lead to a more serious condition. There is a remote chance that infection with or vaccination against chickenpox, smallpox or whooping cough may also cause encephalitis, possibly through an allergic reaction from the brain. The same sometimes occurs in children after measles. This is one of the reasons for innoculation against these diseases. Bacterial infection of the brain is always encapusulated, and causes a cerebral abscess.

Some cases of encephalitis are caused by fungus and parasites, most notoriously toxoplasmosis in an unborn child, which can cause severe brain damage through calcification. Symptoms of encephalitis can vary considerably. In the most frequent mild infection the patient has a fever, headache and slight neck cramp as a result of the meningitis. There are no faculty, failures, and the patient recovers in 1 to 2 weeks.

Endocarditis. Inflammation of the inner membranous lining of the heart, usually the heart valves.

Symptoms are slight to moderate fever headache, fatigue and muscular pain. They worsen over the weeks and months, until the patient is mortally ill; damage may be caused to the heart valves covered by the affected membrane, resulting in leakage. Treatment is by large quantities of antibiotics and long-term bed rest. If a cardiac valve is seriously affected, it can be replaced by an artificial one.

Endometriosis. Presence of uterine mucous membrane outside the womb, occurring particularly in childless women between the ages of 30 and 40. In rare cases the condition is primary, that is to say it originates during embryonic development, when it can be in the lungs and cause monthly coughing up of blood. It is more usually caused by the detachment of endometrial tissue during menstruation or surgery. The tissue can lodge in an ovary, Fallopian tube, uterine muscular tissue, abdominal cavity, on the bladder or in the rectum. It is affected by the sexual hormone cycle, and itself menstruates. Blood in the abdominal

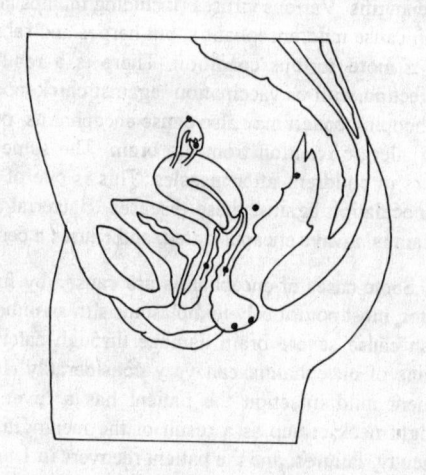

Endometriosis is the presence of endometrium (uterine mucous membrane) in places other than the womb.

cavity causes severe pain, and the principal symptom is monthly recurrence of such pain; the patient also experiences pain during intercourse, and infertility can result. Diagnosis is by laparoscopy, and treatment with hormones to suppress the menstrual cycle.

Endometritis. Inflammation of the endometrium (membrane lining the womb) which usually occurs during childbirth, particularly if the membrane was damaged long before birth (puerperal fever). It may occur outside childbirth if an intrauterine device (coil) has been used frequently. If only the endometrium is inflamed there may be few symptoms such as some pain and fever; pus may be produced and menstruation may be more copious. If there is pain and fever, antibiotics are often prescribed and bed rest is essential. If pus remains in the womb medication may be prescribed to induce contractions.

Endometrium, cancer of. Malignant tumour originating from the mucous membrane lining the womb, three times less frequent

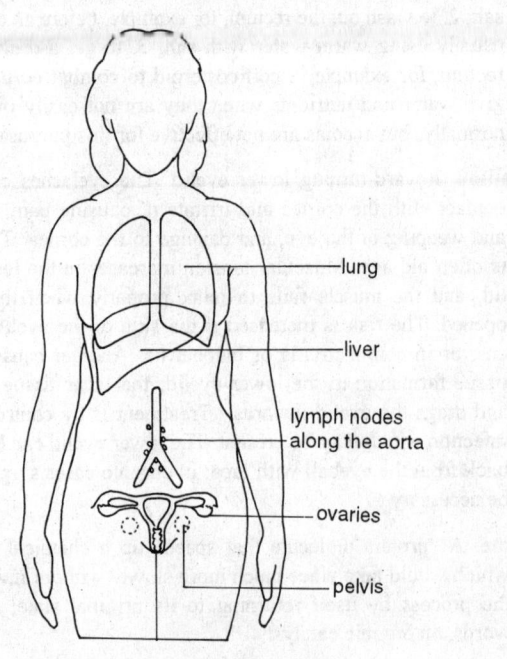

Cancer of the endometrium metastasizes most frequently to the parts of the body indicated.

than cervical cancer. It occurs relatively more often in over-weight women who have not had children, menstruate copiously and had a late menopause, probably because of excessive stimulus by the hormone oestrogen.

Symptoms are abnormal blood loss from the vagina and a watery discharge containing blood, which before the menopause could have a number of causes, but are more suspect after it. The extent of the cancer is significant in the treatment and its success.

Enema. A liquid injected into the rectum, usually containing a drug. Enemas may serve one of four purposes: 1. To relieve severe constipation, when the liquid is usually warm water containing salt; 2. to wash out the rectum, for example, before an operation, usually using warm water with salt; 3. to get a drug into the rectum, for example, a corticosteroid to combat *colitis;* 4. to give water and nutrients when they are not easily introduced normally, but enemas are not effective for this purpose.

Entropion. Inward-turning lower eyelid. The eyelashes come into contact with the cornea and irritate it, causing pain, redness and weeping of the eye, and damage to the cornea. The cause is often old age. Muscular tension increases in the lower eyelid, and the muscle fails to relax properly when the eye is opened. The risk is increased if the skin of the eyelids slackens, or in conjunctivitis or blepharitis. Another cause is scar tissue formation in the lower eyelid; the scar tissue shrinks, and drags the eyelid inwards. Treatment is by control of any infection which may be present. The lower eyelid can be pulled back from the eyeball with tape; in chronic cases surgery may be necessary .

Enzyme. A protein molecule that speeds up a chemical reaction which would take place much more slowly without it, but ends the process by itself returning to its original state; in other words, an organic catalyst.

Enzymes work because they are large molecules made up of many atoms which attract or repel each other, causing the whole molecule to take on a unique configuration. At one place in this tangle like a rubber band rubbed between the hands, two or a small number of atoms are brought into close juxtaposition. The forces between them can capture another molecule and assist it to change its chemical structure. The second molecule is called a substrate. In the process, the enzyme may itself change its configuration. But the change in the substrate or in the enzyme or both changes the relationship of atoms at the binding site. The substrate is released, and the enzyme returns to its original form.

Enzymes may change substrates in four general ways: 1. by splitting them into one or more segments; the split is always between the same atoms; 2. by linking the substrate or part of it to another molecule; 3. by removing or adding atoms, often atoms of oxygen or hydrogen; 4. by causing the substrate to change its own configuration and, therefore, its function. Each enzyme performs only one or a very small number of actions on one or a small number of subtrates.

The enzymes are direct products of the genes, that is, a gene governs the sequence of atoms forming an enzyme. Thus, the great majority of enzymes in the body are newly synthesized under instructions form the genes. Just as each of us has thousands of genes, so we each have a large number of enzymes not all of which have yet been identified. What is more, the difference between cells in the eye and cells in the arm muscle, for example, is the respective enzymes contained by each. Many are the same in all cells, but many more are unique to eyes or muscle and determine the functions of those cells. How exactly differentiation develops and how the number of enzyme molecules in a cell at any given time is fixed remain subjects of active research.

Epidermoid cyst. Small skin in tumour that results when skin cells are pushed under the skin by an injury. The wound heals normally and is usually forgotten, but the cells under the skin become a cavity (cyst), formed by tiny sweat and sebaceous glands which have also been pushed under the skin, in which fluid accumulates. A few months after the healing of the wound the cyst may be large enough to be noticed; it may be several millimetres in diameter, and positioned on the site of the wound. A distinction should be made between a sebaceous cyst and a ganglion. Epidermoid cysts can easily be removed by surgery, because they are loosely bedded in tissue.

Epididymal cyst. A cyst in the epididymis, attached to the testicle, felt as a swelling in the scrotum. The cyst is usually filled with cloudy white fluid, translucent if illuminated. The fluid contains stream which are largely incapable of life. The condition sometimes occurs in boys, but more usually in men, and causes little discomfort. If it occurs on both testicles, the patient is often rendered sterile. If the cyst becomes excessively large it can be drained after a few months with a needle. In children the cyst can be removed by surgery if necessary.

Epididymitis. Inflammation of the epididymis of the testicle on one or both sides, usually associated with an infection of the urethra or prostate gland. It usually runs its course very rapidly. The inflamed and swollen area is extremely painful to the touch, and patients are often extremely ill, with fever, cold shivers and vomiting. The condition should be treated in hospital with bed rest, scrotal support, antibiotics and pain killers.

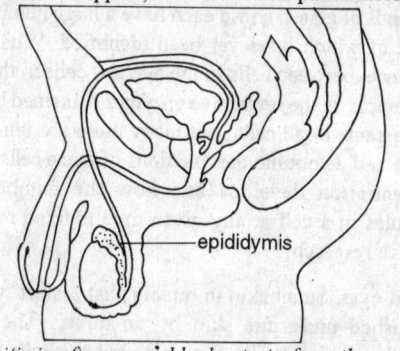

epididymis

Epididymitis is often caused by bacteria from the ureters.

Epiglottitis. Inflammation of the epiglottis at the back of the throat, usually associated with inflammation of surrounding tissue and severe swelling, which can block the air passages. It is caused by a bacterium, *Haemophilus influenzae*, and usually affects the whole larynx, with redness and swelling of the epiglottis as the principal symptoms. It is often associated with inflammation of the throat, but can occur independently. The symptoms are similar to those of preudo-croup.

Epilepsy. Disorder in which abnormal electrical activity in the brain cells caused convulsions.

Epilepsy can be congenital and have no recognizable cause. Acquired epilepsy can occur after brain damage, for example after a birth injury, serious concussion or as a result of circulatory disorders (stroke). Other causes are stimulus from a brain tumour or encephalitis.

Epilepsy manifests itself in various ways; sometimes the patient and those around him notice little; in other cases the attacks are so severe that they could cause serious brain damage, but fortunately such attacks can often be controlled or prevented by medication. The best-known and most dramatic type of epileptic seizure is the grand mal, in which all the brain cells are stimulated by the abnormal electrical discharge.

Treatment of epilepsy is largely by medication to make the nervous system less sensitive to stimuli. The effect of treatment varies from patient to patient, who should try to lead a steady life to avoid overstimulation of the nervous system. Many activities are forbidden to epileptics; they are not permitted to drive a car or ride a motor cycle until their EEG is normal, and after two years free from attacks.

Epiphysiolysis. Detachment of the epiphysis, the end of a growing bone, from the rest of the bone in a growing child. If the epiphysis is part of a joint, the function of the joint is severely disturbed. Between the epiphysis and the diaphysis (the central section of the bone) is a cartilaginous plate, the epiphyseal cartilage, which is responsible for longitudinal growth of the bone. Epiphysiolysis can occur only while growth still persists; the plates 'close' when growth stops. The cause can be external injury, or processes in the bone affecting the plates, such as inflammation of the bone marrow, a bone tumour or osteochondritis. If the epiphyseal plate is damaged, the result can be restricted bone growth, and thus legs of differing lengths.

Treatment is by re-attachment of the epiphysis and a plaster cast.

Epispadias. Abnormal opening of the urethra on the upper side of the penis. The condition is congenital, and often associated with exterior growth of bladder tissue; the front edge of the bladder is open. The abnormal opening results from the non-closure of the urethra on the upper side during embryonic development and can be anywhere between the root and the tip of the penis. The condition is sometimes associated with urinary incontinence and inability to introduce semen into the vagina on ejaculation; a condom with the tip removed can prevent this.

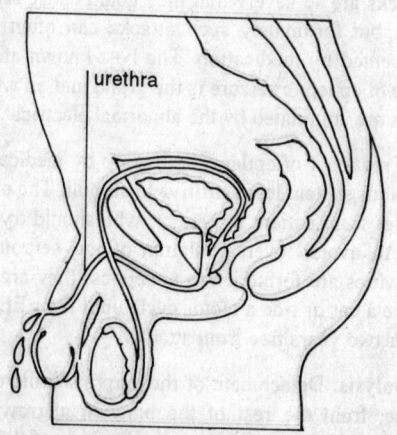

In epispadias the end of the urethra is misplaced, so that urine is discharged from the upper part of the penis instead of the glans.

Erysipelas. Acute, progressive infection of the skin by streptococcal bacteria, frequently accompanied by a high temperature. This condition occurs after an infection of a small wound, which may even be be too small to be detectable.

Erysipelas begins suddenly with a reddening, and sometimes as swelling, of the skin at the site in question. This is
accompanied by a high temperature, sometimes with cold
shivers which are so severe that the whole bed shakes. Nausea
and sometimes vomiting also occur. Complications in erysipelas
are usually caused by bacterial products. As a result, serious
kidney disorders or rheumatic fever may set in. Serious damage to the kidneys and cardiac valves may result, although
this is rare. Erysipelas is treated by absolute rest in bed and by
antibiotics. After the condition has healed, the skin at the site
of the erysipelas peels off.

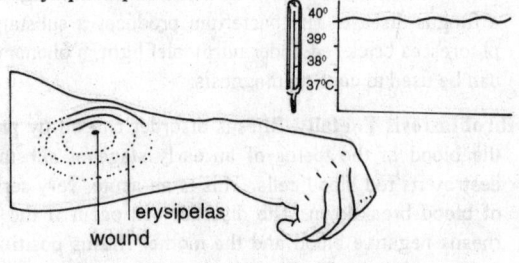

*Erysipelas is an infection which spreads from a small wound; it
is associated with high fever.*

Erythema multiforme. Rare skin disease with patches resembling
a target and consisting of a small central blister surrounded by
a slightly swollen pale area, itself often with a red rim. The
patches usually occur on the arms and legs.

No cause is known, and the condition is treated with soothing ointments; aspirin is efficacious in some cases. There are
similar conditions caused by allergy to certain medicines.

Erythema nodosum. Very painful skin condition which occurs particularly in young adults, equally in men and women. Purplishred
patches appear on the skin; they are very painful, somewhat
swollen and warm to the touch, and between 1 and 5 cm in

diameter. They are usually on the front of the lower leg, but occasionally on the upper part of the leg or even the arms. The patient usually has slight fever. Blood tests show little abnormality. At one time a tubercular centre in the lung was found to be a cause, but since TB has been all but eradicated this is no longer the case.

Erythrasma. Skin condition generally free from problems, more common in men, but also occurring in women. A reddish brown area appears in moist areas such as the genital area, around the anus or between the toes; the skin rubs off in scales. The patch rarely spreads, and is not usually itchy.

    The condition is caused by a bacterium, although much like a fungus disease. The bacterium produces a substance which pluoresces brick red under ultraviolet light, a phenomenon that can be used to confirm diagnosis.

Erythroblastosis Foetalis. Rhesus disorder caused by presence in the blood of the foetus of an early stage of substances that destroy its red blood cells. This is an acute, very serious form of blood breakdown. The disorder can occur if the baby has rhesus negative blood and the mother rhesus positive (rhesus incompatibility). The mother produces antibodies which are disadvantageous to the baby. The first baby is usually healthy, unless the mother had produced antibodies before the pregnancy-for example through a blood transfusion is which the child's factor was present.

    Symptoms run from severe anaemia to serious oedema (hydrops foetalis). In some cases the condition is so serere that the baby is born dead. Anaemia sets in because of the breakdown of red blood cells, jaundice appears within 24 hours, and rapidly increases in intensity. Liver and spleen are often enlarged, the child is drowsy, and does not take milk. If treatment is delayed the brain may be attacked by bilirubin, and the baby, if it survives, permanently brain damaged.

Euphoria. Feeling of physical and mental well-being associated with a positive mood, even when there is no cause. In normal life this is a normal reaction shortly after passing an examination, or if one has just fallen in love, for example. The condition also occurs in various illnesses, and then mood and reality are out of phase, even though the patient feels that the mood is normal. Sufferers from multiple sclerosis are prone to the condition.

Exhibitionism. Irresistible urge in men to achieve sexual excitement and satisfaction by showing their naked genitals to women. Exhibitionism is considered a perversion and is punishable by law. People wishing to expose themselves usually make preparations by wearing clothing which can be quickly opened, and they choose places where no-one they know is likely to appear, but at which there are nevertheless many people. Quite often they are married or formerly married men whose partners knew nothing of the problem. The exposure of the genitals, particularly the erect penis, is associated with great tension and sexual excitement. Satisfaction is more likely if the victim reacts with fear. Exhibitionists almost never commit assault or rape, in fact they are likely to be incapable of normal heterosexual contact.

Exophthalmos. Eyeball placed relatively far forward in the skull, resulting in a protruding eye. The condition can be unilateral or bilateral, and may be caused in various ways, commonly by inflammation is the region of the eye, usually sinusitis, a tooth abscess or facial boil. The tissue around the eye swells as a result of the inflammation and forces the eyeball outwards. The eyelids are often swollen, preventing the eye from opening. Treatment is by controlling the inflammation, sometimes by lancing the abscess. Possible complications are encephalitis of inflammation of the cerebral blood vessels.

Eye, foreign body in. Sometimes in the eye causes pain, redness, hepersensitivity to light and weeping, often with cramp in the eyelid so that the eye can be opened only with difficulty. The foreign body is usually flushed out by tears, but this is not always the case if the object has hit the eye at some speed and becomes embedded in the cornea or conjunctiva (such as steel splinters). In such cases the irritation is more acute than if, say, a grain of sand is blown into the eye. It is advisable to remove an object which has lodged in the eye within a short time, or the cornea may be damaged. With a steel splinter there is the additional danger that a ring of rust could form around it. It is best for an doctor to remove the object, because he will be able to check whether the cornea is damaged and requires special treatment. Antibiotic eye drops or ointment are usually put in the eye to prevent inflammation.

Eye, inflammation of. Characterized by redness and often pain and a feeling that the patient has sand in his eye; also by hypersensitivity to light and weeping. The commonest inflammation of the eye is the largely harmless conjunctivitis usually caused by viral or bacterial infection, sometimes by allergic reaction. Iritis is a less common condition, usually caused by reaction to infection elsewhere in the body or by a rheumatic disorder sometimes by bacterial infection. Inflammation of the vascular membrane is caused in the same way as iritis.

Eye injuries. May be inflicted a blunt or a sharp object. Damage by a sharp object (pin, fingernail, metal splinter, etc.) damages either the cornea or the conjunctiva. Such wounds are painful. Any foreign body remaining in the eye must be removed by a doctor, and antibiotic ointment applied to prevent infection. If the object has cut right through the cornea or conjunctive, rapid treatment is necessary to prevent clouding of the eye. There is also a risk of inflammation of the eye itself, which could lead to its loss.

Eyelid Disorders. Any skin condition of the face can also affect the eyelids. The skin of the eyelid is rather more loosely textured than that of the rest of the face, and therefore more liable to swelling. Blepharitis produces symptoms of redness and scaliness or crust formation; a chalazion is a painless swelling caused by blockage of a sebaceous gland in the eyelid. Sties are accumulations of fat in the skin of the upper or lower eyelid, taking the form of small yellow swellings.

Eye tumour. Benign or malignant tumour of the eye or eyelid. Eye
tumours are rare, the commonest being the retinoblastoma, a
malignant tumour that originates in the retina, usually in children under the age of three. Tumours of the eyelid are more
common; a basilioma is often found on the eyelids of elderly
people, particularly in places much exposed to the sun and in
people with pale skin. Another tumour-like disorder is a
chalazion, which resembles a raised wart. It requires to treatment other than for cosmetic reasons. Swelling of the eyelid is
usually caused by inflammation or a blocked exit from a lymph
node. Tumours originating in a lymph gland in the upper or
lower eyelid are extremely rare. Sometimes a small tumour of
the blood vessels occurs in the eye socket behind the eye. The
family doctor should be consulted about any lump on or on the
eyes or eyelids.

F

Fainting (syncope) Sudden brief loss of consciousness, varying from a few seconds to several minutes. The cause is a reduction in the blood supply to the brain, which is very sensitive to oxygen deficiency; as soon as blood supply is fully restored consciousness returns.

Fainting can be caused by violent emotion, very warm surroundings, standing for long periods, anaemia or low blood pressure. If the patient lies flat, possibly with the legs raised, blood pressure rises again and consciousness is quickly restored. Fainting can also be caused by a brief interruption of heart function, usually a break in rhythm so that the heart beats too slowly, and the blood pressure drops, Certain abnormalities of the aortal valve can also cause inadequate blood supply to the brain.

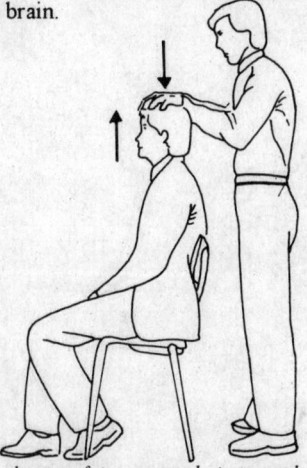

If someone is about to faint a remedy is to apply as much counter-pressure as possible to head and neck, by pressing on the head.

Fallot's tetralogy. Congenital heart condition consisting of an opening in the septum between the left and right ventricles, abnormal placing of the aorta, constriction of the first section of the pulmonary artery and thickening of the wall of the right ventricle. Its most important effect is that too little blood reaches

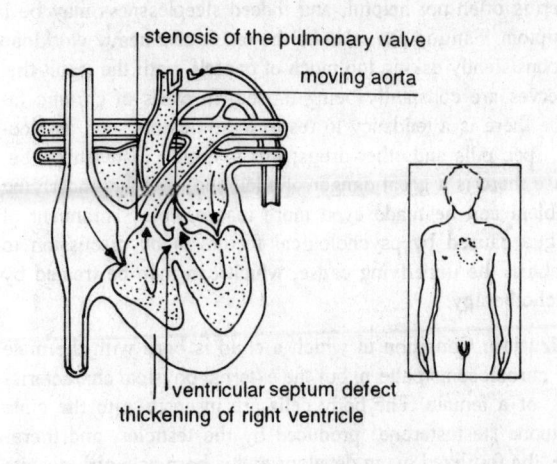

stenosis of the pulmonary valve

moving aorta

ventricular septum defect
thickening of right ventricle

Fallot's tetralogy consists of four heart abnormalities causing symptoms needing surgery.

the lungs, thus reducing oxygen supply to the body. The child looks blue (cyanosis), does not grow properly and is quickly tired and short of breath. Without treatment he is unlikely to survive beyond the age of 15.

Farmer's Lung. Hypersensitivity to fungal spores found in mouldy hay occurring in persons who have been in contact with hay for a number of years. In the initial stages the symptoms disappear completely after an attack, but persistent contact with mouldy hay leads to chronic illness. Attacks follow a set pattern: four to eight hours after inhaling the fungus the patient feels constricted and coughs. There is also fever caused by the violent process of inflammation taking place in the lungs. The symptoms of constriction persist for months or years, combined with chronic coughing, emaciation and periods of fever.

Fatigue. Lack of energy that cannot be explained by physical exertion or a bodily disorder. Psychological fatigue often occurs in depression and neurosis, usually as a result of the suppression of problems by a defence mechanism. In such cases extra sleep is often not helpful, and indeed sleeplessness may be a symptom. Fatigue can also be the result of a heavy workload or consistently asking too much of oneself, with the result that reserves are constantly being tapped. In cases of chronic fatigue there is a tendency to resort to stimulants such as alcohol, pep pills and other drugs; this is highly inadvisable, because there is a great danger of addiction, and the underlying problem can be made even more inaccessible. Treatment of fatigue caused by psychological factors is by discussion to establish the underlying cause, which can then be treated by psychotherapy.

Femininization. Condition in which a child is born with the male XY chromosome pattern, but the external physical characteristics of a female. The body cells are insensitive to the male hormone (testosterone) produced by the testicles, and therefore, the fertilized ovum develops and is born as a girl, despite the presence of testicles.

At puberty the family doctor is usually consulted because menstruation has not started, and he establishes that the patient has a normal female exterior, normal breast development, a feminine figure, but no pubic or underarm hair. Usually there is a normal vagina, ending blind (because the womb is missing), and often an inguinal hernia on both sides containing small, non-functioning testicles. These should be removed to prevent malignant degeneration.

Fetishism. Sexual deviation in which satisfaction is possible only from compulsive attraction to an object or part of the body. To a certain extent everybody has fetishistic traits, and understands excitement caused by a certain smell, the feel of a certain material, or seeing certain parts of the body; a fetishist is completely dependent on such things for sexual satisfaction, however, and the fetish is not part of ordinary sex play with a partner, but the sole object of sexual interest. The object may produce orgasm by seeing, touching or smelling, and is often used in masturbation. Direct sexual contact with other people is often avoided, and fetishists are often impotent if they make such contacts. Some researchers maintain that fetishism is caused by particularly strong sexual excitement or satisfaction gained from a part of the body or object in early youth, and others suggest that it arises from fear of a normal relationship with another person.

Fever. Body temperature above 38°C. Body temperature refers to the internal temperature. It is fairly stable, and is regulated by the temperature centre in the hypothalamus. Skin temperature can be many degrees lower, and is determined by the blood supply to the skin, the ambient temperature and the body's heat production. Measuring rectal temperature or taking it in the mouth gives a good indication of body temperature, normally between 36 and 37°C. Measuring the temperature under the armpit gives a result which is usually 0.5-1°C lower. Temperature is dependent on the time at which it is measured and is at its lowest between 6 and 7 a.m. and highest between 6 and 7 p.m. In women temperature is dependent on the menstrual cycle: body temperature is 0.5 to 1°C higher immediately after ovulation. The body temperature also rises during and after physical exertion, especially in children (1 to 2°C).

Fibrillation, Ventricular. Potentially fatal heart rhythm disorder in which blood no longer circulates from the heart. Under normal circumstances all the muscular cells in the left and right ventricles contract together when they receive the necessary impulse, and this co-ordinated contraction pumps blood out of the ventricles. In ventricle fibrillation the cells contract, but without co-ordination: each cell adopts its own rhythm. The heart stops pumping, and the patient rapidly loses consciousness (heart failure). Usually ventricular fibrillation is the result of coronary infarction, although it can also be caused by an electric shock or being struck by lightning.

Fibroadenoma. Benign, painless swelling in the breast, usually discovered by chance by doctor or patient during an examination,
generally in women between the ages of 20 and 40. Certain
diagnosis is possible only after microscopic examination of the
tissue (biopsy); any tumour of the breast must be taken seriously. A biopsy is taken, usually in an outpatients department,
and if fibroadenoma is diagnosed, surgery is not necessary. A
related condition is a large cyst, also benign, but which must
be removed because it can exert painful pressure on the surrounding area, and also recur. In such cases a short stay in
hospital is necessary.

Fifth disease (erythema infectiosum)   An infectious disease that
occurs in childhood. The cause is unknown, a virus being the
most likely agent. It is a rare disease which normally occurs in
closed communities, the incubation period is usually 5 to 6
days, sometimes longer. The most important symptoms are a
skin rash with bright red, slightly raised spots. The rash begins on the face and spreads along the limbs and finally the
trunk. The spots are then white in colour. New red spots also
appear, so that the skin becomes highly mottled. There are no
other symptoms of the disease, and there is no fever. The rash
disappears after about a week. Complications do not arise, and
no treatment is necessary.

Filariae. Thin worms varying in length from a few cm to 60 cm.
They live in tissue, blood vessels and lymph vessels, and occur
in the tropics and sub tropics. The female worms bear larvae,
which move into the bloodstream at certain periods of the day
or night, them return to the tissues; they can be transmitted
from one human being to another by blood-sucking insects,
which thus function only as intermediate host or vector. In
man the larvae can grow into adult worms.

Fistula. Abnormal connection between two hollow organs (e.g., bladder and intestine), or between a hollow organ and the skin (as
in anal fistula). Fistulas can occur for no clear reason, but
some conditions are known for a tendency to fistula formation,
particularly intestinal cancers diverticulitis, Crohn's disease

and intestinal tuberculosis. The symptoms of these disorders predominate, and effects of the fistula depend on the nature of the connection which it forms. Fistulas between bladder and intestine can cause faeces in the urine, and vice-versa. A fistula from intestime to vagina can introduce pus or contents of the intestine into the vagina. Anal fistulas usually exude pus on to the skin.

Treatment is by surgical removal; recovery can be slow and fistuals tend to recur.

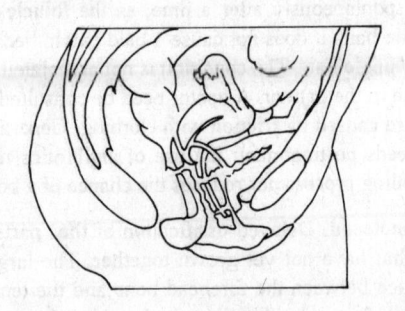

Fistulas are abnormal connections between organs, which can be caused by ulceration.

Fleas. Laterally-compressed jumping insects a few millimetres in size. They feed on the blood of humans and animals (dogs, cats, mice, rats). The larvae are 2 and 4 mm long and look like small caterpillars. They develop into fully grown fleas after about four weeks. If a human is bitten by a flea, small, red, very itchy lumps form on the skin. Fleas can also be conveyors of diseases: the rat-flea (*Xenopsylla cheopsis*) is notorious as a conveyor of plague and typhus. The sand-flea (*Tunga penetrans*) occurs in Central and South America. Africa and Asia. These fleas live in sand and dig into the skin of humans and domestic animals, usually in the foot. An itchy swelling then forms around the flea which lays its eggs towards the outside. The swelling can be removed surgically. Flea bites are treated by powder or ointment to ease the itching. Fleas can be exterminated by means of pesticides.

Folliculitis. Inflammation of a follicle, the 'bulb' from which a hair
grows. It can occur anywhere on the skin where there is hair,
in other words anywhere except the palms of the hands and the
soles of the feet. The condition is caused by the bacterium
Staphylococcus aureus, which is also responsible for
hidradenitis (inflammation of the sweat glands). Boils may be
considered complications of folliculitis. In the first place a pimple
appears, an area of swelling and redness around the hair. This
heals spontaneously after a time, as the follicle is forced out
with the hair. It does not cause a bald patch, because it affects
only a single hair. The condition is not associated with fever or
malaise in the patient. A doctor need be consulted only if problems are caused by friction with clothing. Generally the condition needs no treatment; the use of antibiotics neither speeds
the healing process nor reduces the chance of a boil forming.

Fontanel, unclosed. Delayed ossification of the parts of a baby's
skull that have not yet grown together. The large fontanel is
the space between the forehead bone and the temporal bones;
the small fontanel is between the bones. A fontanel consists of
rigid periosteum, which protects the blood vessels and brain
beneath it.

Food Poisoning. Intestinal disorders caused by bacterial products
(toxins), not by the growth of bacteria in the intestine. Toxins
may originate from within the bacterium, the bacterial wall, or
can be actively produced by the bacterium. The term 'food
poisoning' is often used incorrectly to describe gastroenteritis*,
which usually results from a salmonella bacterium that multiplies to cause an ordinary infection. Most cases of food poisoning are caused by staphylococcal toxins, usually from meat,
fish or milk. Even pasteurized milk can sporadically lead to
food poisoning, because although the bacteria are killed in
pasteurization their toxin can remain intact.

Foot disorders. Usually take the form of abnormalities in the shape
of the foot. These are often congenital, but can also arise in

later years caused, for example, by shoes which are too tight. A club-foot is congenital. The foot is turned inwards and tilted, so that only the outer edge of the foot touches the ground. Club-feet occur in either or both feet in about 1 in 1000 newborn babies; boys have them twice as frequently as girls. Treatment must be commenced as soon as possible and consists of repeated applications of plaster to impose normal posture gradually. A surgical operation can be performed if necessary. A hollow foot has a characteristic strong upward curvature caused by a disturbance in the normal balance between various groups of muscles, Paralysis or weakness of certain muscles is often the cause; an operation is usually the only solution. In flat feet, the arch of the foot has fallen so that the whole sole of the foot touches the ground. Flat feet frequently occur in overweight people, pregnant women and workers in professions involving an abnormal amount of standing. Young children can suffer from flat feet by walking too early and too often. Symptoms include pain and fatigue in walking and standing. Back complaints also often occur. Treatment is by means of muscle exercises and arch supports. In addition to abnormalities of shape, fractures of one or more bones in the foot also occur as a result of injury or even walking for long distances. Foot ailments may be accompanied by back complaints caused by abnormalities in the walking pattern or by abnormalities which occur in standing. Inflammation of the foot joints is also common, as the result of a wound or part of a rheumatic disorder. Disturbances in the supply of blood to the foot especially the toes, frequently occur in scleroderma, diabetes, or fatty degeneration of the arteries (atherosclerosis). Death of tissue occurs as a consequence. The dead tissue forms an ideal culture medium for bacteria, and wet necrosis or gangrene can be the result.

Fracture. Break or split in a bone. A distinction can be made between simple and compound fractures. In simple fractures the skin remains intact; in compound fractures of more pieces of bone protrude through the skin. In a comminuted fracture the bone is broken into several pieces or fragments.

A division can also be made into complete or incomplete fractures. In a complete fracture the bone is broken into two or more pieces, whereas in incomplete fracture it is still intact in one place. An example of the latter is a 'greenstick' fracture, which can occur in children: because the young bone is so pliable and the periosteum so strong the bone does not break completely. A crack or fissure is also an incomplete fracture.

Fractures are caused by force. They can, however, also occur as a result of normal pressure on the bone, if the bone is diseased (for example in osteoporosis); this is known as a spontaneous fracture.

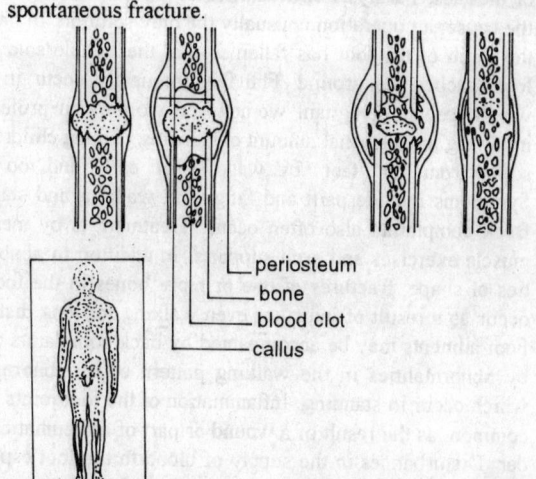

periosteum
bone
blood clot
callus

A fractured bone heals when tissue forms in the blood clot(callus), and then calcifies.

Fractures are also classified by form: in a transverse fracture the line of break runs almost perpendicular to the length of the bone, in a slanting fracture the line slants throat the bone and a fracture caused by twisting is a spiral fracture.

Symptoms of a fracture are pain, swelling, abnormal position, abnormal movement and inability to move the affected limb oneself. Muscles go into spasm as a result of fracture, and if the fracture is complete the pieces of bone are forced to overlap.

It is important to limit movement of the affected limbs during transport by means of a splint.

Framboesia. Tropical infection caused by the spirochaete bacterium *Treponema pertenue*, related to *Treponema pallidium* which causes syphilis, which framboesia closely resembles.

Framboesia occurs mainly in warm, damp regions with poor hygiene. It is above all a disease of the young, two thirds of the cases occur in patients under fifteen. The illness begins two to three weeks after infection with painless yellow-red raised patches on the skin. After a few months similar small swellings can occur all over the body, which enlarge, at which point the skin can break to reveal a pink mass. These 'strawberries', which give the disease its name appear on the lips, elbows and buttocks. The abnormalities of the skin usually heal spontaneously in a few months sometimes leaving small scars. Years later abnormalities of the skin and mucous membranes can occur, but bones and joints can also be affected, leading to malformation and disability. The bacteria are spread by direct contact with the affected skin, entering the body via a wound. Treatment is by antibiotics, or by operation is cases of disability.

Freckles. Flecks of pigment in the face, particularly in patients with a fair skin, usually on the cheeks and nose, but possibly also all over the face and arms as well. Redheads generally have more freckles than other people, because pigmentation is different for them. It is not possible to remove freckles, only to make them less conspicuous. It is important to protect the skin against ultraviolet light with a suntan cream with a high protection factor. Freckles can be made somewhat paler with weak acids such as lemon juice.

Friedreich's Ataxia. Hereditary condition of the nervous system, involving decay of lateral and posterior columns of the spinal cord, and abnormalities in the cerebellum. The disorder begins gradually in childhood and the most important symptom is ataxia, i.e. disturbed muscular coordination resulting from loss of a sense of depth.

The first symptoms are insecure walking, with broader, jerkier steps, followed after some years by increasing unsureness in the use of the hands and indistinct, irregular speech. Finally paralysis can occur, sometimes associated with failure of the nerves of face, throat and eyes; sometimes there are abnormalities of the heart and skeleton (club foot, scoliosis). In mild cases the condition is compatible with a normal life; in other cases the patient may well become an invalid. Life can be shortened by the associated heart abnormalities and by the increased chance of pneumonia (as a result of choking, among other things). Diagnosis is by the characteristic symptoms; the picture can be much like multiple sclerosis. There is no direct treatment; physiotherapy is of lasting value.

Frigidity. Somewhat old fashioned term for the condition of women who do not experience orgasm, and have few or no passionate feelings during sexual intercourse. In serious cases there may be aversion to sex, possibly associated with vaginismus.

Frostbite. Damage to the skin caused by excessively low temperatures, mostly affecting the tip of the nose, the fingers and the toes. In the polar regions freezing may affect tissues deeper in the body. The cold closes the blood vessels in the affected area, to prevent the blood, and therefore the body, cooling down too much, and consequently the affected area can drop below freezing point, when the skin literally freezes. Ice crystals form in the frozen skin cells, and can rupture and destroy them. The small quantity of blood left in the blood vessels freezes and causes thrombosis; these two changes cause damage to the tissue when it thaws out again. Frozen skin is pale, sometimes white, and can feel stiff. The victim feels stabbing pain in the affected area. The damage after thawing is sometimes indistinguishable from a burn and the same distinction in degree is made, first degree freezing being the most superficial.

Frozen shoulder. Serious restriction of shoulder movement caused by inflammation or injury. Inflammation of joint tissue can cause growths and calcium deposits, but one of the commonest causes of frozen shoulder is wastage of capsule and ligaments caused by keeping the shoulder still for a long period, either to avoid pain in shoulder conditions or by wearing a sling or plaster for too long. To avoid frozen shoulder it is thus important to use painkillers and remove dressings which restrict movement as soon as possible. Frozen shoulder is difficult to treat; extensive physiotherapy including heat treatment, massage and exercises can be used to try to extend movement gradually.

Fungus infections. Infection with fungal micro-organisms. Fungi are plants without leaves that depend for their existence on other plants or animals; some of them are useful to man-in the preparation of antibiotics for example, edible mushrooms, and yeasts used in the manufacture of bread and beer. On the other hand fungi can attack edible plants, cause food to decay and induce infection in man. Fungi take various forms : multicellular organisms which grow by forming long threads or inter-woven structures (mycelium), and unicellular fungi (yeasts) which reproduce themselves by bud formation. It is possible that in nature the 'myceliar form' is produced and in man the 'yeast form', e.g. in histoplasmosis. A fungus spreads by means of spores, from which new fungi develop.

Functional. 1. With reference to function as distinct from the structure performing the function. 2. In a medical context, a functional disorder is a disorder of a function, for example walking or thinking, but not of a structure. A structural disorder would be a broken bone or dementia, the former causing a disturbance of walking and the latter of thinking (among other mental activities). Structural disorders have come to be called organic because they have a demonstrable organic cause. 3. Thus, the most common use of functional is in reference to a mental disorder, for example, *anxiety, depression* or *schizophrenia*, which has no identifiable or demonstrable structural cause. That this designation is far from satisfactory can be seen by a glance at mental deficiency associated with a remote but demonstrably related birth defect such as *phenylketonuria*. No one knows what organic connection exists between the missing enzyme in that disease and the mental disorder, but nevertheless, it is classified as organic. Conversely, mental deficiency can be caused by an unknown birth trauma and be termed functional because it has no identifiable structural component. In these examples, functional neither describes accurately a causal relationship nor helps the study, treatment, or cure of the condition. The word derives from an older science in which function was separated from structure to promote the study and recording of accurate detail, but the incorrectness of the division is well illustrated by the word functional itself.

G

Galactorrhoea. Secretion of milk outside the breast-feeding period. In new-born children it can occur because of the removal of the hormonal function of the placenta. In women of child-bearing age such secretion may have a number of causes, such as inflamed or wet eczema, which affects both breasts; it can also result from an increased quantity of the hormone prolactin, caused by a benign tumour in the pituitary gland, again with secretion from both breasts. The condition also occurs in some forms of breast cancer, usually in one breast only. Further examination is necessary. Treatment after diagnosis may be by surgery or medication.

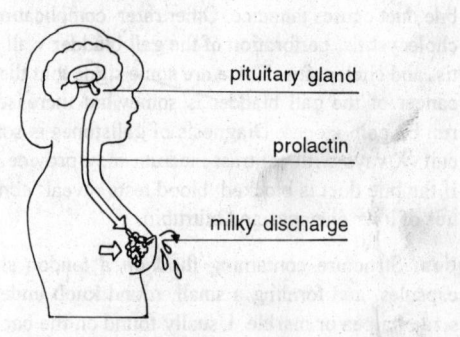

pituitary gland

prolactin

milky discharge

Abnormal discharge from the breast can be caused by a local stimulus or increased hormone activity.

Gall bladder, cancer of. A relatively rare malignant tumour, more common in women than men. There may be a connection with gallstones, but this is not certain. It tends to be discovered at a late stage, because symptoms are slow to show. The first symptom is usually increasingly severe jaundice, because the tumour

inhibits the flow of bile. This is associated with pain in the
upper abdomen, poor appetite and loss of weight, and possibly
fever and cold shivers.

Gallstones. Common condition in overweight, middle-aged women;
it is often hereditary. The stones usually consist of a mixture of
chloresterol, bile pigment and calcium, often in differing proportions; stones consisting purely of cholesterol and bile pigment are rare. Gallstones occur in the gall bladder or sometimes in the bile duct. They can remain in the gall bladder, but
may block its exit or pass into the bile duct.

Symptoms can vary considerably: it is possible for a stone
to cause no difficulties for years and simply to remain at rest in
the gall bladder. Often however they move as described above,
causing typically colic, violent pain in the area of stomach and
gall bladder, radiating to the right and to the back, nausea and
vomiting. The pain may disappear after several hours, but if
the stone remains, it can cause cholecystitis. Blockage of the
bile duct causes jaundice. Other rarer complications are chronic
cholecystitis, perforation of the gall bladder wall with peritonitis, and cholangitis. There are some signs that the possibility of
cancer of the gall bladder is somewhat increased in the long
run by gall stones. Diagnosis of gallstones is sometimes difficult: X-rays with contrast medium may provide an indication.
If the bile duct is blocked, blood tests reveal abnormal quantities of liver enzymes and bilirubin.

Ganglion. Structure containing fluid on a tendon sheath or joint
capsules, and forming a small, round knob under the skin the
size of a pea or marble. Usually found on the back of the hand,
the wrists, the ankles or behind the knee, ganglia are not painful, but can hinder movement. The fluid contained is bright to
light red and watery. A ganglion is formed by tissue degeneration of the tendon sheath or joint capsule as a result of
irritation of this tissue, for example during or after tenosynovitis,
or in rheumatic conditions of the joints. They often occur without clear cause.

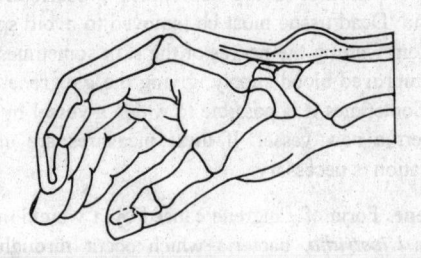

A ganglion is a moisture-filled lump originating in the tendon sheath.

Gangrene. Death of tissue through shortage of oxygen.

There are two kinds of gangrene. In the dry form the tissue dies because of interruption of the blood supply. There is no infection, and the affected part dries up and wastes away. In the wet form, infection sets in after the tissue has died. The affected area looks damp, and often smells very unpleasant because of the infection. The feet are particularly susceptible to diseases linked with restricted oxygen supply to the tissue, caused by interruption of the blood supply as in the case of diabetes, thrombosis, severe atherosclerosis and Buerger's disease. The first symptom of interrupted blood supply is pain when walking, subsequently persisting when the patient is at rest. The affected area is cold and pale, no arterial pulse can be detected, the tissue is starved of oxygen and dies. In the early stages of gangrene the skin is blue, later darker and then black. Wounds in areas with poor blood supply heal only with difficulty, and gradually become infected, resulting in gangrene. Diabetes affects the nerves, and patients do not feel wounds, so they are often infected before the patient notices. This occurs most usually in the feet (diabetic foot), but only after a number of years. It is then essential to avoid wounds, by not wearing shoes that are too tight, not walking on bare feet and practising adequate hygiene. The feet should be checked for wounds every day. If infection does occur, the area should be kept as dry as possible. Antibiotics are sometimes prescribed to kill the bacteria. Dead tissue must be removed to avoid spreading the infection. Cutting the nerves of the skin sometimes provides it with improved blood supply, giving the gangrene a chance to heal. Sometimes it is possible to widen a vessel by surgery, or to insert a new vessel. If these measures are unsuccessful, amputation is necessary.

Gas gangrene. Form of gangrene caused by a wound infected with certain *Clostridia,* bacteria which occur throughout nature. Spores of the bacteria that cause the condition are found in soil, street refuse and human and animal excrement. Gas gangrene occurs principally in deep, very dirty wounds (war wounds).

Treatment is by removal of dead tissue and administration of antibiotics. Treatment in an oxygen tent is effective because the bacteria are not resistant to oxygen in large quantities.

Gastric flu. Intestinal disorder due to an infection, commonly by a virus, and usually not severe: it can lead to gastroenteritis however. Sometimes gastric flu is caused by a virus including coxsackie viruses, echoviruses and adenoviruses) and sometimes by a bacterium (such as salmonella).

Gastroenteritis. Collective name for inflammation of the mucous membrane of stomach and intestine usually caused by a virus (gastric flu). less often by a bacterium (paratyphoid) or bacterial poisoning (toxins food poisoning), and sometimes poisonous substances (alcohol, medicines, fungi, lead). The condition can vary from slight inflammation causing little discomfort to a dangerous condition which can lead to dehydration, especially in children. Characteristic signs are nausea and vomiting cramp, watery diarrhoea, sensitive abdomen, sometimes dehydration and even shock, especially in children. Recovery is usually spontaneous after a few days.

Gene. A segment of a chromosome which contains an instruction that can be converted by the cell into a genetic characteristic. The genetic characteristic is a protein, usually but not always an enzyme. Exceptions include the proteins that make up haemoglobin, the gas-carrying molecule that gives colour to red blood cells.

The gene itself consists of a series of linked nucleic acids, each one attached to a molecule of a simple sugar, deoxyribose. The nucleic acids are not all the same, but come in four varieties. The sequence of these different kinds of nucleic acids along the gene is of the utmost importance: it spells out in genetic language the sequence of amino acids that will be used by the cell to make the protein specified by the gene.

The four amino acids are identified by means of those parts of them that differ, their bases, as a adenine (A) Cytosine (C) guanine (G) and thymine (T). As noted, they are arranged in a sequence which spells out a genetic "word", the individual letters being codons. Three nucleic acids in sequence make up a codon. Thus because there are four nucleic acids, combinations of three of them permit a total alphabet of 64 codons: AAA, ACG CGT, ACT and so on.

These deoxyribonucleic acids (DNAs) are first translated into a nucleic acid combined with ribose sugar or ribonucleic acid (RNA). For reasons having to do with the different atoms in ribose, the four nucleic acids in RNA are adenine (A), cytosine (C), guanine (G) and uracil (U). As in DNA, however, three nucleic acids comprise a codon, the same three as in the DNA from which the translation was made, with the difference that thymine is replaced in RNA by uracil.

RNA leaves the nucleus of the cell and is taken up by a ribosome, a cellular machine for manufacturing protein. The ribosome engages the RNA as a template into which it fits the appropriate amino acid. Since a protein is made up of combinations of only 20 amino acids, some of the amino acids are identified by more than one letter in the genetic alphabet; that is, more than one codon specifies a single amino acid.

Other codons tell the ribosome when to start or when to stop. The functions of one or two codons is still unclear.

The proteins made in response to instructions by a gene perform functions which give cells their characteristics, as nerve or muscle cells, or as cells in blue as opposed to brown eyes.

Genital herpes. Venereal disease caused by the herpes simplex virus type II. Herpes simplex type I is transmitted by kissing and usually only caused sores and blisters around the mouth, the condition known as cold sores, which can sometimes affect the genitals by oral contact. Herpes simplex II affects the genitals in the first place, and sometimes the lips and mouth by oral contact.

Symptoms usually begin 4 to 6 days after infection. One or more painful, moisture-filled blisters form around the penis or vagina; the blisters burst after a few days, followed by itching and smarting. During this active phase the patient may have high fever and muscular pain, and the lympth nodes in and around the genitals may swell. The patient is infectious to sexual partners until two to three weeks after the sores have healed, after which the virus remains inactive in the skin, and no longer presents danger of infection. In some people the condition never recurs, whereas other patients are repeatedly affected by the active phase. There is no drug against the virus; the only therapy is pain killers and speeding up the drying of the blisters. It is important to avoid sexual contact during attacks, and to beware of infecting the eyes via the hands.

Genu varum (bow leg) Condition in which the ankles touch when the legs are outstretched, but there is still a space between the knees. The result of outward curvature of thigh and shin bones, it is present in about 75 per cent of babies and young children, and usually disappears at around the age of 3. However, if the bones remain too flexible through calcium or vitamin D deficiency (rickets), bow legs may persist or even become worse. Bow legs can also occur in older people as a result of osteomalacia or Paget's disease. In growing children the condition can be corrected by the use of splints and support shoes. If the distance between the knees is greater than about 10 cm the epiphyseal cartridge on the outside of the leg bones can be fixed in position (epiphysiodesis), thus checking bone growth on the outer-edge, and reducing crookedness.

German measles (rubella) Acute and highly infectious viral invention, with an incubation period of two to three weeks. The lymph nodes in the neck and behind the ears swell without previous symptoms of illness. The temperature rises to 38.5°C and a skin eruption appears: the spots are pinkish and small, appearing first on the face, and covering the whole of the trunk and limbs within 24 hours; most of them disappear by the end of the first day. The child is not usually seriously ill, and the disorder confers life-long immunity; complications are rare. The illness is harmless for children, and requires no treatment.

Giardiasis (lambliasis). Infection caused by a cosmopolitan flagellated protozoan parasite (*Giardia lamblia*). In some countries more than 10 per cent of the population carry it, and it is particularly widespread among children in the tropics. Europeans who have visited the tropics may also become infested. *Giardia lamblia* is able to travel through the intestine and it attaches itself to the wall of the duodenum or the small intestine with a sucker, and lives on the liquid contents of the intestine.

Giardiasis is infestation with a parasite which causes diarrhoea. A cycle occurs via contaminated water and vegetable.

The parasite can be surrounded by a solid wall (cyst) and be passed with the faeces, and can thus find its way into food and drinking water. The parasite is highly resistant to chlorine, so that even apparently pure water can be a source of infection. Many infected patients show no symptoms, but in more serious cases the small intestine is coated with parasites, causing abdominal pain, nausea, loss of appetite and diarrhoea. Sometimes incomplete digestion of fat leads to malabsorption.

The disease can be confirmed by examining faeces for cysts of the parasite. Treatment by drugs is possible.

Gigantism. Rare growth in children and young adults resulting from over-production of growth hormone, caused by a tumour of the pituitary gland. Because the growth hormones stimulates activity in the epiphyseal plates in the bones, ultimate bone length-and thus body length-is much greater than normal; a height 2.3 metres can be reached. The condition is detected by measurements to establish the amount of growth hormone in the blood, and the skull is X-rayed to check for the presence of a pituitary tumour. Treatment is by surgery to remove the tumour, and radiation therapy. Medication can also used to limit excess growth hormone formation.

Gilles de la Tourette syndrome. Rare condition characterized by brief spells of involuntary movement of the face, head, and later possibly of the limbs. Groans, obscenities and swearwords may also be uttered. The patient is not able to suppress the symptoms; the condition is made worse by emotion and tension. It is often thought that the syndrome is caused by an underlying psychological disorder, but this is not the case. In principle the patient functions quite normally, although the nature of the symptoms places him under psychological pressure.

Gingivitis (inflammation of the gums) General acute inflammation of the gums is characterized by redness, pain, swelling and minor bleeding from the mucous membrane around the teeth. Inflammation can result, for example, from poor oral hygiene, a diet which lacks certain essential foodstuffs, alcoholism or invention of the mouth by bacteria, viruses or fungi.

Glandular fever (mononucleosis) Infectious disease caused by the Epstein-Barr herpes virus, transmitted in saliva by direct contact (hence the old name 'kissing disease') or by coughing in the faces of other people. One to six weeks can pass between infection and outbreak of the disease. Later stages vary from person to person. There is often a general feeling of malaise, associated with sore throat; swelling of the lymph nodes of the neck, armpits and groin and gradually increasing fever. The spleen may be enlarged and the liver may be affected, possibly causing jaundice. Other symptoms are headache, stiff neck, inflammation of the eyes, nausea, vomiting and sometimes a red skin eruption. The disease can last for several weeks or months; fever and swelling usually disappear after a few weeks, but the patient may feel tired and listless for a longer period. In extreme cases depression can occur because the patient has been feeling unwell for so long. Other possible complications are anaemia, meningitis and inflammation of the heart or kidneys.

Glaucoma. Abnormally high fluid pressure within the eyeball. Pressure is determined by the balance between formation of aqueous tumour and its removal. Normal pressure is between 15 and 20 mm of mercury.

There are three distinct forms of glaucoma. In congenital glaucoma the removal of aqueous tumour is restricted by a

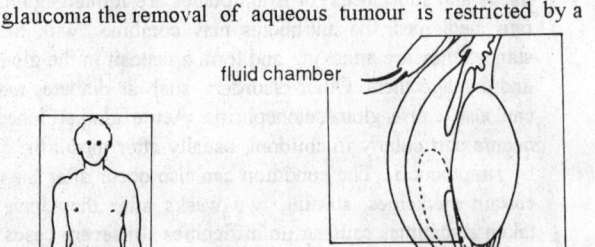

fluid chamber

In glaucoma the drainage of aqueous humour from the eye is restricted, thus increasing pressure in the eyeball.

congenital abnormality, and the new-born infant has a uni-
formly enlarged eye, with excess pressure in the eyeball. Primary glaucoma is caused by an abnormality of the drainage
form. Secondary glaucoma is a complication of another condition such as inflammation, damage or a tumour, which affects
the removal of aqueous humour.

Glioma. Tumour originating in the cerebral nerve cell support tissue
(and sometimes in the spinal column). The condition occurs
mainly in childhood or around the age of 50. There are various kinds, with different growth rates, and different degrees of
benignity. Gliomas grow offshoots between the normal brain
tissue, which makes them difficult to remove completely.

Growth of the tumour puts brain tissue under pressure, producing such symptoms as function failure, headache, nausea
and vomiting. Radiation treatment may be used in addition to
surgery; dome Gliomas produce cerebral haemorrhage, with
accompanying deterioration of the clinical picture.

Glomerulonephritis (Bright's disease) Form of kidney inflammation that affects the glomeruli (blood filters) of both kidneys,
usually as a result of an immune reaction. After inflammation
elsewhere in the body in an autoimmune disease (condition in
which the body produces antibodies that act against its own
tissue and substances) or if antibodies are formed against certain medicines, the antibodies may combine with the substances they are attacking and form a deposit in the glomeruli,
and damage them. Other disorders, such as diabetes mellitus,
can also cause glomerulonephritis. Acute glomerulonephritis
occurs particularly in children, usually after tonsillitis, caused
by streptococci. The condition can also occur after the use of
certain medicines, starting two weeks after they have been
taken sometimes causing no difficulties. In severe cases urine
production declines, blood appears in the urine (uraemia) and
tissue swells through fluid accumulation (oedema), particularly in the face. Recovery is complete in most cases, but the
condition sometimes persists-particularly in adults—and becomes chronic, leading to progressive damage to the kidneys

and eventual kidney failure.

Glossitis. Inflammation of the tongue, usually as a secondary condition. Thus vitamin deficiency, dietary insufficiency, anaemia and irritation, caused for example by chemical substances, can reduce local resistance and lead to glossitis. Glossitis can be accompanied by inflammation of the mucous membrane in the mouth.

Glue ear. Chronic inflammation of the mucous membrane of the cavity behind the eardrum and the Eustachian tube, causing an accumulation of fluid in the middle ear. The cause is usually a cold in the nose or infection of the upper respiratory tract. The condition usually occurs in children aged between 5 and 8, because the Eustachian tube is short and almost horizontal in infants and young children, and easily infected. The first signs of the condition are usually slight earache, whistling or bubbling sounds, and slight hearing loss. If the fluid behind the eardrum is pus, the condition is known as purulent otitis media. Inspection of the ear shows a discoloured, indrawn eardrum, and hearing tests confirm hearing loss. Deafness and other abnormalities of the inner ear are possible consequences of poor treatment of glue ear.

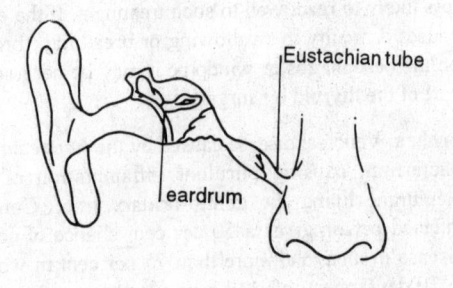

In glue ear the Eustachian tube is blocked and the eardrum drawn inwards.

Treatment is by the introduction of a small, plastic tube (grommet) into the eardrum, which removes the fluid and balances the pressure on each side of it. While the grommet is in position, care must be taken to prevent water getting into the ear (when washing the hair, or swimming).

Goitre. Enlargement of the thyroid, usually associated with malfunction of the gland. If the thyroid is functioning normally the condition is usually caused by iodine deficiency. This occurs particularly in countries a long way from the sea (endemic goitre). If a person's diet contains too little iodine, the thyroid has to overwork to produce enough thyroid hormone. The condition can also occur in periods when the body requires additional thyroid hormone : in puberty, pregnancy and the period after it, when a baby is being breast-fed. Table salt containing iodine, sea salt and fish products can provide enough iodine and prevent this form of goitre. If the thyroid is enlarged it is important to establish whether the swelling is even (diffuse) or whether certain areas feel abnormal (thyroid nodules). In the latter case it is possible that a malignant growth is developing, and extensive examination is necessary. Before a diffuse goitre is treated artificial thyroid hormones are usually administered. The swollen gland is thus rested, and may return to its normal size, but if the condition has been present for a long time it is less likely to react well to such treatment. If the enlarged gland causes difficulty in swallowing or breathing through pressure on the oesophagus or windpipe it may be necessary to remove part of the thyroid by surgery.

Gonorrhoea. Venereal disease caused by the *Neisseria gonorrhoeae* bacterium, causing purulent inflammation of the mucous membrane lining the genito-urinary tract. Contact with an infected person gives a 50 per cent chance of contracting the disease in men, and more than 75 per cent in women. After 2 to 10 days most infected men experience a burning sensation when urinating and a milky discharge from the penis; the discharge becomes thicker after a few days. Sometimes the lymph ducts in the groin swell. Symptoms may disappear without treatment, but the man is still a source of infection for his sexual partner(s), and is in danger of inflammation of the epididymis and the prostate, with sterility as a possible complication.

Gout (podagra) Metabolic disorder in which uric acid crystals accumulate in the joints. Hereditary factors are sometimes important; it can be passed by a daughter to her children, although she herself does not contract the disease. It is much more common in men than women. Uric acid is a normal breakdown product of cell protein, usually removed from the body by the kidneys; an attack of gout is often preceded by a (temporary) increase in blood-uric acid content, sometimes attributable to excessive uric acid production, sometimes to a kidney malfunction that makes them less able to excrete uric acid. The cause of over-production is usually not clear, but it is known that the treatment of cancer with cell-killing drugs can cause gout, because many cell proteins are broken down in the process. Accumulation of uric acid crystals in the joints causes an acute, painful inflammation reaction. In principle it can occur in any joint, but the most usual site is the big toes, possibly because the temperature is somewhat lower there. The pain occurs suddenly, and within a short time the joint is so sensitive that even the pressure of a blanket is painful. The skin is warm, red, shiny and swollen, and body temperature may rise.

Granuloma inguinale. Venereal disease caused by the *Donovania granulomatis* bacterium. The disorder occurs mainly in the tropics, and more in men than women, and is transmitted by sexual contact, although some researchers maintain that it can also be caused by poor hygiene. Symptoms usually occur a few days after infection, but sometimes not until weeks later. Small wounds with the appearance of round abrasions appear on the genitals and anus. Sometimes the groins, thighs and face are also affected. If untreated the wounds develop into ulcers, and the underlying tissue becomes damaged. In the long term arthritis and anaemia can set in.

Diagnosis is by skin tissue tests; treatment is with antibiotics.

Growing pains. Pains that occur in children during periods of rapid growth, usually localized in the legs, and affecting the child at night. Pain is caused by differing growth rates in different tissues and probably stems from painful stretching of nerves and blood vessels in and around the muscles. It is important in such cases to bear in mind other possible sources of muscular pain, such as excessive exertion. There are also a number of disorders of the muscles and some rheumatic disorders associated with muscular pain. Growing pains generally need no treatment.

Growth, abnormal. Growth disturbances leading to anomalies in a person's height occur in two forms: too fast and too slow. Growth in children should be checked by regular measurement compared with the growth curve of contemporaries of the same sex.

Slow growth can be linked with hereditary factors such as short parents, with malnutrition or chronic illness (such as bronchial asthma or kidney disorders). Genuine dwarfism is less common, and caused by hereditary metabolic disturbances, bone and cartilage conditions or growth hormone deficiency. Infection can cause temporary slowing down of growth, but this is usually quickly made up after recovery. Hereditary factors also play a part in rapid growth-at the onset of puberty, for example, and its associated growth spurt. If puberty begins early, a child can shoot up above his or her contemporaries; this usually happens earlier in girls than in boys, because puberty is later in boys. Growth differences in puberty are quickly made up; the production of more sex hormones at the end of puberty checks the growth spurt. In girls the mmenarche (beginning of menstruation) is a sign of the end of the growth spurt; body length increases only by a few centimetres after that. Girls who are taller than their contemporaries can often be reassured by the fact that their mother had an early menarche; this is likely also to be the case with the daughter, and suggests that she will ultimately be of normal height.

Gullain-bare syndrome. Paralysis or sensory difficulties caused by inflammation of the nerve roots in the spinal column. The cause is not yet fully known, but it is probably associated with an allergic reaction of the nervous system after a virus infection, because the syndrome usually follows an attack of influenza.

Gumboil. Abscess on the root of a tooth, usually caused by inflammation after bacteria have been introduced into the root canal by dental caries. If the inflammation is not treated and becomes chronic, the accumulation of bacteria and dead white blood cells forms pus. The resultant abscess causes swelling, sensitivity to pressure, and pain. The usual treatment is by drainage, i.e. lancing, supplemented by antibiotics. Often the tooth has to be removed.

Gynaecomastia. Development of mammary glands in a boy or man; glandular tissue can be felt under the nipple. The condition usually occurs in puberty, and can affect one or both breasts. The cause is unknown. The condition can be somewhat painful, but the patient suffers most from embarrassment, because he is often the butt of teasing at swimming or other sports. In younger patients the condition disappears spontaneously after a few years; surgery is resorted to only if the boy is undergoing acute psychological distress.

H

Haemangioma. Tumour-like growth of small blood vessels in and beneath the skin, nearly always found in children. There are three main kinds: the strawberry mark or naevus, capillary haemangioma and cavernous haemangioma.

Strawberry marks almost always occur on the face or the neck, are present at birth and result from severe dilation of the capillaries, causing a pale to dark pink patch not raised above the skin; they can cover a large area. Unfortunately little can be done about them.

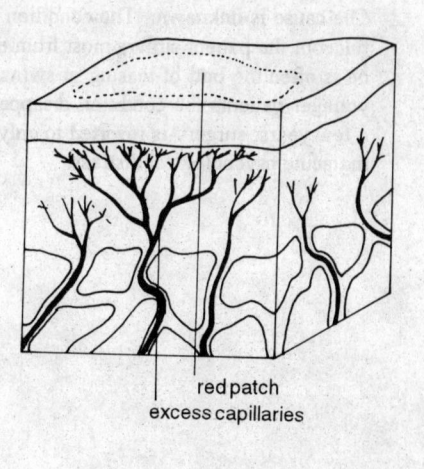

red patch
excess capillaries

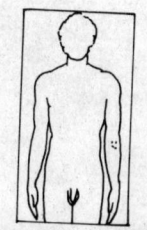

Excess capillaries cause a red patch like a port wine stain on the surface of the skin.

Haematemesis (vomiting blood) Associated with a condition in the upper part of the alimentary tract, usually the oesophagus, stomach or duodenum. It is important to differentiate between vomiting blood and coughing blood (haemoptysis). In vomiting the blood is almost always partly digested and looks brown. It is bright red only in the case of a sudden, severe haemorrhage. A possible difference can be that in haematemesis acid gastric juices are mixed with the blood, whereas if it comes from the lungs it is often foaming. Also in haematemesis the quantity is usually greater than if the blood comes from the lungs. In a condition of the alimentary tract blood is often visible in the faeces.

Haematoma. A bruise, caused by damage to a blood vessel beneath the skin leading to accumulation of blood in the surrounding tissue before a clot can form and the blood coagulate. The condition persists for some days until the blood is broken down and completely removed; the stages of this process can be seen from the changing colour of the skin. Blood shows through the skin as blue, and the breakdown products show subsequently as green, yellow and brown the normal sequence in the healing of a bruise.

Haematoma, cephalic. Haemorrhage under the periosteum of one of the bones of the skull of a newborn baby and visible as a fairly severe swelling which feels soft and as though it contains fluid. It is caused by friction of forceps or a vacuum extractor against the skull, or friction of the skull against the mother's abdominal wall before birth.

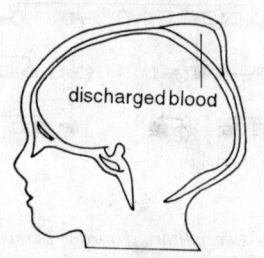

discharged blood

Cephalic haematoma is a discharge of blood between the skin and cranium of a newborn baby; it disappears within a few weeks.

Apart from a temporary strangeness of appearance there
should be no adverse consequences for the child. The blood is
completely reabsorbed, sometimes slowly, sometimes quickly.
Bone may be deposited, causing hardening of the swelling, but
a cephalic haematoma disappears completely in the short or
long run.

Haemochromatosis. Accumulation of excess iron in the skin or
internal organs, usually caused by a hereditary metabolic disorder, sometimes after a number of blood transfusions. Each
time a litre of blood is administered 0.5 grams of iron enters
the body as a component of haemoglobin. Symptoms can be
bronze discoloration of the skin, diabetes mellitus caused by
the effect on the pancreas, malfunction of the liver through
cirrhosis of the liver, heart failure and pain in the joints.

Hemophilia. Congenital blood deficiency involving lack of a clotting factor. Haemorrhage is arrested naturally in two stages:
staunching and coagulation. Staunching is the formation of a
clot by the platelets, and is followed by coagulation to occur
there must be proteins in the plasma known as coagulation
factors. Coagulation is necessary to give the clot sufficient
rigidity, and if one or more coagulation factors are missing the
condition is known as haemophilia. The commonest form of

*Heamophilia is a hereditary disorder passed on via the X- chro-
mosome. The disease spread from Queen Victoria to males in a
number of European royal houses because of intermarriage.*

haemophilia is linked with the X-chromosome, meaning that the disease can be transmitted by women to the next generation, but only men can suffer from it. The most important symptom is recurrent haemorrhage; a wound will stop bleeding, because the platelets function normally in forming a clot, but the clot is weak, and becomes detached, allowing the wound to start bleeding again.

Haemorrhage, epidural. Haemorrhage between the skull and the outermost layer of the membrane enveloping the brain and spinal cord (dura), usually caused by an accident. Cranial fracture may also be present. The characteristic feature is that the patient recovers after a short period of unconsciousness, but then gradually becomes more dazed from pressure on the brain as a result of the haemorrhage. Constriction of brain tissue leads to an increasingly deep coma, associated with a wide-open pupil which no longer reacts to light on the same side as the haemorrhage, and paralysis of the opposite side of the body.

Haemorrhage, Subarachnoid. Haemorrhage in the space between the innermost and the middle cerebral membrane (the arachnoid mater), as a result of an abnormality of a blood vessel.

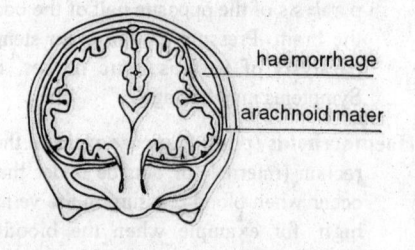

haemorrhage

arachnoid mater

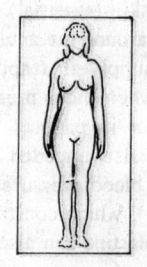

Subarachnoid haemorrhage occurs in the cavity beneath the arachnoid mater membrane.

This can be an aneurysm (balloon-like dilation of a blood vessel) or a cluster of dilated vessels. These are vulnerable conditions, and can occur in adulthood without particular cause. The symptoms are very sudden headache associated with nausea and vomiting as a result of irritation of the cerebral membrane, and sometimes a short period of unconsciousness followed by confusion. The vessels of the brain become narrower because of the loss of blood and this sometimes also causes cerebral infarction and paralysis on one side. In the case of a torn cluster of vessels aphasia or epilepsy can occur as a result of irritation of the cerebral cortex.

Haemorrhage, subdural. Haemorrhage from a blood vessel between the middle and the outer cerebral membrane (the dura), caused by injury to the skull, sometimes quite slight, commoner in older people because the blood vessels are easier to squash. The possibility is also increased in patients subject to epileptic convulsions, alcoholics and patients using medication to thin the blood (anticoagulants). Pressure on the brain increases slowly, so that symptoms, psychological changes such as decreased activity, apathy and sleepiness also develop slowly. The picture can be similar to dementia. Subdural haemorrhage can exert pressure on the brain in such a way as to cause paralysis of the opposite half of the body to the affected half of the brain. Pressure on the brain stem can finally also cause paralysis of various optic nerves, causing double vision. Symptoms may be vague.

Haemorrhoids (piles) Varicose veins in the anus, either inside the rectum (internal) or outside under the skin (external). They occur when blood pressure in the veins around the anus is too high, for example when the blood supply is trapped by excessively long retention of faeces, or when undue pressure is needed for evacuation; they often occur in patients with a sedentary life-style. Blood supply is also impeded during pregnancy and childbirth, and by high blood pressure in the portal vein (e.g. in cirrhosis of the liver), which constricts all intestinal veins. Swelling of the large intestine can also cause haemorrhoids, but often there is no identifiable cause. Small internal haemorrhoids are imperceptible and should cause no discomfort, but larger haemorrhoids can result in itching, smarting and blood in the faeces. A possible complication is prolapse, which if it persists, can cause chronic loss of blood and anal fissure. Haemorrhoids can also become blocked or thrombosed, and cause swelling and severe pain. Inflamed, the thrombosed or prolapsed haemorrhoids are directly visible on external examination, but haemorrhoids without complications can be detected only by rectoscopy, often necessary in elderly people to distinguish haemorrhoidal blood loss from loss resulting from other conditions. If haemorrhoids cause little or no discomfort surgery is not usually necessary, although a varied diet is advisable to keep faeces soft, thus avoiding the need for strain during defecation. The patient should also take exercise, and defecate regularly. Haemorrhoidal cream or suppositories suppress pain, but do not cure the condition. In the case of discomfort or complications various treatments are possible, such as sclerotherapy (injection into the vessel to seal it), cryosurgery (treatment by cold), widening the anus (dilation), or rubber-band treatment (nipping off the haemorrhoids with a rubber band). Removal by surgery (haemorrhoidectomy) is necessary only in 10 per cent of cases.

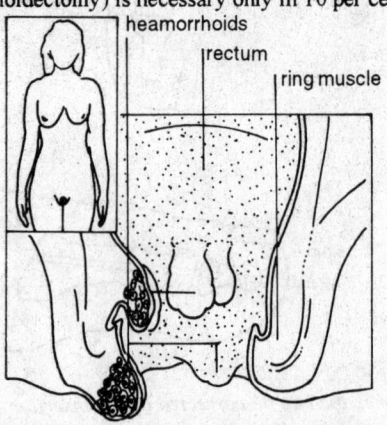

Haemorrhoids are varicose veins in the mucous membrane of the rectum

Hallucination. Sensory perception of something that does not exist. Hallucinations can affect any of the senses; the patient is certain that what he perceives is the truth. Hallucinations should be distinguished from 'illusory falsifications', in which one believes something to be the case because it is what one expects and hopes-as in missing spelling mistakes because one believes them to be correct.

Hammer toe. Condition, often affecting the second toe, in which the rearmost of the three toe bones is tilted upwards and the two foremost ones turned down, causing the tip of the toe to touch the ground. Hammer toes are usually caused by ill-fitting or unduly small shoes. They can cause pain when walking or corns through pressure from the shoe. Treatment is by surgical removal of the foremost part of the rear bone of the toe to create room for the three bones to lie in line with each other.

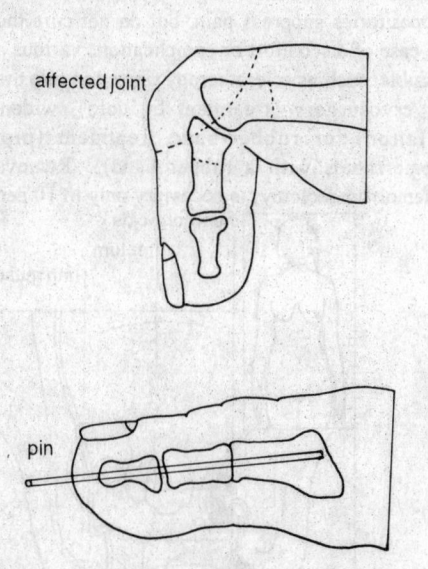

A hammer toe can be corrected by the insertion of a temporary pin through the affected joint of the first toe phalanx.

Hare lip. Congenital split in the upper lip, sometimes associated with a split in the upper jaw and cleft palate. Hare lip is established in the first weeks of pregnancy as a result of a growth disorder in the lip cleft. It occurs in roughly 1 birth per 1,000, more in boys than girls. The cause is unknown; hereditary factors are significant. Chances of hare lip increase with the age of the mother, and vary according to population group. The outlook and seriousness of the condition are very varied. Associated particle cleavage of the nose can occur, but is rare; other variants are oblique, bilateral and single hare lip. It is understandable that children with the condition often have difficulties with drinking, and breast-feeding in particular can be a serious problem; generally a bottle is used, with a large teat open at the side, or the child may be spoon fed.

Hay fever (allergic rhinitis) Allergic condition classified with asthma, hives, and some forms of eczema. Allergic reactions are in fact defensive responses to substances, usually harmless, in the environment; they are also known as atopic reactions. The substances responsible are often the pollens of grasses and other plants, but others include flakes of animal skin, dust, fungal spores and feathers, It is estimated that 10 to 15 per cent of people have an atopic constitution, i.e. could develop and allergy on contact with an allergen. Most grass pollens are relatively large (0.025-0.4 mm) and stick to the nasal mucous membrane on inhalation. Very few penetrate to the small branches of the air passages.

Headache. May be caused by disorders of the face, abnormalities elsewhere in the body or within the head.

Causes of headache in the region of the face include otitis media, sinusitis, jaw abscess, dental problems, ill-fitting dentures, colds and focusing difficulties in the eyes. This form of headache is generally nagging, dull or stabbing, but not usually throbbing.

Headache can also be caused by all sorts of diseases and disorders elsewhere in the body. These include high blood pressure, kidney disorders, hangover after alcohol abuse, allergy, fever, depression, constipation, anaemia and some nervous disorders. Such headaches can be dull, throbbing or pounding, are usually present on waking, and are associated with other symptoms that indicate the underlying condition.

Heart block. Disturbance in the transmission of the electrical stimuli that cause contraction of the cardiac muscle. The stimuli originate in the walls of the right auricle and normally pass to the ventricles via the cardiac septum. If damage to a heart muscle impairs the functioning of this system, impulses from the auricles do not reach the ventricles, which slowly contract independently of the auricles, slowing down the heart beat, and possibly causing the patient to faint. Treatment is by implantation of an artificial pacemaker to regulate the heart beat.

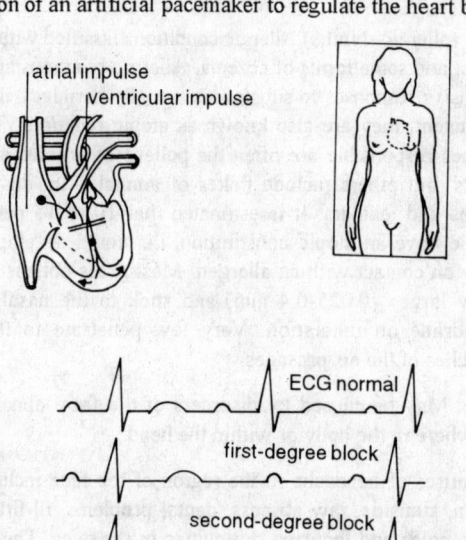

atrial impulse
ventricular impulse

ECG normal

first-degree block

second-degree block

Heart block is caused by an interruption in the transfer of impulses from the atrium to the ventricle. In the course of time the ventricle then produces on impulse itself.

Heartburn (pyrosis) Sharp burning feeling behind the breastbone resulting from the mucous membrane of the oesophagus coming in contact with gastric juices from the stomach. In contrast to the gastric mucous membrane, which is resistant to the very strong gastric acids, the mucous membrane of the oesophagus is not. Everyone suffers from heartburn occasionally, for example after a heavy meal, or even without a definite cause. If heartburn recurs regularly, it will usually be the result of a malfunction of sphincter at the entrance to the stomach, and as a result gastric juices can flow into the oesophagus (reflux), especially when the person is lying down. Rupture of the diaphragm is an important cause of reflux. Another is increased pressure in the abdominal cavity, with gastric acid being squeezed upwards in consequence; this occurs for example, in cases of obesity and during pregnancy.

Heart failure (cardiac decompensation) Inability of the heart to maintain normal circulation of the blood; there are various

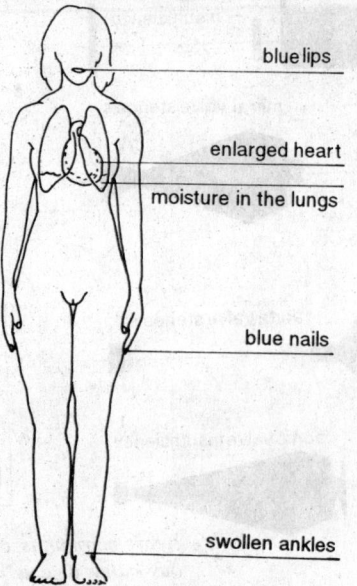

Heart failure is accompanied by a number of symptoms; they can often be eased by medication.

causes, but the consequences are always the same. Decompensation on the left-hand side can be caused by abnormalities of the aortal and mitral valves, high blood pressure and cardiac infarction, causing failure of part of the heart muscle of the left ventricle. Right-hand decompensation occurs in conditions of the tricuspid and pulmonary valves, and in pulmonary heart disease. If all heat muscle cells are affected (as in rheumatic fever) both halves of the heart may fail.

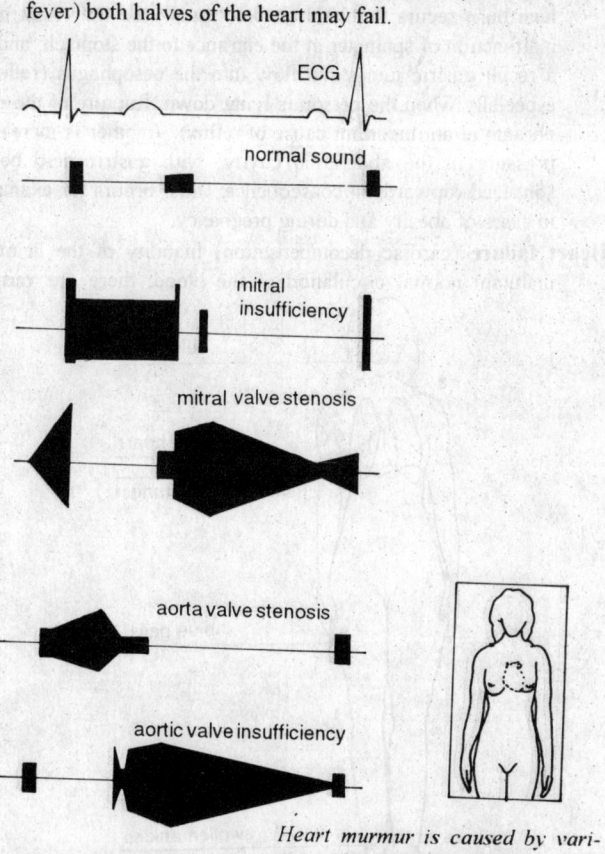

ECG

normal sound

mitral insufficiency

mitral valve stenosis

aorta valve stenosis

aortic valve insufficiency

Heart murmur is caused by various value defects, each of which has a characteristic sound.

Heart murmur. Noise accompanying the heart beat that indicates abnormal turbulences in the bloodstream within the heart. In a healthy, normal heart the blood flows with some turbulence; defects such as leakage through a valve or a hole in the heart alter the flow pattern, thus causing an abnormal noise. Any valve abnormality causes a characteristic noise, identified by the moment and the place at which it is best heard with a stehoscope. If a valve is constricted, the sound is produced as the blood passes through it-in the systole (contraction) therefore if the aortal or pulmonary valves are constricted, and in the diastole (relaxation) if the problem lies in the mitral or tricuspid valves.

A leaking valve causes noise when it should be tightly closed: in the diastole for the aortal or pulmonary valves, and in the systole for the mitral or tricuspid valves. A hole in the atrial or ventrical septum produces noise in the systole. By no means every noise is a sign of heart abnormality; in children in particular, quite innocent noises may be produced.

Heart rhythm, disorders of. Abnormally fast, slow or irregular heart beat, caused by disturbed impulses from the central node or irregularities in their transmission. Under certain circumstances impulses may be produced in parts of the heart other than the sinoatrial node, in which case the regular rhythm is disturbed by extra beats (extrasytole). Abnormalities in the transmission system impair the passage of impulses from the auricles to the ventricles, and in serious cases they can be entirely blocked (heart block), meaning that the ventricles do not contract, or contract only at a very slow pace.

Heart valve defects. A normal heart valve allows blood to flow unrestricted in one direction, but closes to prevent it flowing back. There are two possible abnormalities, constriction and leakage. In constriction blood cannot pass freely, so the heart has to work unduly hard; if the valve leaks, some blood can flow back through the valve, reducing the efficiency of the heart's pumping action. Both conditions can occur at the same time. The most important cause of valve problems is rheumatic fever, but valves can also be affected by endocarditis and degeneration with age, and may in a small number of cases be congenital. Defects cause symptoms only if they are so severe that the function of the heart is affected (heart failure). The symptoms can often be treated by drugs, although sometimes an artificial valve has to be fitted.

Hemianopia. Loss of half the field of vision. Homonymous hemianopia affects the left or right side of each eye. Bitemporal hemianopia is failure of the outer field of vision in each eye. Failure of the innermost fields division is extremely rare. Homonymous hemianopia is caused by a condition of a part of the cerebral cortex or of associated nerve tracts, possibly the result of a stroke or brain tumour. The patient tends to bump into things to one side, and has problems with reading. Bitemporal Hemianopia is caused by pressure on the junction of the optic nerves generally the result of a pituitary tumour close to this junction. Vision becomes increasingly indistinct, and it may be some time before the patient or those around him notice this. Because the central field of vision is seldom affected, and the eyes can still be directed at individuals or objects.

Hemiparesis and Hemiplegia. Decline in strength (hemiparesis) or paralysis (hemiplegia) in one half of the body, common in older people. Physical movement is controlled by the cerebral cortex. Nerve fibres run from there to the muscles and cross over before entering the spinal cord, so that the muscles in the left half of the body are served by nerves in the right half of the brain, and vice versa. If the right half of the brain is affected, hemiplegia in the left half of the body occurs as a result. The centres of speech are usually in the left half of the brain, and therefore hemiplegia is accompanied by speech and comprehension disorders only if the right half of the body is paralyzed. The most frequent cause of hemiplegia is a cerebral haemorrhage. Other caused are a brain tumour or severe concussion, but hemiplegia can also occur in such diseases as multiple sclerosis. In conditions which arise suddenly, slack paralysis of the opposite half of the body initially occurs. Speech

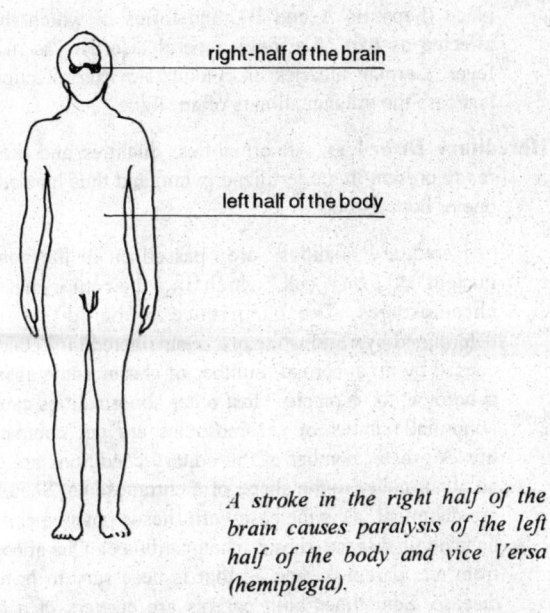

right-half of the brain

left half of the body

A stroke in the right half of the brain causes paralysis of the left half of the body and vice Versa (hemiplegia).

is frequently indistinct because one corner of the mouth hangs down. The disorder often recurs to a greater or lesser degree, but spasticity often occurs. The course taken by the condition is entirely dependent on the nature and extent of the cause. Reasonable recovery is usually possible, especially after a cerebral haemorrhage. Treatment is directed towards the underlying condition. Therapeutic exercises are also important in order to keep the muscles in optimum condition. The clinical picture may improve in the first two years after the condition commences.

Hepatitis. Liver disorder in which the liver is inflamed and swollen: cell death can also occur. There are numerous causes, which can be divided into two groups: infections caused by a virus or other micro-organism and inflammation caused by toxins. Both groups can be sup-divided. The infective hepatitis group is divided into forms in which the liver is affected in the first place (hepatitis A and B), and forms in which the liver is affected as part of a more general disorder (as in glandular fever, German measles or cytomegalovirus infection). In the last case the inflammation is often slight.

Hereditary Disorders. Abnormalities, qualities and disorders already present in the fertilized ovum, and thus handed down by one or both parents.

Hereditary qualities are passed on in the genes in the nucleus of every cell, which in their turn are bound to chromosomes. The occurrence of hereditary disorders determined by various factors. Some hereditary conditions are caused by an abnormal number of chromosome as in Down's syndrome, for example. Most other abnormalities caused by an abnormal number of chromosomes are not compatible with life. A greater number of hereditary conditions are caused by an abnormality in the shape of a chromosome. Some disorders are dominant, as is the case with rhesus positive children with haemolytic disease (rhesus incompatibility). One abnormal gene from one parent is then all that is necessary to bring out the disease. Sometimes both parents are carriers of a hereditary disorder of which they show no symptoms (recessive traits), but a child receiving a pair of the affected genes contracts the disease. This is sometimes the case in mucoviscosidosis, some cases of muscular dystrophy and many metabolic disorders. Some hereditary disorders are sex-linked, such as haemophilia, colour blindness, Turner's syndrome and Klinefelter's syndrome. Academic research is constantly discovering new hereditary disorders.

Diagnosis is by external symptoms laboratory tests, amniocentesis and chromosome tests.

Hermaphroditism. In genuine Hermaphroditism, the person in question possesses both a testicle and an ovary. The phenomenon is extremely rare.

What more frequently occurs is that the external equal characteristics and organs do not correspond to the internal ones.

This phenomenon is known as pseudo-hermaphroditism and can occur both in men and women.

Male Pseudo-hermaphroditism is the form in which testicles exist in an individual who has female external sexual organs and characteristics. One example is testicular feminization. Female pseudo-hermaphroditism is the form in which ovaries exist internally in a person having a male outward appearance. One example of this is the adrenogenital syndrome.

Hernia. Protrusion of tissue through a hitherto non-existent opening, affecting various kinds of tissue, usually in the abdomen. A slipped disc is also known as a hernia (herniated or prolapsed

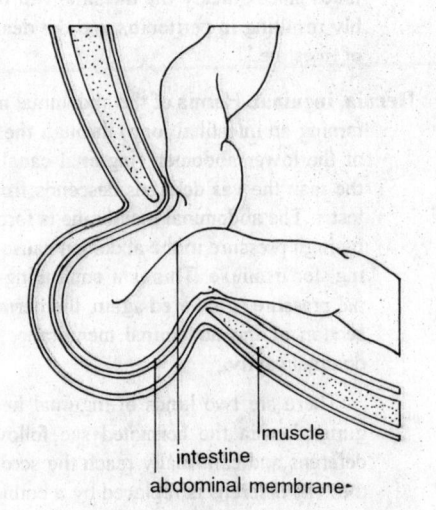

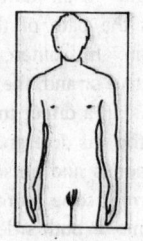

muscle
intestine
abdominal membrane

In strangulated hernia there is a danger that the trapped intestine could die because the blood supply is interrupted.

nucleus pulposus). Hernias are named after their location; common forms include inguinal hernia (in the groin), umbilical hernia (in the umbilicious) and hiatus hernia (of the diaphragm). A hernia can be congenital, but more often occurs in later life. It is always caused by an unduly wide opening, or by a weak spot in the abdominal wall, or by regular raising of the pressure in the abdomen-for example by straining during defecation, chronic coughing, or awkward lifting.

Symptoms depend on the location and content of the hernia. If the herniated sac contains intestine there may be problems with digestion and defecation. In intestine is actually trapped in the herniated sac (stangulated hernia) it is associated with severe pain and local inflammation, and unless an operation takes place quickly the intestine will be blocked (ileus), possibly resulting in peritonitis and the death of the trapped section of intestine.

Hernia, inguinal. Hernia of the abdominal membrane (possibly containing an intestinal loop) through the muscle and tendon wall of the lower abdomen (inguinal canal), the point at which in the man the vas deferens descends from the abdomen into the testis. The abdominal membrane is forced through this passage by high pressure in the abdomen caused by straining or coughing, for example. This is a continuing process; when abdominal pressure is lowered again, the herniated sac, the protruding section of the abdominal membrane, slips back into the abdominal cavity.

There are two kinds of inguinal hernia. In an indirect inguinal hernia the herniated sac follows the path of the vas deferens and can finally reach the scrotum. In women, where the vas deferens is replaced by a connective strand, the herniated sac can descend to the labia majora. In a direct inguinal hernia the herniated sac does not follow the vas deference, but protrudes directly through the slack tendons and muscles of the lower abdomen. Indirect inguinal hernia is the more common form. The condition can occur on one or both sides, and be congenital or caused by weakening of the tissue.

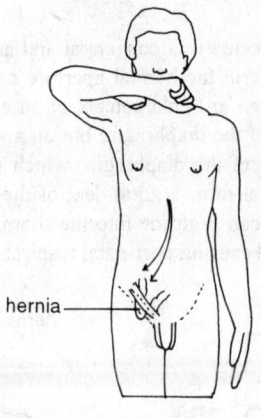

hernia —

The presence of an inguinal hernia can be detected by pressure on the hand.

Hernia, umbilical. Weakness of the abdominal wall at the navel, allowing membrane or possibly also intestine to bulge out of the abdominal cavity (although probably remaining under the skin). Before birth the umbilical cord was joined to the child's body at this point and the navel is a naturally weak point in the abdominal wall of new-born babies; thus umbilical hernia is most common a few weeks after birth, via the navel scar. In later life it is no longer a weak point. A characteristic of umbilical hernia is a swelling at the navel which increases in size with an increase of pressure in the abdomen (when the child laughs or cries, for example). In some rare congenital forms, the herniated sac can be large, and contain a large quantity of the contents of the abdomen.

Hiatus Hernia. Aperture in the diaphragm, through weakening of the diaphragm or widening of an existing aperture, by which means an abdominal organ (such as the stomach) protrudes upwards into the chest cavity. The reverse (displacement of lung or heart into the abdominal cavity) never occurs because pressure in the abdominal cavity is generally higher (there is low pressure in the lungs during respiration to draw in the air).

The condition occurs in a congenital and an acquired form. In the congenital form the hernial aperture can occur in various places. It is often an enlargement of an existing aperture on the lower side of the diaphragm, but an aperture can occur in the upper dome of the diaphragm, which is normally closed. In this congenital form a great deal of the content of the abdominal cavity can protrude into the thorax, putting pressure on the lungs and causing post-natal respiratory difficulties.

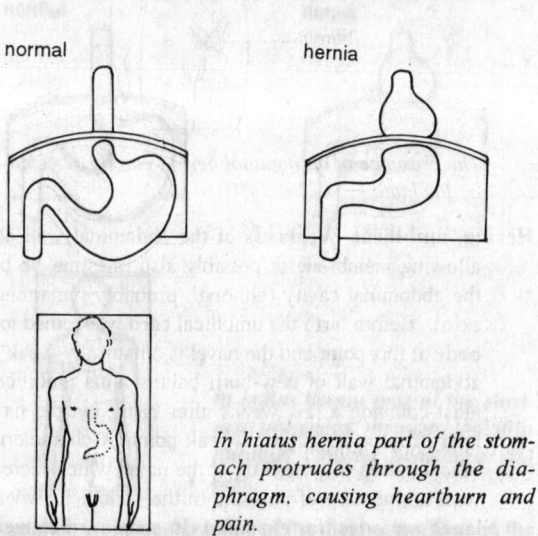

normal   hernia

In hiatus hernia part of the stomach protrudes through the diaphragm, causing heartburn and pain.

Hiccups. Repeated, violent contraction of the diaphragm, forcing the glottis to close. First air is drawn very rapidly into the lungs, then blocked by the closure of the glottis, causing a characteristic sound. Hiccups is caused by stimulation of the nerve that causes the diaphragm to contract, and is almost always a perfectly harmless condition. It may be provoked by eating too fast, or by eating hot or spicy food. There may be a physiological cause if hiccups occurs frequently, at length and stubbornly; it may result from a condition of the oesophagus, pneumonia, the consumption of alcohol, pregnancy, or kidney disorders with a high urea level in the blood; or thoracic or abdominal surgery can cause stubborn hiccups.

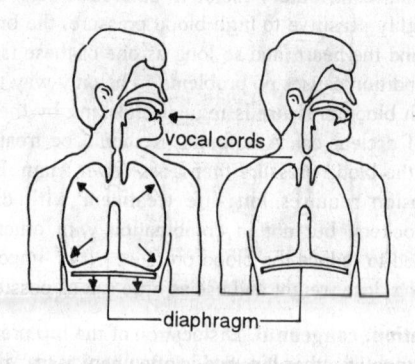

Hiccups is an involuntary contraction of the diaphragm causing air to be forced inwards through the vocal cords, and interrupting the flow of air by contraction of the vocal cords.

Hiccups can usually be surprised by raising the carbon dioxide content of the blood by holding the breath or by breathing into a paper bag for a few minutes. Other methods are: drinking a glass of water rapidly, eating dry bread, or careful pressure on the eyeballs. Extremely stubborn cases can be treated by medication, and as a last resort the nerve may be anesthetized or severed.

High blood pressure (hypertension) Blood pressure higher than normal. Blood pressure in excess of 130/90 carries an increased health risk and is usually regarded as hypertensive. In about 90 per cent of patients with high blood pressure no cause for the abnormality can be found, and it is then known as 'essential hypertension'. It is possible that factors such as a salty diet, excess weight and stress are involved, but this has yet to be proved. A clear cause is present in less than 10 per cent of cases, and often that is a disorder of the kidney. Other causes are excess corticosteroid production and abnormalities in the part of the nervous system responsible for regulating the blood pressure. In some women blood pressure rises during pregnancy, causing pre-eclampsia. If high blood pressure persists for a long time it affects arterial walls and is thus an important contributory factor in atherosclerosis. Some organs are highly sensitive to high blood pressure: the brain, the kidneys and the heart, and so long as one of these is not affected the condition causes no problems. The only way to keep track of high blood pressure is regular checking by the family doctor. If a clear cause is found, it should be treated: in many cases the blood pressure then goes down again. Essential hypertension requires long-life treatment with diuretics and betablockers, but not in combination with other medication intended to reduce the blood pressure. It is important to stop smoking, lose weight and use as little salt as possible.

Hip dislocation, congenital. Dislocation of the hip present at birth. It can involve either hip, and is often hereditary: affecting birth in 1,000. It is caused by an imperfectly formed hip joint, in which the head of the thigh bone (femur) dose not fit into the socket of the hip, and so can slip out. If the condition is discovered early (before the baby is three months old) excellent results can be achieved by very simple treatment, but it is not always easy to detect the condition so early. Careful attention should be paid if it is common in the family. The condition is more common in girls than boys, in breech births and in first births. Early recognition is not only important for successful treatment, but also for good development of muscular movement. A baby who does not move well is also likely to have difficulties in psychological development. Checks should be made for asymmetrical posture or apparent shortness of one leg. Sometimes the cleft in the buttocks is abnormal; sometimes hip movement is restricted. There are various techniques for detecting the fault; in cases of doubt, or if the condition exists in the family, X-rays should be taken. Before the third month a thick nappy, special trunks or a splint are often adequate; later, treatment is more time-consuming. Splints, plaster or surgery usually give good results.

Hip disorders. The hip is the largest ball-and-socket joint in the body. The ball (the head of the thigh bone) is surrounded to a large extent by the socket in the pelvis, which gives it great stability but means that the ligaments in the hip are not as robust as one would expect in a joint of the size. Hip disorders are an important cause of temporary or permanent disablement, particularly in older patients. Extra strain on the hip joint may then lead to arthrosis; fractures of the oblique upper part of the thigh bone are also common in the elderly as a result of osteoporosis. Younger people suffer from congenital hip displacement. Perthes disease and certain forms of rheumatic inflammation.

Hirschsprung's disease. Congenital condition of the large intestine; constipation is the most important symptom, caused by nerve cells missing in part of the intestinal wall which normally provides peristaltic movement. There can be symptoms shortly after birth, when the baby passes no meconium, or passes it with difficulty; others suffer later from persistent constipation. Because the abnormality usually occurs at the end of the large intestine, faeces accumulate in the preceding section, causing it to distend; the condition is worsened by the accumulation of intenstinal gas. Affected children sometimes have a distended, hard abdomen, with peristalsis visible in the healthy section of the intestine. In some cases the condition can lead to ileus (intestinal obstruction), a serious condition requiring immediate treatment.

Hirsutism. Undesirable hair growth on the face, arms, legs, and the chest of women; the border between normality and hirsutism is not always clear however.

The condition can have various causes, particular conditions resulting in an excess of male hormone such as an ovarian or adrenal tumour and the Stein-Leventhal syndrome, or medication that has side-effects similar to those of male hormone. Treatment is by surgery, radiation therapy or medication, depending on the precise cause. There is also a form of hirsutism for which no cause can be found, known as ideopathic hirsutism; only the symposiums can be treated, by cutting off the hair, depilation or bleaching.

Histoplasmosis. Infection with the fungus Histoplasma *capsulatum*, especially common in North and Central America and in many South American countries, and introduced to Western Europe from these countries. In America more than half a million people are infected each year, half of whom display no symptoms. The fungus lives in soil fouled with chicken, bird or bat droppings, and inhalation of the fungal spores can cause infection in man, particularly in the lungs.

Hoarseness. Failure of the vocal cords to close properly when speaking. There can be various causes, such as pharyngitis in the case of a cold or influenza. Factors other than infection are important, such as a smoky, stuffy environment. Inhalation of steam, resting the voice and a ban on smoking are usually sufficient treatment. If the condition is chronic, abuse of the voice is a much more important factor, as in singers, market traders and teachers. Resting the voice and a ban on smoking are also the treatment, possibly combined with voice lessons. Any underlying condition should be treated. Abuse of the voice can also cause nodes on the vocal chords, small benign lumps opposite each other on both vocal chords, preventing them from closing. They can usually be eliminated by resting the voice and voice lessons surgery is rarely necessary. Malignant tumours of the vocal cords occur particularly in middle-aged men, possibly encouraged by smoking and alcohol abuse.

Hodgkin's disease. Form of cancer of the lymph nodes (lymphoma), with unchecked growth of cells in the nodes. The cause is unknown, and it is more common in men than women. The first symptom is usually painless swelling of the lymph nodes in the neck, armpits and groins. As the disease develops, more lymph nodes are affected, with associated fatigue, itching, sweating, loss of appetite and sometimes periods of fever.

Hooked nail (onychogryphosis) Very hard deformed nail which can protrude a long way; it usually affects the big toe, very rarely the fingers. The nail is usually too hard to cut, and pressure from the shoe makes it grow hooked, so that it resembles the claw of a bird of prey. The size of the nail quickly causes discomfort; growth must be controlled by filing. The only real treatment is complete removal of the nail, along with its bed, to prevent recurrence of the condition.

Hook worm. Parasitic infestation with the nematode worm *Ancylostoma duodenale* or *Ancylostoma americanum*. About 200 million people are infested with hookworm, most of them in the tropics or sub-tropics. Hookworms are 1-1.5 cm long, and feed on the mucous membrane of the small intestine. They live for about 8 years, producing eggs which are excreted with the faces and develop in the soil, requiring moisture and warmth (about 27°C). The eggs develop into larvae which enter man via the skin and eventually establish themselves in the intestine. Infection with the larva is contracted by walking with bare feet and legs. Infestation with large number of hookworm (to a maximum of 5,000) can cause stomach and intestinal disorders, abdominal cramp and diarrhoea. Anaemia because of blood loss from small wounds in the intestinal wall is another possibility. Many people are infested with the worms without any symptoms at all.

Worm cure treatment is necessary only if the patient suffers discomfort. It is important to prevent infestation in the tropics by wearing stout shoes and covering the lower legs.

Hormone. A chemical synthesized by a cell or group of cells which diffuses through the body fluids to change the functions of a cell or cells which may be nearby or elsewhere in the body. The classical definition of a hormone as a chemical released into the blood by cells in one organ to change the functions of cells in other organs is now considered to be a special case of the general definition applying only to some hormones. The general definition, moreover, does not absolutely distinguish hormones from nervous transmitters. It does distinguish between hormones and enzymes, however, an enzyme alters chemicals inside or outside cells whereas a hormone alters the functioning of a cell.

The hormone acts by becoming attached to a receptor molecule on or inside a cell. It thereby initiates a sequence of
chemical changes which in most cases either suppress or activate genes in the cell. The effect is to change the cell's function. The same end is achieved by some hormones which ini-
tiate a sequence of intracellular chemical events landing to a
change directly in the structure of a cell. Examples include
chemicals which act both as hormones and as the transmitters
of signals between nerve cells.

Faulty hormone production may be the cause of disease, in
disorders of the thyroid gland and *diabetes*. For that reason,
hormones are used as drugs to correct or control pathological
conditions.

Horner's syndrome. Abnormality caused by failure of sympathetic
nerves to the eye. There are three signs: a drooping upper lid
(ptosis), contraction of the pupil (miosis) and backward displacement of the eyeball (enophthalmos). If the two eyes are
compared, a clear difference can be seen. Sometimes no sweat
is produced on the affected side of the face. If the sympathetic
element of ocular nerve provision fails, the parasympathetic
element becomes dominant. In some cases the condition is
congenital; usually the cause is unknown. Sometimes the sympathetic nerve is damaged by a tumour in the neck, a tumour
of the thyroid gland or an abnormality of the carotid artery.
The symptoms cannot be treated.

Horseshoe kidney. Connection of the two kidneys along the body's
central line, producing a horsehoe shape. Connection can be
by the upper lobes, but is usually by the lower ones. It produces a single, large kidney, which usually functions normally,
although the abnormal shape can trap other organs or tissue,
causing discomfort. The position of the ureters means that they
can become trapped by blood vessels for example-causing urine
obstruction, possibly leading to pyelitis, stone formation or
hydronephrosis.

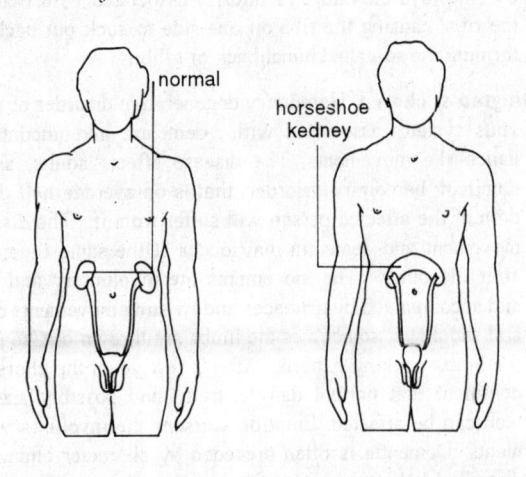

Horseshoe kidney is a condition in which the two kidneys have for one reason or another grown into one, which usually functions normally.

Hot flushes. Irksome condition that occurs during the menopause, and sometimes also in younger women receiving antihormonal treatment or after an ovariectomy. Hot flushes begin with a sudden feeling of heat in the chest which spreads over the whole body. The face reddens, and sudden sweating and accelerated heartbeat may occur; sudden pallor and dizziness are also possible. Hot flushes can occur at night as well as during the day, sometimes several times within an hour. They usually disappear after one or two years, but some women suffer from them for many years. They are caused by hormonal changes in the menopause which affect the sympathetic nervous system. If they are problematical and frequent they can be treated with hormonal preparations containing oestrogen, which cause renewed bleeding of the uterine muious membrane. He flushes can also be caused by emotional tension, in which case discussion and group therapy may reduce the symptoms.

Hunchback (gibbus) Abnormal elevation of the back, associated with backward curvature of the spinal column (kyphosis) or by sideways curvature (scoliosis) associated with twisting of the ribs, causing the ribs on one side to stick out backwards, forming the so-called hunchback or gibbus.

Huntington's chorea. Hereditary degenerative disorder of the nervous system, associated with dementia and uncontrollable dance-like movements. The disease affects adults, and is a dominant hereditary disorder, that is on average half the children of the affected person will suffer from it. The disordered movement and dementia may occur at the same time, or one after the other. The movements are involuntary and abrupt, and accompanied by grimaces and twisting movements of trunk and shoulders; sometimes the limbs are thrown out, sometimes the limbs walking pattern. After a few years the chorea is so dominant that normal daily activity and possibly speech as well can be affected. Emotion worsens the involuntary movements. Dementia is often preceded by character changes and disturbed behaviours, and the condition is sometimes associated with psychiatric disorders such as delusions. The speed at which the patient deteriorates varies, but the pattern is often the same within a particular family. Family the patient is reduced to complete helplessness by dementia and disability. There is no treatment; certain medicines can reduce the severity of the symptoms, but the cannot influence the course of the disease.

Hydatidiform Mole. Abnormal development of the placenta. The foetus dies at a very early stage, but the placental cells continue to grow, then swell, and form vesicles about the size of a grape. A hydatidiform pregnancy seems normal in the early stages, but morning sickness is more frequent, and the womb grows rapidly in proportion to the length of the pregnancy; the uterus is soft, and neither the child's limbs nor a heartbeat can be felt; no foetus shows on an ultrasound scam. Abnormal production of the pregnancy hormone HCG is another strong indication of a hydatida form mole (this is the hormone found in the mother's urine in a positive pregnancy test). Growth usually declines between the 10th and 20th weeks, and there

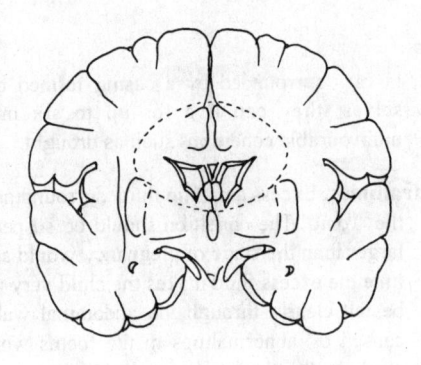

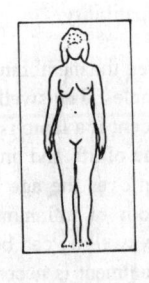

*In Huntington's chorea the areas
of the brain around the cerebral
cavity are the most affected.*

is often severe hemorrhage, giving the impression of a miscarriage. If a hydatidiform pregnancy is suspected, it should be
terminated, particularly as there is a chance of the hydatidi
form mole developing into a malignant tumour
(choriococarcinoma). Labour should be induced, followed by a
curettage to remove any remaining fragments. The urine should
afterwards be regularly checked for pregnancy hormone. To
avoid complications, at least a year should elapse before the
next pregnancy.

Hydatid disease (echinococcosis) Serious form of tapeworm infestation, which occurs at a particular developmental stage of the
tapeworm. The larval worm develops from the ovum (egg) of
the tapeworm. The ova of the tapeworm are actually encysted

larvae surrounded by a casing formed by the larvae themselves, they can live for up to six months, even under
unfavourable conditions such as drought.

Hydramnios. Excess amniotic fluid surrounding an unborn baby in
the womb. The condition should be suspected if the uterus is
larger than the stage of pregnancy would suggest. At the same
time the excess fluid makes the child very mobile, and this can
be felt clearly through the abdominal wall. The condition is
caused by abnormalities in the foetus which prevent it from
drinking the fluid, such as lack of a swallowing reflex or a
closed sophagus. The condition also sometimes accompanies
diabetes mellitus and rhesus incompatibility.

Hydrocele. Accumulation of fluid between the membranes surrounding the spermatic cord and the testicles. The swelling contains
a pale yellow liquid and is translucent if a lamp is shone on it.
The condition can arise at any time of life and on one or both
sides, but it usually occurs in men over the age of 20. It is
sometimes a side-effect of a tumour of inflammation of the
epididymis and/or the testicle. The swelling can be fairly considerable in young boys, but no treatment is necessary at that
age because the condition disappears of its own accord within
a few years. In adults, it can become troublesome because of
its size and weight. Siphoning off the liquid with a hollow
needle is a temporary measure; an operation is the most effective course and is permanent.

Hydrocephalus (water on the brain) Accumulation of cerebrospinal
fluid inside the skull as a result of a blockage. The cranial
sutures of babies do not close before the age of one or two,
and as a result an increase of cerebrospinal fluid in the ventricles causes the skull to become enlarged. However, once
the cranial sutures have knitted together the skull can no longer
swell in this way and therefore the pressure inside the skull is
increased; this is known as internal hydrocephalus.

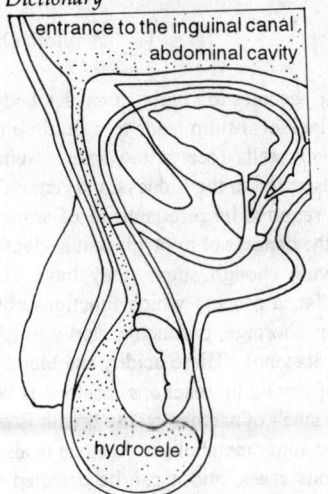

entrance to the inguinal canal
abdominal cavity

hydrocele

Hydrocele is fluid which descends into the scrotum, remaining in contact with the abdominal cavity.

Hydronephrosis. Dilation of the pelvis of the kidney, caused by a blockage in the flow of urine.

In each kidney, the urine passes through the renal calix into the renal pelvis, and from there into the bladder via the ureter. The bladder opens to the exterior through the urethra. A blockage anywhere in these ducts can result in hydronephrosis because urine backs up above the obstruction. If the emptying of the bladder is impeded, it is known as urine retention. An accumulation of urine in the bladder makes it difficult to discharge the urine from the kidneys through the ureters to the bladder, and the result is that urine builds up in the two renal pelvises. A ureter can be blocked by a stone inflammation or a tumour. A kink in a ureter, such as may occur with a floating kidney or a congenital predisposition in one or both ureters, can also cause hydornephrosis.

Hyperglycaemia. Excess glucose in the blood, usually caused by diabetes mellitus. Blood sugar (glucose) content is regulated by a number of hormones, but only one of them, insulin, can reduce the level if it becomes too high. It causes body cells to absorb sugar, thus lack of insulin leads to a fluid up of excess blood sugar, but body cells receive too little. Some of the excess sugar is transported to the kidneys and removed via the urine; this process requires large quantities of water making dehydration one of the dangers of hyperglycemia. Because body cells are not receiving enough sugar, they have to produce energy by burning fat, a process which functions abnormally because of the sugar shortage, producing acid waste products (ketones, including acetone). These acidify the blood and thus prevent a number of metabolic reactions: acetone is present in exhaled air, and the smell of acetone on the breath is an important sign of disturbed sugar metabolism. Acetone is also present in the urine in serious cases, and it can be detected with test papers.

Hypermetropia (long- sightedness) Abnormality of the eye in which long-distance vision is keen, but not short-range vision. Long-sightedness can have two causes: excessive weakness of the eye's refractory system, or too short an axis of the eye. The latter is the more frequent cause. In both cases, perception of objects in the distance is hazy when the lens of the eye is relaxed, but when the patient makes a conscious effort to focus the object can be perceived very sharply. A long-sighted person who does not wear glasses has to accommodate continuously in order to have sharp vision. This is tiring and can lead to headaches. As the subject's age increases, sharp short-range vision becomes more difficult. Long-sightedness is corrected by means of a positive lens in spectacles or contact lenses. The strength of this must be such that the long-sighted person can see into the distance without accommodation. It is best for a long-sighted person to wear his spectacles continuously, because he does not then have to strain his eyes. A long-sighted person has a somewhat greater chance of contracting glaucoma, because the longitudinal axis of the eye is shortened.

Hypernephroma. Extremely malignant kidney tumour predominantly in patients over forty and commoner in men than women. The tumour itself does not cause discomfort until a late stage, so that secondary tumours produced by metastasis are likely to make their presence felt sooner. Symptoms are fever, weight loss, and finally blood in the urine (haematuria) in 90 per cent of patients. Growth of such tumours can vary considerably, from rapid growth and metastasis to slow growth without symptoms.

Hyperthyroidism. Condition in which thyroid hormones are over-produced. It is one of the most common hormone disorders, occurring five times as often in women as men. Under normal circumstances, thyroid function is regulated by the pituitary gland, which produces substances that stimulate the thyroid to release hormones into the blood. In hyperthyroidism this regulatory mechanism is disturbed, and the thyroid begins to produce large quantities of hormones unnecessarily. Sometimes

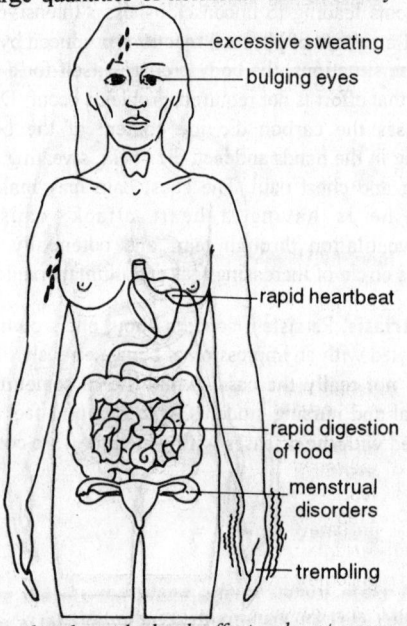

excessive sweating

bulging eyes

rapid heartbeat

rapid digestion of food

menstrual disorders

trembling

Because the thyroid gland affects almost every organ in the body the symptoms of hyperthyroidism are very varied.

this causes the gland to swell (goitre), in other cases it is only partially active (thyroid tumour). The most important task of thyroid hormones is the acceleration of a number of metabolic processes; overproduction of hormones means excessive acceleration. Mentally this results in ability and tiredness, but also sleeplessness. Because the metabolic processes release heat, the patient is too hot even in cold weather, and sweats continuously. Other symptoms are trembling hands, and a rapid, sometimes irregular, heartbeat. An accelerated metabolism also causes increased appetite, because a great deal of energy is needed, but despite this the patient loses weight. This is partly a result of diarrhoea, because the intestines process food more rapidly: in women menstruation is often irregular or completely absent.

Hyperventilation. Excessively rapid and deep respiration can cause symptoms leading to unconsciousness. Intensive breathing is part of a pattern of physical reactions produced by fear, anxiety or tense situations; the body prepares itself for a major effort, and if that effort is not required, problems occur. Deep breathing increases the carbon dioxide content of the body, causing tingling in the hands and feet, dizziness, sweating, a constricted feeling and chest pain. The chest pain may make the patient think he is having a heart attack, causing further hyperventilation through fear, and potentially leading to a vicious circle of increasing fear and ultimate panic.

Hypochondriasis. Persistent concern about one's own health, often associated with an impression of being seriously ill even though this is not really the case. A mild form sometimes occurs in medical and nursing students, who begin to feel that they are afflicted with the diseases with which they are confronted.

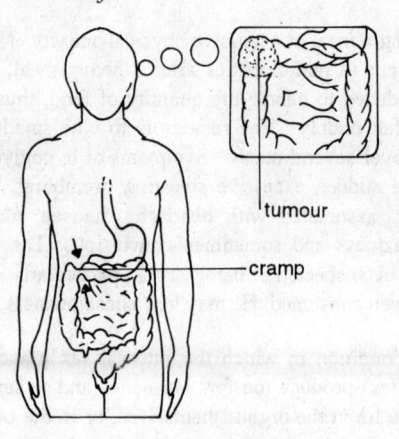

Hypochondria is the condition in which a patient blows up an insignificant symptom in his mind into a dreadful disease. and then believes that he is really suffering from it.

Hypoglycaemia. Low level of glucose in the blood, particularly in diabetes being treated with insulin or tablets to lower blood sugar levels. The cause is excessive insulin injection, too many

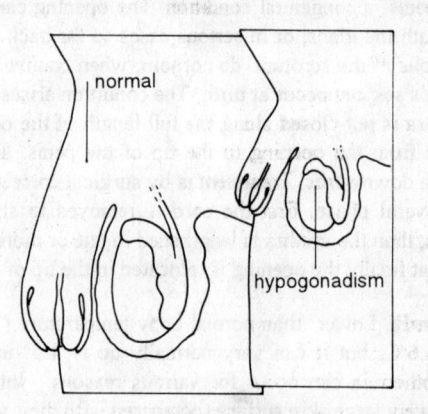

There are various reasons for underdevelopment of the genital organs: the condition is usually associated with infertility.

tablets, missing a meal or excessive physical activity. The condition can occur in non-diabetics after a heavy meal; excess insulin is produced to handle the quantity of food, thus blood sugar levels fall unduly. The remedy is to take smaller portions spread over several meals. Symptoms of hypoglycaemia in adults are sudden excessive sweating, trembling, hunger and yawning, associated with headache, nausea, muscular weakness, haziness and sometimes convulsions. The patient may unjustly be suspected of being drunk, particularly if some alcohol has been consumed. He may lose consciousness.

Hypogonadism. Condition in which the internal sex glands (testicles or ovaries) produce too few hormones and/or sex cells. The cause can lie in the organs themselves, or in the pituitary gland, which is responsible for stimulation of the sex organs. The condition can be congenital, or can arise from later genital disorders such as infection of cysts or tumours of the testicles or ovaries. A special form of the condition occurs if the pituitary gland produces too few stimulating hormones.

Hypospadias. Abnormal opening of the urethra on the underside of the penis, a congenital condition. The opening can be directly beneath the glans, or in serious cases so far back that the two sections of the scrotum do not join, when confusion about the child's sex can occur at birth. The condition arises because the urethra is not closed along the full length of the penis. A cord leads from the opening to the tip of the penis, and pulls the organ downwards. Treatment is by surgical correction, usually in several phase; first the cord is removed to straighten the penis, then the urethra is lengthened in one or more operations, so that finally the opening is relocated in the tip of the penis.

Hypothermia. Lower than normal body temperature (the average is 36.6°C, but it can vary normally up to 1.5° up or down). Hypothermia can occur for various reasons. Infants have a relatively large skin surface (compared with their volume), and thus can lose warmth rapidly at low temperatures. Adults lose warmth when they drink alcohol, as a result of blood vessel dilation. Body temperature can also drop rapidly through immersion in cold water. Finally old people are prone to heat loss if they do not move around enough. In very rare cases hypothermia is caused by a disorder of the hypothalamus of the brain, which contains the temperature regulation centre.

Hypothyroidism. Condition in which too few thyroid hormones are produced, especially common in middle-aged women; in very young children or infants it is known as cretinism. Hypothyroidism can be caused by pituitary disorders, in which too few thyroid stimulants are formed. Other possible causes are iodine deficiency, excessively drastic treatment of hyperthyroidism or inflammation of the thyroid gland. Lowered content of thyroid hormone in the blood slows down the metabolism causing some symptoms precisely opposed to those of hyperthyroidism. The patient feels listless and tired, and has difficulty in concentrating. The voice is low and hoarse, and hearing declines. The skin feels dry and cold, and sometimes shows puffy swelling (myxoedema). Nails are thin and fragile, and hair loses its normal gloss. The patient is sensitive to cold; the ambient temperature is never high enough, and extra blankets are needed on the bed even in summer. The heart beats slowly, the patient is often anemic, and constipated bake of intestinal relaxation. In women, menstrual bleeding is heavier and more persistent. In exceptional cases, for example as a result of infection, cooling or the use of drugs to aid sleep, loss of consciousness may occur.

Hysteria. Neurotic disorder characterized by theatricality, inauthentic feelings and the expression of them, egocentricity and infantilism. Often the patient attempts to manage those around him, and is inclined to attract unhappiness, bad luck and trouble. Almost everyone will recognize something of themselves in the above, but in true neurotics these traits occur in exaggerated form; they are designated as hysterical when they are predominant. Hysterical people often irritate their fellows, who do not understand that the behaviour is unconscious. The following symptoms are common in this neurosis; conversions,

brief loss of consciousness, anxiety in many forms, disturbances of sexual function and depersonalization. Hysterics are
more likely than others to resort to repression as a defence
mechanism.

I

IASIS. A process or the condition resulting from the process, especially a disease.

Ichthyosis. Skin condition associated with dryness, stiffness and characteristic fish-like scales, caused by thickening of the horn layer of the skin and thinning of the normal skin layers. The condition is hereditary and more common in men than women. The cause of Ichthyosis cannot be treated. The abnormal horn layer can be treated only locally with horn solvents, because general application has too many side-effects.

Idiocy. Most severe form of mental deficiency with an IQ of less than 25. Idiot children are not accustomed to feeding themselves, and almost always have to be admitted to an institution where they can receive specialized care. Such children are more than usually prone to infectious diseases. The mental age of an adult idiot is comparable with that of a child of two or younger. Generally the cause is severe abnormality of the brain, linked with physical abnormalities. The children are often spastic and epileptic.

Ileus. Cessation of intestinal function. There are two major forms, mechanical or obstruction ileus (see intestinal obstruction) and dynamic ileus, in which the intestine ceases to function through lack of peristalsis, the motive force in the intestine (paralytic ileus or intestinal paralysis). The latter condition can arise from peritonitis, or the nerves regulating intestinal function can be (temporarily) switched off by neurological disorders, kidney failure a blood clot in the intestinal blood vessels or a gallstone or kidney stone attack. Extensive surgery can also cause intestinal paralysis; thus no solid food should be taken after an operation until wind is broken, a sign that intestinal function is restored. Symptoms of intestinal paralysis are

affected by the underlying condition. Paralytic ileus itself can
lead to vague abdominal pain, distended abdomen, no passage
of faeces and possible vomiting. Abdominal examination by
stethoscope reveals silence, or absence of the sounds of peristalsis. An X-ray often shows fluid surfaces, distended intestinal loops with gastric juices and air above them.

Imbecility. Form of mental deficiency in which the IQ is between
25   and 50. Imbecile children are difficult to feed, but may
well learn some behavioural norms. There are often psychological problems, because mental defectives do not have the
insight to solve problems. They have often to be permanently
admitted to institutions. The mental age of an adult imbecile is
comparable with that of a child of 2 to 7. If problems are
approached properly an imbecile often appears affectionate and
compliant.

Immune defence system. The whole array of cells and chemicals
that protect the body against damage by foreign chemicals,
viruses and organisms. The skin and mucous membranes that
line all outward-facing surfaces of the body are only the most
familiar elements in this complex system.

We are born with the potentiality for two interrelated
immune defence systems: natural (or non-specific) and
adaptive. The non-specific system exists in all normal infants
at birth, but the adaptive system develops and changes
throughout life.

Perhaps the most pronounced evidence of the non-specific
immune response is *inflammation*. The *swelling*, heat and redness of inflammation are caused by chemicals released by mast
cells which exist throughout the body for this purpose. In addition, there are two classes of white blood cells which eat parts
or all of invasive organisms and neutralize or destroy them.
Various other chemicals are produced by other kinds of cells;
for example, all cells seem to possess the ability to synthesize
an antiviral chemical called interferon and an antibacterial called
lysozyme in response to an appropriate challenge. In addition,

the blood contains a related sequence of chemicals called collectively, complement, because they are complementary to the cellular immune defence machinery. These cells and substances will be activated either by a local invasive challenge or by a threat anywhere in the body.

The adaptive immune defences consist of two classes of cells and the chemicals these cells produce. Both classes of cells are called lymphocytes because they are found in the lymph system although they originate in the bone marrow like red and white blood cells.

The cells that produce antibodies are called B-cells. They were named after the bursa of a chicken, a kind of crop which does not exist in mammals, where they were first identified. B-cells become active in response to the presence of an antigen which stimulates one or a small number of cells probably in the part of the body where the antigen is first introduced. These cells make two responses to the antigen: they tailor-make antibodies against it, and they multiply, forming a clone of B-cells which now have the knowledge of the kind of antibody needed to attack that antigen if it ever reappears. B-cells are the basis for the success of vaccination, a vaccine consists either of an antigen which is separated by physical means from the disease-causing elements of the organism, or of an organism (inclusive of antigen) which has been weakened or attenuated organically, usually by growing in a non-human host. A clone of B-cells develops in response to the antigen so that if the infectious organism reappears, they will be available immediately to produce antibodies against it.

To achieve full activation, however, B-cells require the co-operation of the second class of adaptive immune defence cells, T-cells. The T stands for thymus, a gland in the lower neck, where T-cells formed in bone marrow are matured, at least during the early years of life. There are several varieties of T-cells, each with different functions. For example, T4-cells are called "helper" cells because they are needed to obtain a satisfactory response by B-cells to new antigens, and because they also activate other T-cells. Some T-cells destroy organisms, tumour cells and body cells infected by viruses. T-cells are responsible for the delayed hypersensitivity reaction which is an inflammatory response to an antigen that has appeared in the body at least once before (see *allergy*). Not only are T-cells "assigned" these functions when they mature in the thymus, but they are also modified in a way that allows them to distinguish between cells of their own body and other cells.

In part as a response to antigen, T-cells recognize other immune cells and release chemicals called lymphokines which enhance or suppress their activities. The other immune cells may be other T-cells or B-cells. Because T-cells are engaged in these linking and coordinating functions, they are the core of what is called cell-mediated immunity. B-cells are responsible for the humoural immune response because they produce antibodies which move through body fluids.

The complex inter reactions of the immune defence system serve to protect the body while not causing damage to it. Cells interreact chemically, recognizing molecules which are a far cry from the kind of sensory recognition of which the whole organism is capable. These cells exhibit kinds of chemical memory and learning reminiscent of the functions performed by nerve cells in the brain, but how far this analogy can be taken remains uncertain.

Immune deficiency. Deficient resistance by the body to disease. The defence system consists of two parts: white blood cells and proteins in the blood (antibodies). Immune deficiency can result from a shortage of either. White cell shortage or malfunction can occur in leukemia and Hodgkin's disease. If only the antibodies are in short supply the condition is known as agammaglobulinaemia. The general characteristic of immune deficiency is increased susceptibility to infection; a normally harmless virus or bacterium can cause dangerous illnesses such as severe pneumonia or meningitis.

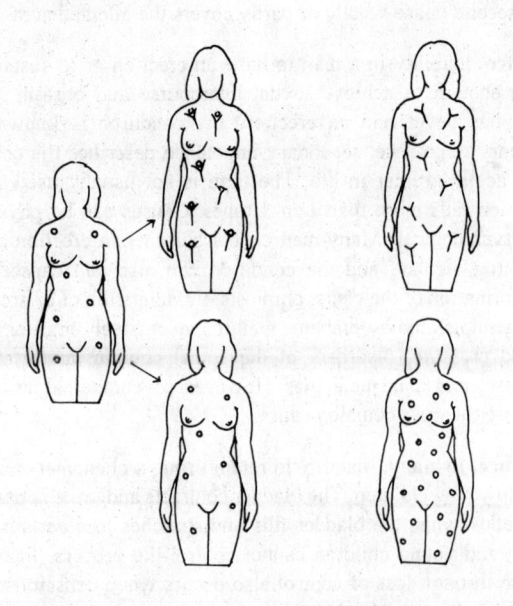

Normally the body produces antibodies when infected with micro-organisms. In immune deficiency this is not the case, and the micro-organisms continue to multiply.

Treatment depends on the cause of the immune deficiency. Infection must be avoided as much as possible and, if it occurs, must be treated immediately with antibiotics.

Impetigo. Bacterial inflammation of the skin, most common in children but occurring also in adults in unfavourable circumstances. The disease is highly infectious, particularly if hygiene is deficient, although modern improvements in this field have much reduced the incidence of the disease.

The first phase usually consists of small, suppurating blisters on the face which burst quickly. The most characteristic symptom of impetigo is the honeycoloured crust which during the second phase wholly or partly covers the affected area.

Importance. Inability in a man to have an erection or to sustain it long enough to achieve sexual intercourse and orgasm. If a man has never had an erection, the condition is known as primary impotence; secondary impotence describes the condition acquired later in life. The term is not usually used until erection fails more than 1 in 4 times. Causes can be physical or psychological. Many men cannot sustain an erection after drinking alcohol, and the condition can also be caused by malformation of the penis, phimosis, inflammation of or around the genitals, and by diabetes mellitus, excessively high or low blood pressure, disorders of the spinal column, many other diseases and some medicines. However, psychological difficulties are the most common cause.

Incontinence, urinary. Inability to retain urine, a phenomenon normal in young children. The bladder contracts and urine is passed by reflex when the bladder fills and stretches to a certain degree, and young children cannot control the process. Incontinence through loss of control also occurs when consciousness is lowered or completely lost.

In adults, control can be lost through spinal cord disorders or injury to the sphincter, the latter mainly in women who have had children.

Indigestion. Slight, temporary digestive disorder, usually caused by mild infection in the alimentary canal, by overeating or hurried meals, or by eating combinations of food that the intestine cannot process. Characteristics are that the intestine shows no or only mild abnormalities, and that the symptoms are slight. The condition can cause abdominal pain, a build-up of wind, thin faeces and possibly diarrhoea. Sometimes there is heartburn. Extensive examination is not necessary, and a doctor need not be consulted.

Inferiority complex. Continuous sense of inferiority and inadequacy, unrelated to reality. Such feelings are a factor in almost every neurosis , possibly because the neurosis causes the patient to function less well than he should; an excessively strict conscience is another factor. If one expects more from oneself than is humanly possible, then failure is inevitable. The slightest clumsiness or slip is torment to a perfectionist. The feeling probably originates from a childhood in which only perfection was esteemed, or in which extremely severe punishments were meted out. If a child knows that a small misdemeanour is going to incur major punishment, he will develop a conscience which is even stricter than his parents. Another method of upbringing which may lead to an inferiority complex is one which induces guilt feelings in the child; mother is not angry just sorry and disappointed. A child who fells guilty about his mistakes loses a sense of self-esteem; he is only at peace with himself if he makes no mistakes at all. In later years he is likely to establish a demanding lifestyle dependent upon proof and assurance that he is doing well from those around him. Treatment is by psychotherapy directed at storing self-esteem.

Infertility. Inability to conceive (in a woman) or to induce conception (in a man). About 10 to 15 per cent of all married couples are infertile, temporarily or permanently. In 40 per cent of cases the man is responsible, in 40 per cent the woman; in the remaining 20 per cent neither is clearly responsible. In most cases (8 out of 10) there is a physical cause; in the man these include imperfectly functioning testicles, caused by mumps virus infection, for example, venereal disease such as gonorrhoea or congenital testicular deficiency. Sometimes a prostate operation, severe diabetes mellitus or nerve damage can cause semen to enter the bladder on ejaculation, instead of being forced out through the penis. Sperm deficiency is another common cause of male infertility.

hostile mucus

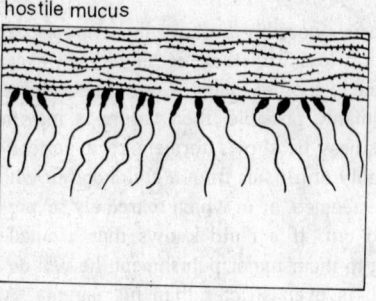

normal

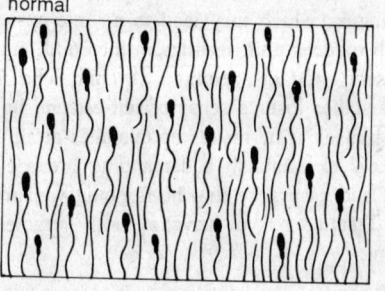

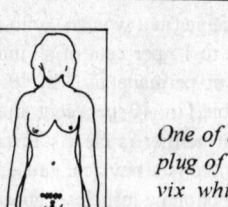

One of the causes of infertility is a plug of 'hostile' mucus in the cervix which prevents spermatozoa from entering the womb.

Influenza. Infectious viral disorder of the air passages. Some people say they have 'flu' if they have only a slight cold, but genuine influenza is seriously debilitating, and can even be dangerous.

Infection is through inhaling infected droplets in the air. One to four days later symptoms such as pain in the back and loins, fever, general malaise, headache and sometimes a dry cough, hoarseness, sore throat, sneezing and nasal discharge suddenly occur. Most symptoms disappear after four days, but fatigue and weakness persist for longer. In a small number of cases the virus can cause life-threatening pneumonia: the patient's condition deteriorates rapidly and there are respiratory difficulties. Another complication is bacterial pneumonia later in the course of the influenza. Both complications usually occur in groups at high risk from influenza, such a patients with chronic lung disorders, heart disease, chronic liver and kidney disease, diabetes mellitus. pregnant women and the elderly. From time to time influenza is pandemic: i.e. affects the entire world in epidemic proportions.

There are three types of influenza virus, A.B. and C, each with its own subtypes. Type A is the principal cause of epidemic influenza and winter pandemics. Type B can cause epidemics in the winter or late spring, but has less severe clinical manifestations. Type C hardly ever causes illness in man. Great epidemics occur every 2 to 3 years. The so-called antigen shift means that the old immunity to the A virus is no longer valid, because the antigen qualities of the virus have changed. The virus is thus able to infect large groups of people very rapidly. The symptoms are also more severe after a shift of this kind.

Ingrowing nail. Usually in the toes. Shoes can push the nail into the membrane of the toe, causing it to press on the pain nerves. The condition is almost exclusively limited to the big toe, because the nails on the other toes are not so robust, so that they distort under pressure rather than growing inwards.

When a nail grows in, a channel forms along the length of it through which bacteria can enter. This causes inflammation, worsening the pain. Most people react to an ingrowing toenail by clipping away the edges; but this makes the nail wedge-shaped, thus increasing the chance of aggravating the condition. It is therefore better to clip the end of the nail off straight, so that the edges protrude in front of the toe. If a toe is inflamed because of an ingrowing nail the foot can be bathed in soda solution. In severe cases it may be necessary to remove the nail under local anaesthetytic.

Insomnia. Discontent with the quantity or pattern of sleep, even though there is opportunity to sleep. It is very rare not to be able to sleep at all, even those who maintain that they 'haven't slept a wink' in fact sleep perfectly well from time to time. It is quite normal to sleep less with age. The term insomnia is usually reserved for patients who cannot function properly during the day. Problems can occur in getting to sleep, or because the patient wakes during the night, or too early, and cannot get back to sleep. Waking too early in the morning can be symptom of endogenous depression. Difficulties in getting to sleep are common if the patient has been particularly active in the course of the evening, and cannot relax enough to sleep. Some people sleep badly after taking coffee, tea or chocolate, or if they have smoked heavily or eaten a big meal shortly before going to bed. Pain or cold also prevent sleep, because muscles cannot relax sufficiently. Interrupted sleep can be caused by the consumption of quantities of alcohol; it is easy enough to get to sleep, but after a few hours the kidneys begin to produce more urine and the patient has to get up, and then often cannot get back to sleep again. Other causes of sleep disorders are anxiety tension or psychosocial problems.

Intercourse, painful (dyspareunia) Pain can occur on initial penetration of the vagina by the penis, or when deeper thrusts are made. There may be various causes for such pain, which can seriously affect sexual enjoyment. In the man it is usually inflammation of the genitals (balanitis) or a tight foreskin (phimosis). In the woman too the commonest cause is inflammation of the genitals (vaginitis), but it can also be excessively rapid penetration by the penis. Sexual arousal and stimulation cause the walls of the vagina to secrete a lubricant, which is a natural means of easing penetration by and movement of the penis, and time is needed before the lubricant is produced in sufficient quantity to allow comfortable penetration. Inexperience, haste, lack of knowledge of each other's body and anxiety can all contribute to the experience of intercourse as painful. The family doctor should check for inflammation, and treat it if found; other sources pain can be corrected by good sexual counselling.

Interferon. A protein formed in all body cells in mammals when the cells are invaded by viruses. Its function is presumably to control further viral development in the cells, but its value as a natural antiviral and as a drug is extremely limited. How exactly interferon interferes with viral growth is not clear and, perhaps for this reason, its limitations are not understood.

Different animals produce different interferons, and even within the human body different cells synthesize slightly different forms of the chemical. The hope that large doses of one of these varieties might control some forms of *cancer* has so far not been fulfilled.

Intermittent claudication. Pain in the legs resulting from thickening of the leg arteries in atherosclerosis. The pain is caused by oxygen deficiency in the leg muscles, itself the result of poor supply of oxygen-rich blood from the thickened arteries. There is usually no discomfort when the patient is sitting or standing still, but when walking pain occurs, causing a limp, and stops again when the patient stands still. The best treatment is surgery (replacement of the thickened artery with a plastic tube, widening the artery etc.); drugs generally have little or no effect.

Interstitial fibrosis. A complication of many chronic conditions of the air passages, which in the long term result in the formation of fibrous tissue around the follicles in the alveoli, which hinders the lungs in their task of extracting sufficient oxygen from the air. The disorder is a complication of many chronic diseases such as CARA, chronically recurring diseases of the air passages, slowly progressing forms of lung cancer, long exposure to irritant substances, and as a side-effect of certain medicines. The extra tissue increases the resistance of the blood vessels in the lungs and thus the right side of the heart has more difficulty in pumping blood through the vessels in the lungs. In the first instance this causes compensatory enlargement of the right side of the heart and this may subsequently result in heart failure. The body then receives too little oxygen indicated by such symptoms as shortness of breath, cyanosis, drumstick fingers, watch glass nails and some increase in the number of red blood corpuscles. The symptoms of interstitial fibrosis can resemble those of various serious lung conditions, heart diseases and severe anaemia.

Intertrigo. Condition occurring in folds of skin, for example under the breasts, in the buttock cleft and the groin. Small suppurating blisters are formed by regular friction in the warm, moist space formed by the fold of skin. They have a red edge and burst and spread quickly, so that the whole area of the fold is quickly affected, and some blisters are also seen at the edge. The disorder is caused by a unicellular fungus which nourishes in warm, moist surroundings. There is also a type of eczema that occurs particularly in folds of skin, and this and intertrigo often occurs simultaneously.

Intestinal atresia. Congenital interruption of the alimentary canal, caused by abnormal development in its blood circulation, so serious in some cases that part of the canal is completely missing. The most frequent position of this abnormality is in the small intestine (1 in 4000 births). All such abnormalities can easily be diagnosed shortly after birth from the symptoms. In the case of atresia of the small intestine the baby spits out food, followed by yellowish-green vomit (bile); the abdomen dilates and meconium is not passed. Atresia of the oesophagus usually occurs in combination with a fistula between the lower part of the oesophagus and the windpipe, in consequence of which food often gets into the air passages, causes the child to become tight in the chest, blow bubbles or breathe stertorously. Pneumonia can result from swallowing the wrong way.

Intestinal cancer. Malignant intestinal tumour (carcinoma of the colon), usually in the large intestine. It is one of the commonest forms of cancer, occurring equally frequently in men and women. It also is one of the most significant causes of death by cancer.

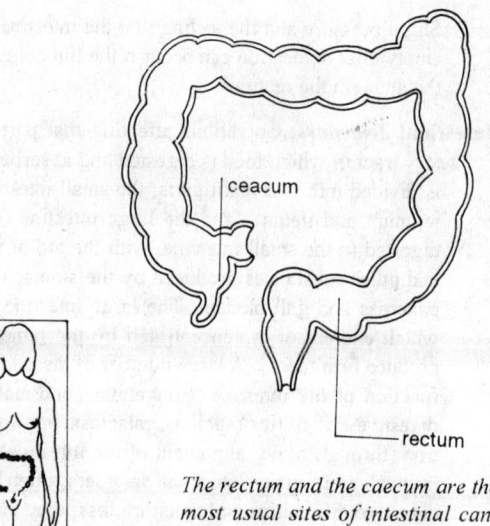

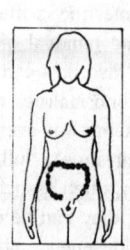

The rectum and the caecum are the most usual sites of intestinal cancer.

Certain illnesses can cause a predisposition to carcinoma of the colon, especially a certain hereditary form of intestinal polyp in the colon, ulcerative colitis and some non-hereditary polyps. Symptoms of intestinal cancer are highly dependent on its site. A tumour in the (narrower) small intestine can cause pain through gradual obstruction, sometimes with the same clinical picture as intestinal obstruction. Sometimes the first symptom is haemorrhage or sudden loss of blood, also a symptom of tumours in the ascending (right-hand) part of the large intestine. Obstruction occurs only at a later stage, because of the width of this part of the intestine. As well as loss of blood there is persistent pain on the right, gradually becoming more severe and colic-like, and associated with malaise and loss of weight. A tumour in the last section of the large intestine causes obstruction much more quickly: the intestine is narrower and the faeces much firmer. This gives rise to pain and changes in the pattern of defecation, with gradually increasing constipation sometimes alternating with diarrhoea. There may also be bright blood in the faeces, possibly mixed with mucus.

Slight pressure and the feeling that the intestine is not properly empty after defecation can occur if the tumour is directly above the anus (in the rectum).

Intestinal disorders. Conditions affecting that part of the alimentary tract in which food is digested and absorbed. The intestine is divided into two main parts: the small intestine (duodenum, jejunum and ileum) and the large intestine (colon). Food is digested in the small intestine, with the aid of juices, enzymes and other substances produced by the stomach intestinal wall, pancreas and gall bladder. The large intestine is the organ in which excrement is concentrated by the removal of water to produce firm faeces. A large number of disorders can affect the function of the intestine. Congenital abnormalities can cause digestive difficulties (such as galactosaemia) or even obstruction (through faulty alignment of the intestine). Inflammation is involved in many intestinal disorders, often associated with digestive difficulties and moisture loss; they can be caused by a virus or bacterium (cholera typhoid dysentery, appendicitis etc.) but may have no specific cause (Crohon's disease and ulcerative colitis). Intestinal function can be completely halted by ileus (intestinal obstruction) or a strangulated hernia. Intestinal tumours (benign and malignant) almost always occur in the large intestine. Many intestinal disorders are the result of a particular pattern of life. A sedentary life and a diet lacking in fibre can cause haemorrhoids, constipation, diverticulosis or spastic colon. Most intestinal conditions are associated with abdominal pain, nausea, vomiting and diarrhoea, together or in combination. Loss of intestinal blood shows in black faeces (melaena; the blood is partially digested) or by passage of brighter blood faeces if the affected area is near the anus (the final section of the large intestine or of the rectum).

Intestinal Obstruction. Inhibition of intestinal function (a form of ileus) caused by mechanical blockage of the intestine or by intestinal strangulation.

Causes of mechanical obstruction include tumours, large gallstones or a hard lump of faeces.

Strangulation of the intestine can be caused by strands of
tissue after abdominal surgery or in Meckel's diverticulum,
volvulus, invagination, or strangulated hernia. Symptoms vary
from vomiting with gradually increasing frequency, dehydration and a swollen feeling associated with delayed production
of faeces in the case of normal obstruction, to rapid onset of
abdominal pain and possible peritonitis if the cause is volvulus.
Intestinal perforation and death of a section of the intestine can
even occur. In ileus, surgery to remove the blockage is often
unavoidable.

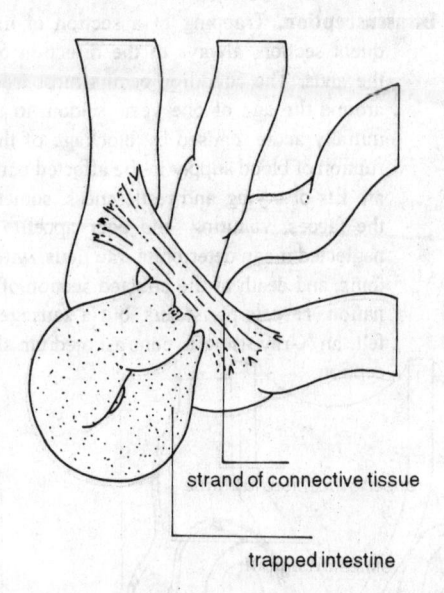

strand of connective tissue

trapped intestine

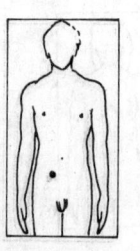

Intestinal blockage can because by
the trapping of a loop of intestine
under a strand of connective tissue.

Intestinal perforation. Hole in the intestinal wall-usually in the
first section of the small intestine, the duodenum. It is usually
caused by a duodenal ulcer which has eaten its way through

the intestinal wall, or by a tumour, a gunshot or stab wound, volvulus, or a sharp foreign body in the intestine. Perforation is usually followed immediately by the symptoms of acute peritonitis and severe pain. Sometimes, in the case of perforation to another organ (fistula) or a covered perforation, the symptoms are less severe and short-lived.

ITIS . A suffix that indicates *inflammation* of the part to which it is attached; for example *tonsillitis*.

Intussusception. Trapping of a section of intestine in the subsequent section, always in the direction of peristalsis, towards the anus. The condition occurs most frequently in baby boys around the age of one year, seldom in adults. Symptoms are initially acute, caused by blockage of the intestine and interruption of blood supply to the affected part. Characteristic signs are fits of crying and restlessness, sometimes a little blood in the faeces, vomiting, and poor appetite. If the condition is neglected it can deteriorate into ileus, with all associated symptoms, and death of the affected section of the intestine. Examination reveals peristalsis, but a sausage-like swelling can be felt; an X-ray using a contrast medium shows up the intussusception.

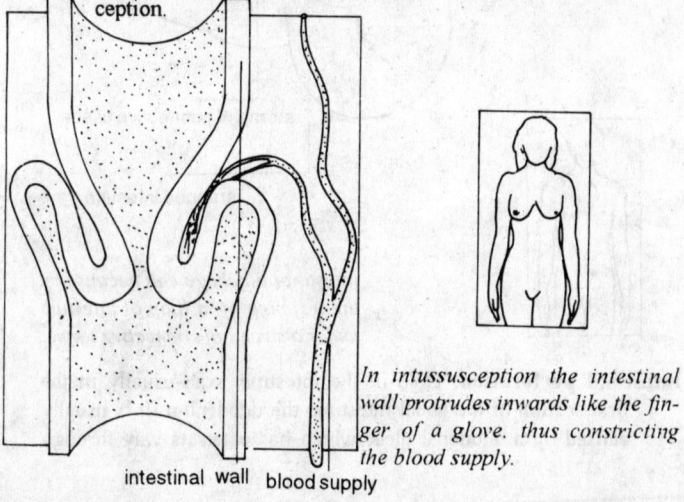

In intussusception the intestinal wall protrudes inwards like the finger of a glove, thus constricting the blood supply.

intestinal wall   blood supply

Iritis. Inflammation of the iris of the eye, possibly associated with inflammation of the ciliary body. It is often the consequence of inflammation elsewhere in the body, such as an intestinal infection, inflammation of the roots of the teeth, nephritis, etc. It can also arise from rheumatic disorders, or in rare cases from tuberculosis or sarcoidosis. Iritis causes irritation of the eye, redness, pain, fuzziness of vision and hypersensitivity to light. The pupil reacts more slowly to light, and testing of this reaction is painful. Swelling often makes the iris paler in colour, the eye is red, and the veins stand out because of increased blood supply. Inflamed cells float between the iris and cornea. Possible complications are: adhesion of the iris to the lens, restricting pupillary movement, or glaucoma because less aqueous homour is removed, thus increasing pressure in the eyeball. Treatment is by an ophthalmologist. The pupil is usually dilated with eye drops to prevent adhesion to the lens, and corticosteroids may be prescribed to suppress the inflammation reaction. If eyeball pressure is high, treatment is as for glaucoma.

Itching (pruritis) Unpleasant symptom of a number of skin disorders, arising because a large number of nerves are slightly irritated simultaneously. Scratching irritates them more, and the itch disappears. Itching is particularly common in constitutional eczema, but can also occur in contact eczema. A birthmark that itches, bleeds or increases in size can be a sign of melanoma (a malignant skin tumour), which requires treatment as soon as possible. Fungus infections of the skin, particularly between the toes (athlete's foot) and fingers, cause pruritis, and these places are difficult to scratch. Bites or stings from insects, gnats or fleas are often itchy, and persistent itching can be a sign of scabies infestation with a mite which lays eggs in the horn layer of the skin. As well as these skin disorders, a number of other diseases can cause pruritis; among them are diabetes mellitus, jaundice and Hodgkin's disease.

J

Jaundice (icterus) Yellow colouring of skin, mucous membrane and bodily fluids by an excess in the bloodstream of bilirubin, the colouring matter of bile. Before it is discharged from the body, bilirubin follows a course which jaundice interrupts in some way. It circulates as follows: bilirubin is a waste product of the breakdown of old red blood cells, which live for approximately 110 days. It is absorbed by the liver and converted into a water-soluble form, then discharged into the bile, which passes through the gall bladder and bile ducts, then to the intestine, where it gives faeces their characteristic brown colour. The most important causes of jaundice are; increased breakdown of blood (haemolysis), with resultant increase in bilirubin level; lack or shortage of liver enzymes, without which bilirubin cannot be converted (certain forms of neonatal jaundice); decreased discharge of bile as a result of liver conditions (such as hepatitis or cirrhosis of the liver); blockage of the bile duct (increasing obstruction by gallstones, cancer of the gall bladder or tumour of the pancreas).

Treatment is directly dependent upon the cause, which must be treated to control the jaundice.

Joint disorders. Generally characterized by pain, stiffness, restricted movement and swelling of the joint. Joints can be damaged by contusion, sprains, dislocation and fractures involving the joint. Damage is caused to ligaments, capsules, and/or the cartilaginous surfaces of the joint. Arthritis (inflammation of a joint) is a common condition, and can be caused by bacteria, viruses or fungus, but also arise from rheumatic disorders, most importantly chronic rheumatoid arthritis. Arthrosis is wear of the cartilage of a joint caused by old age or incorrect stress on a joint.

Joint mouse. Loose piece of bone or cartilage in the cavity of a joint, which can cause pain when the joint is moved, and make the joint jam in a particular position. The condition occurs if a piece of bone or cartilage breaks off, or as a result of bone death caused by circulatory disorders such as osteochondritis. The condition is a apparent on an X-ray of the joint.

Treatment is by surgical removal of the piece as a matter of some urgency, because delay could lead to serious damage to cartilage and possible arthrosis.

Joints, haemorrhage in (haemarthrosis) Discharge of blood in a joint cavity, usually the consequence of damage to the capsule caused by a sprain dislocation or an injury. Such blood usually remains fluid and is broken down slowly and the breakdown products re-absorbed in the bloodsrtream. In the case of large quantities of blood removal by surgery may be necessary, because the enzymes released could affect the cartilage of the joint; damaged tissue may be repaired at the same time. Patients with diabetes mellitus or those using anticoagulants to treat thrombosis, for example, can cause haemorrhage by normal pressure on the joint; ultimately this can cause damage, and lead to immobility of the joint.

K

Kaposi's sarcoma. Rare form of skin cancer, consisting of reddish-purple to brown lumps which sometimes have a wart-like surface. Even though the condition affects the skin in various places, it is thought that this is not metastasis, but simply that the disease tends to affect more than one place at the same time. It spreads slowly, causing some people to think that it is not a cancer but an ordinary skin disease. There is no effective therapy, and because the disorder progresses so slowly, the more aggressive cancer treatments are not applied. Kaposi's sarcoma can also affect AIDS sufferers.

Keloid. Scar tissue that grows rapidly, like a tumour, and protrudes above the surrounding skin; a normal scar is only slightly thicker than the skin. A tendency to the condition is hereditary, and it is commoner in darker-skinned people and following infected wounds. The condition is difficult to treat, because new keloid tissue tends to form in the wound after surgery. Sometimes corticosteroids are injected, but in recent wounds this increases the danger of infection.

Keratitis. Inflammation of the cornea (the transparent membrane at the front of the eyeball), usually superficial, and caused by bacteria, viruses or sometimes fungus. Damage to the cornea by exposure to radiation is also called keratitis. Symptoms are irritation of the eye, pain, redness, weeping and hypersensitivity to light.

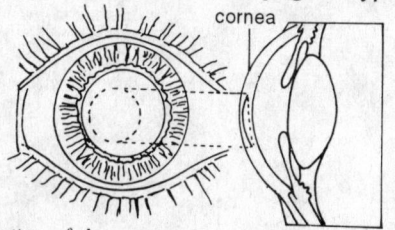

Inflammation of the cornea (keratitis) can cause problems of vision

Bacterial infection can occur after damage to the cornea-by a splinter of metal, for example. The bacteria cause an ulcer, usually restricted to the cornea, although sometimes the ulcer penetrates it and infection spreads to the front chamber of the eye. Inflamed cells cause clouding of the iris, and the cells themselves form a deposit visible as a half moon on the underside of the iris. Treatment is by cleaning the affected part of the cornea, and with antibiotics.

Keratoconus. Conical forward protrusion of the central section of the cornea, making the front of the eye conical or pointed when seen from the side, usually occurring between puberty and the age of 40. Hereditary factors are important, and the condition is common in people with Down's syndrome. In rare cases the condition occurs suddenly as a result of a tear in the membrane that closes the front chamber of the eye, thus allowing aqueous humour to accumulate behind the cornea, which then protrudes. Keratoconus seriously reduces vision; treatment is by wearing a contact lens, but only if the eye is not seriously malformed. Surgery is necessary in severe cases, and a corneal transplant may also be called for.

Keratosis. Excessive scalyness of the skin caused by an accumulation of keratin (the substance that makes up fingernails and horn). It is a symptoms of various skin diseases, particularly eczema and the common wart, at the most important symptom of psoriasis. Scales form on the skin, and indeed the condition lies behind all scaly skin disorders. If there is no underlying condition to be treated, keratosis can often be controlled with medication containing substances that dissolve keratin.

Kidney, cysts in. Fluid-filled cavities in the kidney tissue. The condition often occurs in members of the same family. There are various kinds of kidney cyst; if they appear in the medulla of the kidney they produce symptoms such as high blood perssure, renal poisoning and anaemia in puberty as a consequence of a deficiency in normally functioning kidney tissue.

Kidney, floating. Unstable kidney position caused by detachment of
the organ from its capsule. The kidneys are normally firmly
anchored in connective and fatty tissue at the upper back of the
abdominal cavity, directly below the diaphragm and protected
from the rear by the ribs. Sometimes a kidney is inadequately
attached, and slips loose when the body is in a upright position. It is then known as a floating kidney. The condition
occurs most frequently in women after several pregnancies or
extreme loss of weight. It is possible that a ureter may be
trapped in the process, causing urinary retention in the renal
pelvis, a potential source of Inflammation and even
hydronephrosis. Discomfort is usually restricted to pain in the
renal area, particularly associated with up and down movements such as jumping and horseriding. If severe discomfort
occurs, the kidney can be restored to its normal position by
surgery.

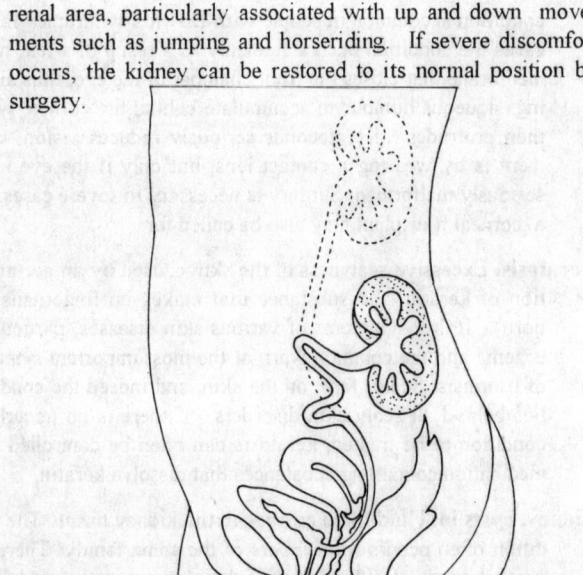

*A kidney can become detached from its capsule and lie loose in
the abdominal cavity, a so-called floating kidney.*

Kidney disorders. The kidneys are responsible for the excretion of waste products. Disorders range from those that are present without symptoms to severe diseases which could be fatal.

Congenital disorders include horseshoe kidney and kidney cysts: a single kidney cyst can also occur later in life. A floating kidney is usually the result of slackening of the tissue in which the kidney is suspended. Kidney stones are usually the result of abnormally large secretions of certain substances or caused by recurrent pyclitis. If a kidney stone sticks in the ureter it can cause kidney stone colic: long-term obstructions of the ureters can cause restricted urinary flow and thus hydronephrosis. The renal pelvis can become so swollen that only a skin of renal tissue remains. Inadequate renal function is known as kidney failure or insufficiency, resulting from conditions such as glomerulonephritis. Kidney failure cause uraemia through the accumulation of poisonous waste products in the blood. There are some highly malignant kidney tumours such as Wilms' tumour in young children and hypernephroma particularly in men over the age of 40. The kidneys can also be involved in diseases that affect the whole body: high blood pressure, diabetes mellitus and many autoimmune diseases. If both kidneys cease to function the condition is potentially fatal. Fortunately modern medicine offers kidney transplants and renal dialysis (kidney machine); however, there is a general shortage of kidneys for transplant purposes.

Kidney failure. Inadequate renal function caused by deficient excretion of waste products, finally resulting in uraemia. A distinction is made between acute and chronic kidney failure; the acute form is usually the result of acute necrosis of the kidney tubules or suddenly reduced blood circulation in the kidneys, because of low blood pressure, for example, or shock, or sometimes by blockage of both ureters. Blockage of one ureter does not usually cause kidney failure. The symptoms are a sudden reduction in urine production (anuria), associated with oedema, and also loss of appetite nausea and listlessness. Recovery is usually spontaneous after a few days or weeks.

Uraemia can occur very quickly in the initial phase, so renal dialysis (kidney machine) may have to be used.

Kidney injury. Damage to the kidney by an external force, of necessity quite considerable if the kidney is healthy, because the organ is well protected in the body. Diseased kidneys are more susceptible to injury. The commonest and least serious injury is a contusion, causing tiny breaks in the kidney tissue which bleed slightly and cause swelling. If the injuries are more serious they can cause total or partial tearing of kidney tissue, and the renal pelvis and capsule can also be damaged, with consequential severe haemorrhage in and around the kidney. The most serious injury of all is crushing of the kidney or tearing of the large blood vessels, leading more rapidly to severe haemorrhage. There is a high risk of shock because other organs are often damaged as well. Symptoms of renal injury are blood in the urine (haematuria), pain in the side and upper abdomen, nausea and vomiting.

Kidney stone. Presence of stone-like deposits of substances hard to dissolve in urine in the renal capsule or renal pelvis. Most of the stones are made up of calcium oxalate and calcium phosphate crystals. Others consist mainly of uric acid or cystine, an amino acid. Often the cause of stone formation is unknown; sometimes it is increased production of the substances named. Calcium, for example, is overproduced in cases of excess corticosteroid hormone and osteoporosis, uric acid in gout and cases of malignant tumour. Excess cystine in the urine usually results from a congenital condition. Other possible factors are limited fluid intake or excessive moisture loss by sweating or diarrhoea, causing higher urine concentration. Local damage caused by inflammation or congenital malformation provides ideal places for the formation of deposits which can grow into stones. Urine acidity is also a factor; urine stones are formed only in very acid urine, and may be dissolved again when acidity is reduced.

Kidney tumour. Can be either benign or malignant; the benign variety are of little significance, because they seldom cause problems. The commonest malignant tumours are hypernephroma, after the age of 40, and Wilms' tumour, before the age of 5. Tumours can also occur in the renal pelvis; they are much the same as polyps and tumours of the bladder.

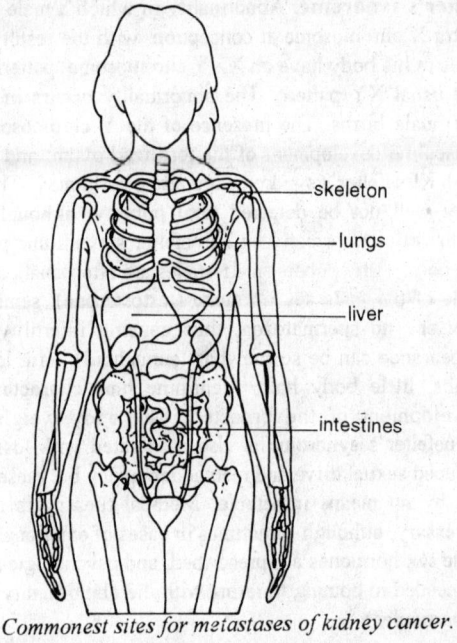

skeleton

lungs

liver

intestines

Commonest sites for metastases of kidney cancer.

Tumours of the kidneys and the renal pelvis almost always cause blood in the urine (haematuria). Hydronephrosis can occur as a result of blockage of or pressure on the ureters, but there may be no specific symptoms in the early stages. General symptoms indicating the presence of malignant tumours are weakness, fatigue, loss of a appetite and loss of weight; these should prompt general examination. A kidney tumour can also be a secondary growth of a cancer elsewhere in the body—the breast or the lung, for example. Kidney tumours can be diagnosed by contrast X-rays of the kidneys and urinary tract (intravenous pyelogram, IVP), contrast X-rays of the renal blood vessels, and sonography.

Treatment is usually by removal of the kidney and associated ureter.

Klinefelter's syndrome. Abnormality in which a male receives an extra X chromosome at conception, with the result that all the cells in his body have an XXY chromosome pattern instead of the usual XY pattern. The abnormality occurs in about 1 in 800 male births. The presence of the Y chromosome ensures masculine development of the fertilized ovum, and individuals with Klinefelter's syndrome are also clearly male. The condition may well not be detected until puberty, although there are some differences between Klinefelter's syndrome patients and the norm. After puberty the testicles are often small, and produce little of the male sex hormone (testosterone): semen contains few or no spermatozoa, thus causing infertility. Outward appearance can be sosmewhat 'eunuchoid', with long slender limbs, little body hair, feminine hair characteristics and development of the breasts if the body weight is high. Klinefelter's syndrome is also associated with loss of libido, reduced sexual drive and mental deficiency but these symptoms are by no means inevitable. Medical thearpy is not usually necessary, although sometimes in cases of emotional instability male sex hormones are prescribed, and psychological help may be needed in coming to terms with the abmormality (infertility in particular).

Knee, torn cartilage. Damage to one/both of the horse-shoeshaped discs of cartilage (meniscus) in the knee, usually in the form of a tear in the meniscus on the inner side of the knee, caused by twisting the bent knee, as a result of which the foot cannot move properly. It often occurs in sports such as football. A ligament may be damaged at the same time. The symptoms are pain and swelling. The swelling is the result of increased production of fluid in the joint and possible haemorrhage (joint haemorrhage) in the knee. The injury can be associated with a feeling of something snapping and the knee sometimes locks in a bent position.

Knee disorders. Include conditions of the kneecap, which itself has a joint with the frontal section of the thigh bone, joining the shin bone at the knee. The joint-forming surfaces of the thigh and shin do not fit precisely together, but are hinged by the inner and outer meniscus, two horse-shoe-shaped plates of cartilage within the joint. There are four important knee ligaments: two on each side of the knee to prevent sideways movement, and two cross ligaments to prevent forward or backward displacement of the joint. Common knee conditions include arthritis, housemaid's knee (synovitis) and rheumatic disorders.

Knock knee (genu valgum) Condition in which there is space between the ankles when the legs are held together and extended. Young children often have knock knees after the third year of life. These usually disappear of their own accord. They may however persist in, for example, cases of flat feet. Because of their wider pelvis, women have knock knees three times more frequently than men. Knock knees may also occur in bone disorders such as rickets and ostemalacia, or in paralysis of the leg muscles. They can also arise by overstraining the ligaments of the joints through obesity or lifting heavy weights.

Korsakoff's syndrome. Clinical picture involving amnesia without the presence of dementia caused by damage to certain deep brain areas through vitamin B deficiency (inadequate nutrition) in alcoholism for example, or Wernicke's disease. The condition can also occur whenever large numbers of brain cells are destroyed.

Kwashiorkor. Combination of symptoms caused by protein shortage in the diect leading to a deficiency in certain amino acids (elements in protein, necessary for building tissues in the body), and possibly also a shortage of minender and vitamins. The condition occurs especially in children, and mostly in developing countries with chronic food shortage. Symptoms are slow growth, abnormal pigmentation and ulceration of the skin, stomatitis (inflammation of the mucous membrane of the mouth), enlarged liver, vomiting, diarrhoea, emacietion with breakdown of muscular tissue and oedema. Diagnosis is on the basis of these symptoms, possibly supplemented by tests such as removal of a piece of liver tissue, which will show characteristci changes (fattiness and formation of connective tissue). The condition should be prevented as much as possibie by good ditary education and hospital treatment of problem cases.

Kyphosis. Curvature of the spinal column, known as a hump back if the condition is clearly visible at chest or shoulder height. Kyphosis may be angular or round. Angular kyphosis is usually

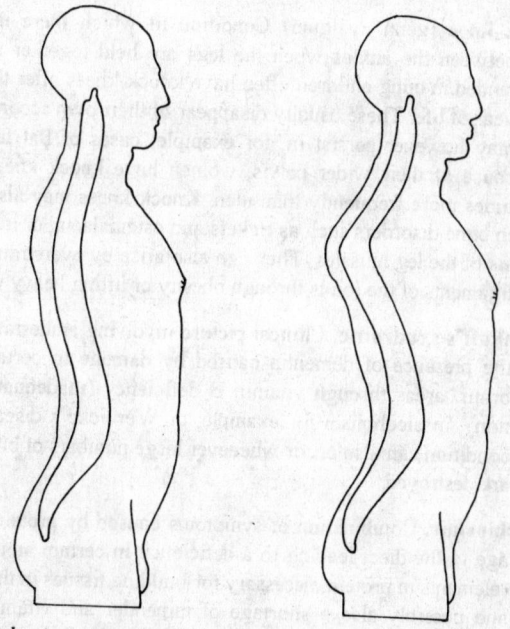

Kyphosis is increased convex curvature of the spinal column at chest height.

the result of deformity of one vertebra; if more than one is affected the curve is more gentle. The condition can be hereditary, or the result of a bone disorder such as osteoporosis or metastasis of tumours. Round kyphosis is the more common; discs are affected as well as vertebrae, and the condition occurs in illnesses such as Scheuermann's disease, rickets and the related condition known as osteomalacia. Kyphosis can also be caused by poor back posture or muscular weakness.

L

Labour, premature. Labour that begins between the 28th and 37th week of pregnancy. Because of the dangers threatening a premature baby such a birth should always take place in hospital, Increasing the child's chances of survival. Reasons for premature labour are often not known. One factor is a disorder of the placenta, in which case conditions outside the womb are probably more favourable to the child. Rhesus incompatibility must also be borne in mind, and abnormality or infection in the child. A defect of the cervix and undue stretching of the uterus, caused by hydremnios or a multiple pregnancy are also possible factors.

Labour, prolonged. Labour lasting for a relatively long time, sometimes even for days. From the moment when a woman believes that labour has begun, she and those around her expect the child to be born within 24 hours. But it can take longer, because the onset of the first period of labour, in which the cervix opens, is difficult to identify. Particularly in a first pregnancy the woman does not know precisely what the should feel, and may interpret the first predictive pains as contractions, and think that labour has begun. The doctor or midwife is important in such cases : false confirmation that labour has begun make it seem to be unduly protracted.

Labyrinthitis. Acute inflammation of the inner ear, which contains the cochlea and the organ of balance. The cause can be viral or bacterial. Possible viral causes are the influenza or mumps virus. Bacterial inflammation, usually resulting from an acute otitis media (inflammation of the middle ear), is much more serious. Viral inflammation of the inner ear, sometimes after influenza or mumps but sometimes in an otherwise healthy patient leads to sudden deafness, often associated with ringing in the ears. Generally symptoms are limited to one side. Sometimes the organ of balance is more affected, causing giddiness, nausea and vomiting. There is no treatment for viral inflammation, and only general measure such as bed rest and medication for giddiness are of any use. The giddiness will pass, but hearing is not usually restored.

Lactose intolerance. Condition in which the intestine reacts against lactose, or milk sugar, caused by shortage or absence in the intestine of lactase, the enzyme that normally breaks down lactose. Lactase deficiency may be congenital, or may come about in later life as a result of conditions such as thrush or other disorders affecting the intestinal mucous membrane. Because lactose cannot be digested normally, it is turned into lactic acid by intestinal bacteria, which irritates the large intestine, causing foaming, watery acid diarrhoea, a bloated feeling burping and abdominal cramp. Diagnosis is by examination of a piece of abdominal tissue (biopsy). Treatment is by a lactose-free diet: babies can be fed with soya milk. The congenital form often develops slowly, and the baby can still be fed with milk.

Laryngitis. Inflammation of the larynx, which connects the throat with the windpipe and consists of a skeleton of cartilage with mucous membrane inside it. The larynx contains the epiglottis, the valve that prove its food entering the air passages, and the vocal cord. Laryngitis is an infection usually resulting from a descending nasal infection or an ascending bronchitis. The inflammation causes a thickly cough and hoarseness. Croup and laryngitis caused by diphtheria are now are. The condition sometimes known as pseudo-croup, however, often occurs in children under the age of five, more in boys than girls, particularly in the months November to April in northern latitudes. Pseudo-croup usually starts with a slight daytime cold in the nose. The child then wakes in the late evening with a sudden feeling of constriction, is alarmed, sits up and coughs with a barking sound. Breathing is obstructed by the swollen mucous membrane, and accompanied by a whistling sound.

The swelling can be so bad that the child can hardly breathe at all and turns blue. The symptoms are quickly reduced by inhalation of water vapour, best achieved by putting the child in a shower cubicle and turning on the warm water.

Larynx. The voice box. In anatomical terms, its principal function is to act as a sphincter which can close the top of the tube leading to the lungs (the trachea), to prevent objects from blocking the breathing tubes. It consists of strong muscles attached to cartilage; the vocal cords are actually ligaments connecting these structures.

Larynx, tumour of. Benign tumours of the larynx often occur in young children and disappear spontaneously at puberty. Such tumours are rare in adults. Persistent strain on the vocal cords can cause modules, but these usually disappear spontaneously when the voice is rested. Malignant tumours usually appear between the ages of 50 and 70, ten times more often in men than women, almost 70 per cent of them on the vocal cords. They give early symptoms in the form of voice changes. Factors which encourage the development of this sort of cancer are smoking (particularly of cigarettes), excessive drinking, inhaling wood and metal dust and possibly abuse of the voice. Any hoarseness or huskiness which persists for more than three weeks should not be dismissed as a persistent cold.

Lassa fever. Viral infection especially prevalent in parts of Africa; it is an introduced disease in Western Europe. Rats are the carriers, excreting the virus in their urine and contaminating food, for example, which leads to infection in man. The virus can also be transmitted from human being to human being. Hospital staff are at risk.

Learning difficulties. Problems suffered at school by normally intelligent children, who are unable to comply with its requirements. The problem is more common than is generally suspected; there are various causes. There can be a medical background such as chronic sickness, causing tiredness and concentration problems; vision or hearing difficulties; or epilepsy.

Environmental factors are often significant-the child may be emotionally neglected, and sometimes the problem lies in teaching methods. As well as difficulty in teaching basic essentials, there may be phenomena such as restlessness, hyperactivity, clumsiness (sometimes indicating minimal brain dysfunction), and fits of temper. Others have more specific difficulties with reading and arthimetic, including dylexia (the inability to read printed letters). The largest group, however, have had gaps at the earliest stage of development which then come to the surface in the form of difficulties at school. Early recognition of learning problems is exceedingly important.

Legionnaires disease. Infectious disease named after an outbreak during a reunion of veterans in the United States in 1976. The disease seems to be caused by a small rod-shaped bacterium (*Legionella pneumophila*) found throughout the world and which can survive well in lukewarm water. The bacteria were spread during the reunion by defective air-conditioning equipment. The illness begins with influenza-type symptoms for 2 to 4 days, with muscular pain and headache. This is followed by high fever up to 40⁰C and cold shivers. The patient is very ill and confused, coughs, is short of breath, sometimes vomits blood and has pains in the chest. Usually this is accompanied by intestinal complaints: nausea, vomiting and watery diarrhoea. Untreated, recovery usually occurs after 10 days, but the disease can also be fatal.

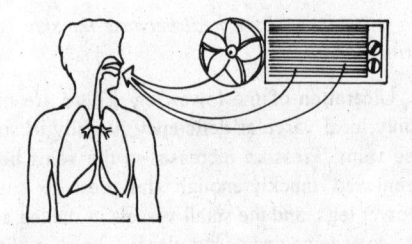

Legionnaires disease is infection with a micro-organism spread by watercooled air-conditioning systems, among other things.

Legs, different length. A common complaint, usually minimal and causing no discomfort, although if more than a centimetre is involved there may be back problems. If the deviation is greater still it causes abdominal slant combined with scoliosis (sideways curvature of the spine). The condition can be congenital, but is usually caused by a fracture, bone or joint inflammation, bone tumours or diseases that lead to damage to the cartilaginous plates during growth; congenital dislocation of the hip joint may also be involved.

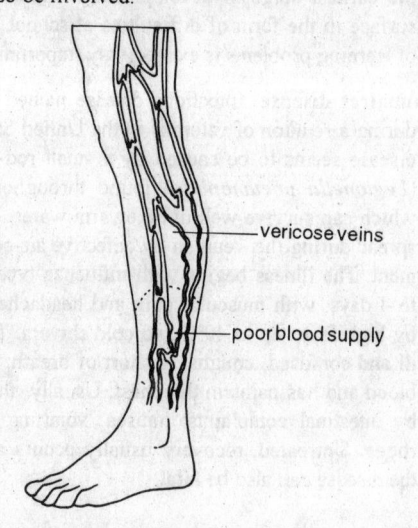

Often a leg ucler will not heal because the skin is poorly supplied with blood

Leg Ulcers. Ulceration of the lower leg. There are many causes, commonly local vascular deficiency, usually in sufferers from varicose veins. Pressure increases in the veins because blood is not removed quickly enough: this pressure causes oedema in the lower legs, and the small vessels in the leg are damaged, leading to eczema and/or leg ulcers. The skin of the lover leg receives insufficient oxygen, and skin cells are destroyed, causing an ulcer (sometimes tens of centimetres in size). Small cuts no longer heal and also form ulcers. The condition is treated with various ointments and bandages, and usually the patient is fitted with made-to-measure classic stockings; they should be worn all the time except when lying in bed with the leg raised.

Leishmaniasis. Infections disease caused by Leishmania donovani, spiral-shaped protozoan parasites which occur in the tropics and subtropics. In Western Europe leishmaniasis is an introduced disease. The parasite develops in the cells of blood-vessel walls and in tissue cells. A small bloodsucking mosquito transmits the parasite from infected people to healthy ones.

Lepsy. From Gr. lepsis=a taking hold, a seizure. Thus *epilepsy* is the outward sign of a seizure.

Leprosy. Infections disease caused by the *Mycobacterium leprae* bacillus. The disease, once known as Hansen's disease, occurs throughout almost the whole of the tropics and subtropics, and there are 15 million sufferers. Infection takes place via the skin and mucous membranes, by contact with infected persons who spread the bacteria by coughing, sneezing and nasal discharge. The chance of infection is increased by poor hygienic conditions and it is usually young people that are affected. Manifestations of the disease vary with the degree of resistance of the patient. The bacillus establishes itself in the skin and nerves in particular. Many cases of leprosy begin three to five years after infection with unusual sensations in certain parts of the body, which become lighter in colour than the rest of the skin. Often the disease confined to several small, clearly delineated areas of skin, and several small nerves are affected. Hair falls out and less sweat is produced in the affected areas. This form of leprosy heals spontaneously in a short time. In patients with reduced resistance the areas of skin are larger and more nerves are affected. The skin abnormalities can then consist of lumps, particularly on hands, feet and face. Finally, the bacteria can spread throughout the body. Mutilation is mainly the result of the affected nerves causing loss of hair and paralysis. The patient does not feel pain, which results in wounds and burns on hands and feet, which are then open to infection by various bacteria, which finally leads to malformation. Tingling and a dead feeling in hands and feet, twisted fingers or toes, ulcers on the palms of the hand and the soles of the feet are all manifestations of leprosy.

Leucoplakia. Local abnormal development of the mucous membrane of the mouth (hyperkeratosis), with a white-colouring. The cause is often long-term irritation of the mucous membrane at a particular point-by badly-fitting dentures or smoking, for example.

Leukemia. Form of cancer that originates in the white blood cells. There are various forms. The first distinction is made between acute and chronic leukaemia. A second subdivision depends on the type of white blood cell that has caused the condition. White blood cells can be divided into two kinds: those which play a part in aspecific immunity (granulocytes) and those which play a part in specific immunity (lymphocytes). The former five rise to myeloid leukaemia, and the latter to lymphatic leukaemia; each of these conditions can be acute or chronic.

The first symptoms of acute leukaemia are fatigue, headache, fever and a sore throat; sometimes the lymph nodes are somewhat swollen. These symptoms are like those of a normal, not too serious infectious disease or glandular fever. It is therefore necessary to prepare a blood smear, in which the white blood cells can be counted and examined. It this does not provide a clear picture, a lumbar puncture can be made to ascertain the number of white blood cells present in the spinal fluid.

Acute lymphatic leukaemia is most common in young children, and is the least serious form.

Generally speaking leukaemia is treated with drugs to inhibit cell division, according to the type being treated. Radiotherapy and bone-marrow transplants may also be prescribed.

Libido, loss of. Loss of desire for sex. It is in fact unclear how these desires come into being; they involve processes in a particular section of the brain, hormones and the nervous system.

Loss of sexual desire can be temporary or permanent. The cause is often difficult to divine. Fear of sex, dread of intimacy, stress, depression and resistance to the partner can all be involved. If the condition is permanent and oppressive, consultation with an expert in sexual matters can be helpful.

Lice. Insects that can infest the skin and hair. Lice occurs frequently throughout the world, and are particularly troublesome under conditions of poor hygiene. They regularly occur in schoolchildren in Western Europe, are resistant to low temperatures, but die quickly at temperatures above 50°C. There are various kinds of louse; the head louse (pediculus humanus capitis) is 2-3 mm long. It is found in the head and beard hair and lives on the host's blood. The female lays eggs 0.5-mm in size (nits), which stick to the hair; they are oval and easy to find.

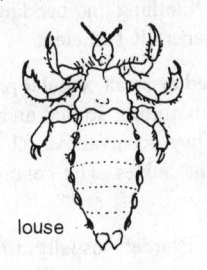

louse

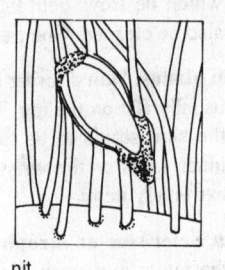

nit

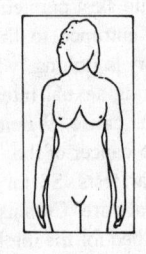

Head louse nits attach themselves to the hair and grow with it.

Lice live for about a month, during which they produce 100-150 nits. When they bite, saliva enters the wound, causing itchy lumps. The body louse (*Pediculus humanus corporis*) closely resembles the head louse, lives in clothing fibres, and can lay about 300 eggs in its lifetime. It is no longer prevalent in Britain.

The crab louse or pubic louse (*Phthirus pubis*) lives principally in the pubic hair, but can also be found in armpit hair, eyebrows and eyelashes. It has a lifespan of roughly one month, and lays 20-50 eggs.

Lice are dependent on the host, and die within a few days if they lose contact. An infested person rarely carries more than 20 lice. The most gradually becomes accustomed to them, and is hardly troubled by them. Lice can transmit diseases such as typhoid and trench fever.

Treatment is by use of an insecticidal lotion or shampoo, which destroys both lice and nits. Clothing and bedding must also be cleaned. One treatment is generally sufficient.

Lichen planus. Skin disorder characterized by small, angular pimples, usually flat on the top. They form in groups, so that an area of the skin seems to be thickened. They occur above all on the inner sides of the wrists and on the ankles. The condition is extremely itchy.

Lichen Sclerosus et atrophicus. Skin disorder usually affecting the vulva in women, but also the groin and anus. The skin of the labia is pale, white and thin. The skin pigment has disappeared locally and sometimes the entrance to the vagina is constricted. The principal discomfort is itching, which can be severe, and there may be pain during sexual intercourse and when urinating. There is no known cause. Women suffering from the condition are more prone to cancer of the vagina, and thus patients should undergo regular tests. So far no therapy has been found which provides a real cure. Creams containing corticosteroids are sometimes prescribed for the intolerable itching. A side effect is that fungus infections often occur. Sometimes subcutaneous injections of lidocaine can control the pain.

Ligament, damaged. Ligaments are the connecting tissue around a joint which largely determine the direction and degree of movement. Damage can result from moving a joint in an abnormal direction or farther than usual in a fall or accident. The damage may be restricted to stretching or slight tearing, or a sprain. In the case of dislocation there is usually tearing of one or more ligaments, causing pain and swelling. In the case of damage to a capsule there can also be bleeding into the joint.

Lipid. A fat. Lipid is generally used to designate a biochemical, whereas fat commonly refers to a substance that might be found in food. In fact, the two words are more or less interchangeable. They are organic compounds, insoluble in water but soluble in alcohol and some other substances. Lipids perform three vital functions in the body: the molecules form an energy store, they serve as cell membranes, the myelin wrappings for some nerves and some other kinds of linings and they are chemical precursors of many hormones.

Lipoma. Benign growth in the fatty tissue under the skin. The fatty tumour takes the shape of a resilient lump below the skin. If a lipoma is not treated, it can grow to a diameter of more than 10 cm and a weight of 1 kg or more. The reason for the formation of lipomas is unknown. In any event, there is no connection with greasy food. Lipomas occur just as frequenty in fat as in thin people. If someone with a lipoma is on a diet, the size of the fatty tumour will not decrease as a result. Lipomas can occur as a single lump or in larger numbers. Some people have some hundreds of lipomas distributed over their whole body. Lipomas practically never cause discomfort unless their site leads to problems such as clothes chafing on the fatty tissue. If discomfort nevertheless arises the growth can be reomved surgically. This is a small operation which some general practitioners carry out themselves. Larger lipomas are left to the surgeon, because there may be many blood vessels running through them. If a patient has a large number of lipomas, it is not feasible to remove all of them, and the surgeon therefore limits himself to those which inconvenience the patient.

Liver, tumour of. Form of cancer that affects the liver. In Africa liver cancer is common in regions where the people eat nuts covered with certain carcinogenic fungi (aflatoxin). In Europe products that might contain this substance (peanut butter, for example) are subject to strict controls. Symptoms of the disease are pain in the area of the liver, enlargement of the liver, loss of weight and general weakness. Suspicious above all is sudden worsening of a cirrhosis of the liver that has been in existence for some time.

Tests in several stages are used to diagnose the condition and to distinguish it from others such as tumours of the bile ducts or pancreas. Liver biopsy (if the tumour can be reached) can be the key; laparoscopy, examination of the abdomen with a special device, by which means a piece of liver tissue can also be removed, is another possibility. Blood tests often show increased liver enzyme production.

Treatment is often difficult because of the extent of the tumour; surgery can be attempted, or drugs to destroy cells (cytostatics) may be prescribed. As well as this cancer, which originates in the liver itself, metastasis frequently occurs in the liver from malignant tumours elsewhere in the body, often the intestine (cancer of the colon, cancer of the stomach), because all the blood from the intestines flows to the liver. Cancer of the genital organs or lungs can also spread to the liver by metastasis.

Liver Disorders. Disorders of the liver, the most important metabolic organ, can affect the whole body. The liver receives almost all the blood from the intestines via the portal vein, which means that foodstuffs absorbed in the intestine pass through the liver first. It plays a major role in the metabolism of sugars (including sugar storage), and in the conversion of amino acids, from which protein is built up. The liver gives out metabolic breakdown products (ammonia), and converts bilirubin, a breakdown product of the red blood cells, into a form in which it can be discharged via the gall bladder in the bile. Other functions are manufacture of coagulant factors, break down of hormones, cholesterol formation and the production of the bile acids, which aid the breakdown of fat in the intestine.

Liver fluke (fascioliasis) Infestation with a *Fasciola* flatworm 2-3 cm long, which lives as a parasite in sheep and cattle. Liver flukes occur throughout the world, but human beings are affected only from time to time. The worm lives in the bile ducts of the liver, where eggs are produced and passed out of the body via the faeces. The larvae emerge from the eggs in water, and develop before attaching themselves to plants which grow on river banks. If the plants are eaten, the liver fluke passes through the intestinal wall to the liver, where it develops into a fully-grown worm. Infestation in man can be caused by eating watercress. The worms cause inflammation of the bile duct, followed by constipation, resulting in pain, fever and jaundice, but infestation can also occur without symptoms. Treatment with drugs, lasting 10 days, is usually effective. It is advisable to avoid eating watercress in areas where liver flukes are prevalent.

Low blood pressure (hypotension) Blood pressure in which the upper value is lower than 90 mm of mercury, often accompanying shock:

A special form of low blood pressure is so-called orthostatic hypotension. If someone quickly stands up from a sitting or lying position, extra blood flows into the legs and lowers blood pressure in the brain for a few seconds, causing slight giddiness. The condition does not require treatment, but sufferers should take it into account when standing up.

Lung abscess. Accumulation of pus in lung tissue, which may have various causes; the condition is rare today. An abscess is a cavity in tissue filled with pus, usually caused by an inflammatory process resulting from bacterial infection. The cavity formed is encapsulated in tissue containing numerous inflammation cells. A lung abscess can result from closure of one of the smaller branches of the air passages by a tumour or foreign body that has gone down the wrong way and come to rest in the lung. Bacterial inflammation can develop in the tissue behind the closure. The normal immune mechanism brings about encapsulation of the inflammation, and an abscess is formed. Bacteria may also be carried to the lungs by the blood from a source of infection elsewhere in the body, thus causing an abscess in this way. Another possible source is tuberculosis. Tuberculosis bacteria may be inhaled and cause abscesses in the lungs; these are encapsulated, forming the caverns typical of tuberculosis. Lung abscesses irritate the lung and cause a ticklish cough. Sometimes the patient coughs up pus or blood, and there may be general symptoms such as fever and malaise.

Lung cancer (bronchial carcinoma) Malignant primary tumour in the lung. The commonest form of lung cancer originates in the air passages; this is bronchial carcinoma, of which the four commonest forms are pavement cell carcinoma (55 per cent), adenocarcinoma (4 per cent), large cell carcinoma (17 per cent) and small cell carcinoma (24 per cent), named after the cells affected. Atmospheric pollution and smoking are linked to all lung conditions, and lung tumours in particular. A direct connection has been shown between lung cancer and the smoking of cigarettes. Cigars and pipe tobacco are less harmful to the lungs because less smoke is inhaled; they do however cause cancers of the mouth and lips. Tobacco smoking became popular at the beginning of this century. The connection between smoking and lung cancer is linked directly to the number of cigarettes smoked and the length of time for which the person has smoked. If nobody smoked at all the occurrence of lung cancer would drop by 90 per cent.

Lupus erythematosus. Disease of which the cause is unknown; it usually affects young women, and men to a lesser extent. It involves inflammation reactions in all parts of the body. Inflammation is normally directed against bacteria or viruses which have penetrated the body. In lupus erythematosus it is directed against cells or parts of cells in the patient's body; it is therefore, classed as an autoimmune disease, but not all patients have auto-antibodies; thus autoimmunity is one, but not the only important factor.

The disease can affect any part of the body and symptoms depend on the area concerned. General symptoms include fever, fatigue and weight loss. Joints are often swollen and painful. A red rash can form on the palms of the hand and fingertips. A symptom specific to lupus erythematosus is a red rash on the cheeks and around the mouth, which can become more severe on exposure to sunlight. The disease is serious if it affects the heart, lungs or kidneys. The kidneys are affected in about half the patients, and they can eventually die as a result of reduced kidney function. Before diagnosis, blood tests are performed and a tissue biopsy may be taken for microscopic examination to establish lupus erythematosus inflammation symptoms.

Lymph. A clear body fluid very similar to blood minus all formed elements such as blood cells. Lymph is formed in and flows through a closed system of vessels called lymphatics. These vessels cover the entire body and are analogous to blood vessels. There is no pump like a heart in the lymph system, however, and therefore, no pressure.

Lymph assists in the distribution of nutrients, especially fats, after they are absorbed from the intestines. It plays a major role in the immune defence system, moreover, because it carries both the immunocompetent cells and the chemicals they synthesize. Some lymphocytes, one of the types of white blood cells, are formed in lymph nodes, parts of the lymphatics.

Lymphadenitis. Inflammation of a lymph node as a reaction to nearby infection, bacterial or viral. Inflammation of the lymph nodes is often associated with inflammation of the lymph ducts running from the infected areas to the node concerned; the inflamed ducts are visible as red stripes on the skin. If a lymph node is inflamed as a result of bacterial infection an abscess

may form, particularly in the groin or armpit. Generally the
inflammation disappears with the infection, although antibiotics are often prescribed in cases of bacterial infection. An abscess in a lymph node should always be lanced, under local or
general anaesthetic.

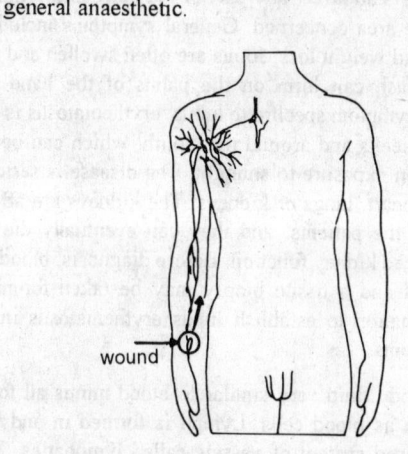

wound

Lymph nodes become inflamed if the local immune mechanisms
fail in the region of a wound.

Lymphangitis. Inflammation of a lymph vessel caused by inflection
in the area that it drains. The condition is sometimes incorrectly called blood poisoning, which term should only be used
if bacteria are present in the blood. Lymphangitis can occur
whenever there is bacterial infection of the skin, because bacteria can enter the lymph duct. Generally the condition is associated with lymphadenitis, because the bacteria are carried in
the lymph to lymph nodes in the area. The characteristic symptom is a painful, red stripe on the skin connecting the site of
the skin infection with the nearest large lymph nodes (in the
groin or armpit, for example). The condition heals spontaneously if the skin infection is treated effectively-by antibiotics,
for example.

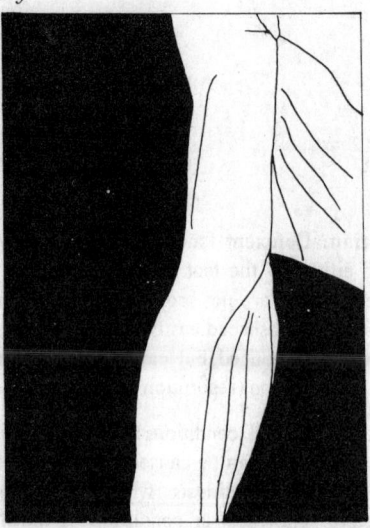

Inflamed lymph ducts in the arm after a wound has become infected.

Lymphogranuloma Venereum. Venereal disease caused by the chlamydia organism, which probably penetrates the skin or mucous membrane during sexual contact. The disease is most common in the tropics, but is not unknown in Europe. In women there are often no symptoms; in men there is a fever ten days after infection, pain in the joints, and a pustule at the point at which the virus penetrated. The pustule usually disappears spontaneously, but after 1 to 3 weeks pus forms in the lymph nodes of the groin causing an abscess.

Diagnosis is by several blood tests and examination of samples of skin and lymph node tissue. If the disease is untreated tumours can appear around the anus, and in women on the labia and clitoris. Treatment is usually with antibiotics.

M

Malabsorption. Deficient food absorption by the intestinal wall, caused either by the fact that large protein, fat and carbohydrate molecules are not broken down into smaller components which can be absorbed easily (maldigestion), or that the components are produced but cannot pass through the intestinal mucous membrane (resorption deficiency.

Many intestinal conditions can lead to malabsorption. Digestive disorders can be caused by conditions of lthe pancreas (such as mucoviscidosis, with a characteristic shortage of pancreatic enzymes) or conditions of the liver or bile ducts (shortage of bile salts).

Resorption difficulties can be caused by surgical removal of a large section of the small intestine, damage to the mucous membrane (by thrush, for example) or inflammation such as Crohn's disease, or by parasites or bacteria, malignant diseases, reduced intestinal blood supply, lymph supply disorders, and various others.

Malaria. Infectious disease caused by *Plasmodium* parasites, transmitted by an *Anopheles* mosquito bite. The mosquito sucks blood from an infected person and tansmits the disease by biting a healthy person. The parasites enter the liver, grow, divide and break up in order to spread. The particles then enter the bloodstream and penetrate the red blood corpuscles, where they develop as small parasites able to affect other red corpuscles.

The parasites develop and are all released from the red blood corpuscles at the same time. This simultaneous release of parasites and their waste products produces produces periodic high fever, preceded by cold shivers. Sometimes the parasites remain in the liver for years, which can result in recurrent attacks of the disease.

There are various kinds of malaria. In malaria caused by *Plasmodium vivax* and *P. ovale*, the patient has fever, with peaks every 48 hours. Malaria caused by *Plasmodium malariae* is characterized by peaks of fever every 72 hours. This clinical picture is rare is Western Europe.

Malaria caused by *Plasmodium falciparum* is the most serious form. Fever is irregular. The red corpuscles containing parasites can block the blood supply to zarious organs, causing death. This form of malaria is sometimes introduced from tropical Africa.

An attack of malaria begins usually with headache, muscular pain, loss of appetite, and sometimes vomiting and diarrhoea. Anaemia can occur because the parasites destroy red blood cells. Not all infected patients become ill; those who do not are carriers of the disease. The number of parasites, their size and the patient's resistance are among factors influencing whether the patient becomes ill or not. Infection can be identified by the presence of larvae or eggs in the faeces. Clinical pictures vary considerably and depend on the parasite concerned. Drug treatment is the usual therapy.

Mallet Finger. Condition in which the topmost finger bone is bent towards the palm of the hand and cannot be aligned with the other bones, caused by tearing of the upper finger tendon by an excessively violent movement of the topmost joint. This often happens in sports such as volleyball when the ball strikes the fingers awkwardly.

Malpresentation. Presentation in which the baby's head is not in or above the entrance to the birth canal after the 32nd week of pregnancy. Presentation is affected by various factors connected with the movements of the foetus and the space available for them. Freedom of movement usually declines after the 32nd week, when a definite position is taken up. The commonest presentation is head presentation (96 per cent), with the baby's

head in or at the entrance to the birth canal. Other presenta-
tions are breech presentation (3.5 per cent) and transverse presentation (0.5 per cent). The baby has a lot of space in cases
of hydramnios (excess amniotic fluid) and slack abdominal
wall, often present after several pregnancies. The baby's position is not stable, and presentation can change at any stage in
the pregnancy.

Mania. Mood which is far more agitated than can be explained by
the circumstances. Genuine mania is a psychosis in which the
sense of self is raised and the motor system accelerated. Self-
criticism and control over reality are disturbed. Mania can be
an element in manic-depressive psychosis or schizophrenia,
but it can also be an independent clinical picture, resulting
from poisoning, or brain disorders such as inflammation and
tumours, or general disorders such as hyperthyroidism. A less
marked form mania is hypomania in which the control of reality is not so disturbed and the patient can still function in a
normal environment. Hypomania or a manic condition can be a
reaction to a particularly pleasing event, or also to something
upleasant: the mania may then serve to mask depression. For
this reason mania often includes fits of weeping.

Manic-depressive psychosis. Clinical picture characterized by repeated periods of mania and depression often occurring within
a family. In the clearest form depressive and manic periods
alternate, with relatively normal periods between them. In other
cases the patient simply undergoes periods of depression, generally associated with physical symptoms and delusions. The
disease is probably rooted in heredity, but a particular event
may set off an attach. Treatment is by medication.

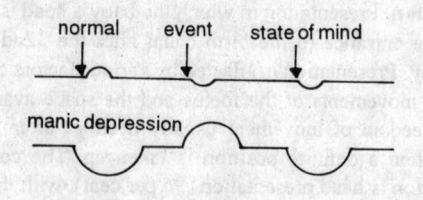

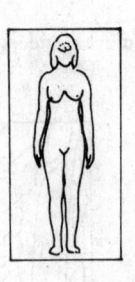

In manic depression the patient's state of mind varies wildly without any particular cause.

Mast Cell. A type of cell defined by its microscopic characteristics found in connective tissue throughout the body and especially in association with *inflammation*. Mast cells synthesize chemicals such as histamine which play a role in the natural immune responses.

Mastitis. Inflammation of the breast. A disorder mainly of mothers breast-feeding their children, it occurs in about 1 per cent of mothers of newly-born infants usually in the second week after the birth. A painful place appears in one of the breasts, associated with high fever and sometimes cold shivers. The cause is usually a bacterium which has entered through a crack in a nipple. Hospitals in particular may house bacteria that have become resistant to antibiotics. If the inflammation does not subside quickly an abscess may occur, which could spread to the armpit, or could break out through the skin or the mammary ducts. Treatment consists of making sure that the breast is thoroughly emptied after each feeding: bacteria grow well in milk. An icepack can give relief. Nipples and any cracks should be thoroughly cleaned. Antibiotics may be administered, particularly if there are cold shivers. If an abscess occurs. It must be allowed to develop and is then lanced under anaesthetic. A bacterial culture may be prepared. Mastitis can be prevented by cleaning the breasts thoroughly after each feeding, touching and holding the body only with clean hands, avoiding nipple cracks and preventing congestion. Nipple caps can be of use.

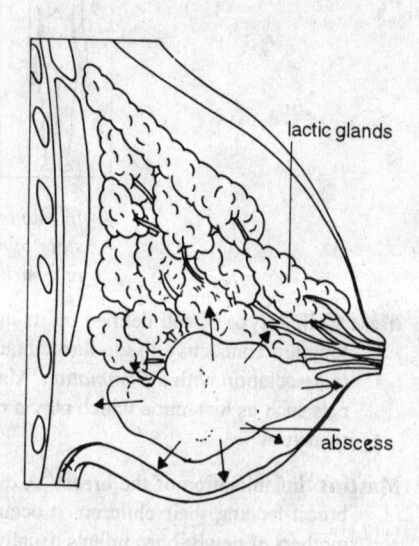

lactic glands

abscess

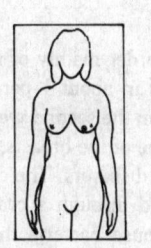

Inflammation of a breast (mastitis) can lead to a breast abscess.

Mastoiditis. Infection of the small chambers containing air in the mastoid bones, which can be felt as bumps behind the ears. The bone contains small cavities lined with mucous membrane and connected with the middle ear. In cases of acute otitis media (inflammation of the middle ear the mucous membrane of these cells is always painful; this is noticeable as pressure pain behind the ear. If the connection between mastoid and middle ear is closed, pus accumulates in the cavities and the bone also becomes inflamed. This condition is known as acute mastoiditis, and it should be suspected if the ear is not dry four weeks after acute otitis, or if swelling occurs behind the ear, associated with severe pressure pain and excessive protrusion of the ear. Other symptoms resemble those of acute inflammation of the middle ear: earache and fever. Undiscovered mastoiditis can sustain otitis, and cause glue ear.

In the early stages the inflammation can sometimes still be treated with antibiotics. Later it is usually necessary to operate: an incision is made behind the ear, and the diseased cells and pus removed.

Mastopathy. Sensitive and painful breasts, in which sometimes small lumps can be felt. It is a common complaint just before menstruation, and even more common in early pregnancy. The condition does not occur after the menopause.

The glandular tissue of the breasts is affected by the sexual hormone cycle; oestrogen in particular causes swelling, which can close the glandular tubules and bring about the formation of cysts, which are felt as lumps and are often painful. Mastopathy declines when menstruation is well under way. The disorder often occurs in both breasts. The lumps are filled with clear fluid and may be transparent under a lamp. After menopause a persistent lump is much more likely to be breast cancer, and for this reason any lump in the breast must be investigated further.

Measles. Infectious viral infection classified as a children's disease. The incubation period is one to two weeks.

The first signs of measles are general malaise, high fever, cold in the nose, inflamed eyes (conjunctivitis) and a dry irritable cough. There are often white patches on the mucous membrane on the inside of the cheek (Koplik's spots). This is the most infectious stage. After three days the temperature drops, and rough round or oval red patches appear behind the ears and on the rest of the body; they run together after one or two days. The child feels very unwell; the irritable cough is tiring, and the inflamed eyes are sensitive to light. There is no specific treatment for measles. Drugs to reduce fever and soothe a cough are useful, and the child should stay in bed. A shady room is recommended for the sensitive eyes. Since the introduction of immunization against measles, the disease is becoming rarer or much milder in form.

Meckel's Diverticulum. Congenital intestinal protrusion, more common in men than women. It consists of a remaining fragment of the connection between the navel and intestine. The protrusion occurs on the final section of the small intestine, before the junction with the colon. The condition is usually unnoticed, and generally causes no discomfort. If there is discomfort it is probably the result of strands connected to the diverticulum: tangling, ileus, intestinal volvulus or intussusception. Discomfort can also be caused by the presence of gastric mucous membrane in the diverticulum, which can be affected by a stomach ulcer. Symptoms of stomach ulcer around the navel which do not react to antacids or the consumption of food can indicate ulcer formation in the diverticulum. If Meckel's diverticulum is causing problems of this kind, it can be removed by surgery.

Meconium, breathing in. Aspiration of the waste products produced by the foetus in the womb. Meconium is the first waste product excreted by a new-born child. It is a greenish-black, viscous, sticky substance which lightens after three days and becomes normal faeces. Aspiration occurs if the baby starts to breathe too soon because it is suffering from oxygen shortage (asphyxia) in the womb. At the same time meconium is discharged, making the amniotic fluid green rather than colourless. Amniotic fluid containing meconium is a danger signal; if it is combined with an irregular heartbeat, labour should be induced rapidly. Symptoms in the new-born child depend on the severity of the asphyxia.

Melaena (blood in the faeces) Blood lost higher up the alimentary canal is partly digested, and appears in the faeces as a black discoloration (melaena). Bright blood is passed in disorders of the rectum and anus. Blood in the faeces may be caused by a number of different conditions. In the first place irksome but essentially harmless conditions of the anus cause loss of blood; they include haemorrhoids, anal fissure and sometimes anal fistula. Inflammation in this area (rectal inflammation) can also cause loss of blood, as can rectal tumours, both benigh (intestinal policy) and malignant (intestinal cancer). Further symptoms are partly related to the cause. Inflammation causes diarrhoea and mucus production, as well as loss of blood. Malignant tumours alter the pattern of defecation, causing mainly constipation. sometimes alternating with diarrhoea. Fissures and haemorrhoids can cause constipation because defecation is painful. It is thus necessary that extensive examination should be carried out if blood is passed in the faeces (particularly in the case of older people), to exclude the possibility of a malignant tumour. The anus should be inspected for fissures and haemorrhoids; a tumour low in the rectum can be felt with a finger. Further examination can be by rectoscopy, coloscopy, or contrast X-ray. Treatment depends on the cause.

Melanoma. The most malignant and least common form of skin cancer, accounting for about 3 per cent of cases. In melanoma the pigment cells of the skin become cancer cells; it the cells continue to make pigment, the cancer is dark-brown to black, but remains pale pink if they lose their pigment-forming capability.

Melanoma usually begins as a birth mark, which starts to grow and itch. Because the normal structure of the skin is attacked by cancer cells, haemorrhage gradually sets in; any birthmark that grows, itches, stings or bleeds should be examined by a doctor. The only sure diagnosis is by microscopic examinatin of the skin disorder. The chance of recovery depends on the point at which treatment can be started. If the tumour is restricted to the skin, the prognosis is good; but if the cancer has penetrated to a greater depth, the treatment is less likely to succeed.

Meniere's disease. Severe attacks of vertigo, usually associated with nausea and vomiting. The disease is prevalent in middle-aged men. The cause is thought to be accumulation of fluid in the semicircular canals of the inner ear; it is not known why the fluid is produced.

Meningioma. Brain tumour originating in the meningeal membranes surrounding the brain. Meningiomas are benign, grow very slowly and do not always cause discomfort. They are encapsulated, which means that complete removal by surgery is usually possible. Problems are sometimes caused during the operation because the tumour is very vascular, and haemorrhage can occur.

Meningitis. Inflammation of the membrane surrounding the brain, usually caused by viruses or bacteria, sometimes however, by a fungus or parasites. The condition often occurs rapidly, after influenza, otitis or pharyngitis. After some days the patient complains of headache and fever, often with nausea and vomiting; consciousness is sometimes lowered. Irritation of the membranes causes a stiff neck. In babies the condition

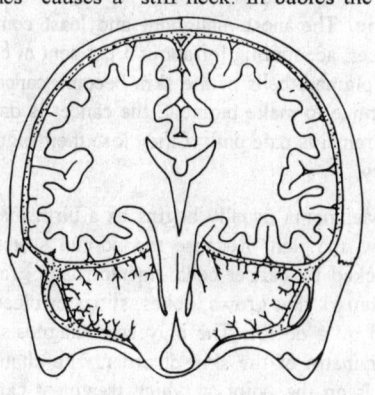

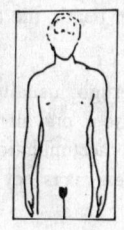

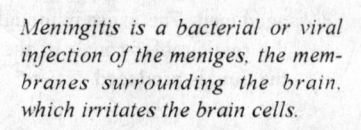

Meningitis is a bacterial or viral infection of the meniges, the membranes surrounding the brain, which irritates the brain cells.

shows in general malaise and nausea and a fontanel which is tense to the touch. Meningeal irritation results in pain if the child's legs are manipulated.

The most notorious bacterium is the highly infectious meninogococcus *Neisseria meningitidis*.

Menopause (change of life) Period of gradual decrease in ovulation and cessation of menstruation, making the approaching end of a woman's reproductive period. Decreased sex hormone production affects women in various ways. The so-called climacteric is the period after the last menstruation, in which certain specific changes also occur. The menopause usually occurs between the age of 46 and 52 . Poor health and nutrition can cause it to begin sooner. Women who had an early first menstruation (menarche) usually have a late menopause; this is linked with high oestrogen production. Some phenomena associated with the menopause can be treated medically. Even before the menopause, menstruation becomes less regular and sometimes heavier (as in puberty) as a result of reduced hormonal function in the ovaries. This can cause anaemia which must be controlled. Hot flushes may occur, possibly a number of times in a given hour; if they occur at night, they can cause chronic lack of sleep and fatigue. In such cases hormonal therapy may be considered. Reduced female sex hormone production reduces the size of the internal sex organs, and the mucous membrane of the vagina becomes dry. The entrance to the vagina may also be reduced in size causing painful sexual intercourse (dyspareunia). In this case oestrogen creams can be useful.

Changes also occur at the emotional level such as headache, depression, dizziness and sleeping problems. These symptoms cannot be treated with hormones, and are more likely to occur in patients already prone to depression. Research in various cultures has shown that these problems hardly occur in women who perform a vigorous social function. Most Western countries have groups that can be attended by women during this period; they have proved very valuable.

After the menopause atherosclerosis, coronary conditions
(coronary thrombosis), cystitis, osteoporosis and changes in
skin and hair occur more frequently, as a result of hormonal
changes. Most of them should be treated by a doctor. In
general it can be said that symptoms increase in direct relationship to the speed of the hormonal changes. Complaints
should always be taken seriously, and good preparation is most
helpful. In some cases hormones can make the changes more
gradual. Many women feel less isolated in this period if they
are able to talk to others with the same problems.

Menstruation, excessive (menorrhagia) Excessive menstrual flow,
generally an individual concept. Doctors consider the flow excessive if it causes anaemia of which it is the commonest
cause in women. There are various reasons for heavy men-

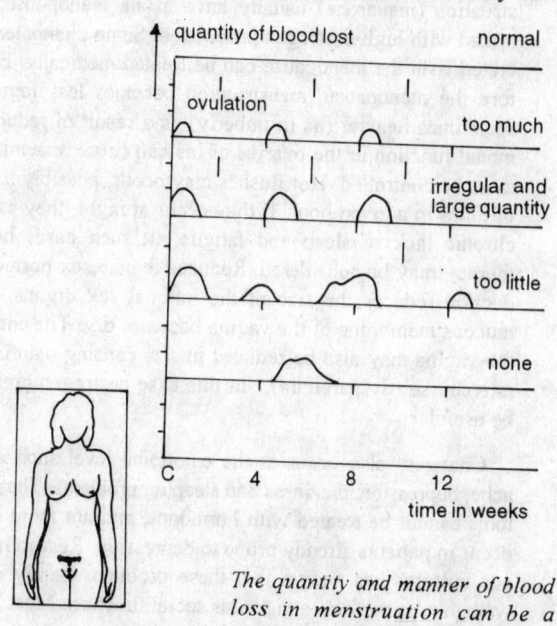

*The quantity and manner of blood
loss in menstruation can be a
pointer to a number of disorders*

struation; it often occurs in young girls is in whom the menstrual pattern is not yet fixed, and in older women near the menopause. The sex hormone level in the blood is not high enough to maintain the balance between build-up and breakdown of the uterine mucous membrane. Uterine myoma, endometriosis and a fixed retroverted womb can cause the womb to be unable to contract during menstruation, leading to excessive blood loss. Overtiredness can also reduce uterine contraction; if the overtiredness is associated with anaemia. It can lead to a vicious circle. Rarer causes are coagulation problems, thyroid hormone deficiencies, congenital abnormalities of the womb, inflammation of the endometrium or polyps. Anaemia is treated in the first place, and uterine contraction can be stimulated with ergotamine tablets. If this is ineffective, a curettage can be performed, which can assist diagnosis and is in itself a treatment.

Menstruation, irregular (metrorrhagia) Menstrual bleeding that does not conform to a regular pattern. A natural process like menstruation will not always occur precisely every 28 days; a cycle which varies between 24 and 34 days is still considered regular. Irregular and often heavy menstruation frequently occurs in young girls because the ovaries are not mature enough to produce adequate hormones to ensure a genuine menstrual cycle. These symptoms disappear in time. The cycle often becomes irregular towards the end of the reproductive period (menopause) as the ovaries are gradually losing their function. The cycle can seem irregular if a little bleeding occurs at the time of ovulation. Irregular menstruation can be caused in various ways. The reason is often disturbed hormonal balance or a disorder of the ovaries. Blood and urine hormone tests can be carried out, a curettage made and the ovaries examined by sonography.

Treatment depends on the nature of the condition. Ovulation can sometimes be induced by drugs; treatment is usually carried out by a gynaecologist.

Menstruation, lack of (amenorrhoea) A symptom, not a disease.

The commonest cause in adults is pregnancy. Primary amenorrhoea is the condition in which a 16-year-old girl has not yet menstruated; in an adult woman the term secondary amenorrhoea is used if menstruation has not occurred for three months, or for six months after ceasing to take the contraceptive pill.

Menstruation, painful (dysmenorrhoea) More than usual menstrual pain, primary if it occurs immediately after first menstruation, and secondary if based on a gynaecological abnormality such as a uterine polyp, endometriosis or closure of the mouth of the womb. In 80 per cent of cases the disorder is primary. Pain usually begins a few hours before menstriation, and persists for one to two days. It is sited in the lower abdomen, like colic, and often associated with premenstrual tension, nausea, vomiting and diarrhoea. The pain often radiated to the vagina and the upper part of the legs. Dysmenorrhoea sometimes disappears after a first child is born. The cause is usually a high prostaglandin level, a substance secreted in all kinds of inflammation reactions.

Treatment can be with aspirin if the pain is moderate, or prostaglandin inhibitors if the pain is severe. These drugs probably have side-effects, and so it is sometimes better to inhibit ovulation, by means of a specially formulated contraceptive pill. Women not wishing to use drugs can by domestic remedies such as warm baths, a hot-water bottle on the back and a warm bath for the feet. Acupuncture sometimes has good results, and can be tried for primary dysmenorrhoea.

Mental deficiency. Mental condition involving a less-than-average IQ. The mental age of an adult mental deficient is comparable with that of a child of 8 to 12 years old. A mentally deficient child cannot cope with normal teaching, and has to be placed in a special school. In this way he or she can be encouraged to develop, and occupy a more or less independent place in society. Children of this kind demand a great deal of attention and control, however, and parents must be aware of the danger that as a result their other children may not receive enough attention.

Mental retardation. Condition in which a person has failed to attain the intelligence quotient (IQ) range appropriate for his or her age.

Symptoms vary from slightly disturbed to mentally defective. There are many causes: hereditary disorders, infection before and after birth, nutritional deficiency, (including iodine and vitamin dificiency), lack of oxygen in the brain (anoxia), and injuries. Environmental factors such as education, physical and mental neglect (affective deficiencies) can also be significant. Often the cause cannot be found, and the symptoms are not always immediately perceptible, so that all too often slight deficiencies are only discovered and dealt with when it is too late. Precise monitoring of the development of babies and young children is important: motor backwardness is often a sign of mental problems. If physical abnormalities are discovered an impression of the degree of backwardness can be gained from IQ and other psychological tests. Support and advice from those around them are important to the parents of a backward child. Placing the child in a home is often difficult, but necessary for child and family.

Metabolic disorders. Disorders caused by defects in the body's metabolism, often due to a deficiency of a dietary factor or an enzyme. Enzymes are necessary for the normal function of the body's numerous metabolic processes; they ensure that the level of metabolic products is not too high by converting them to simple, harmless products or to substances which can easily be excreted via the liver or the kidneys. Because specific enzymes are necessary for each chemical conversion, it follows that shortage of even one enzyme can cause an accumulation of certain materials. Various organs are affected, according to whether the disturbances concern the conversion of amino acids, carbodydrates or fats. Phenylketonuria is the best-known example of an inborn error of metabolism.

Metabolism. The word may mean the total chemical activity of an organism at any one time, but it more often means the chemical processes by which food is converted to energy, body tissue and waste.

The phrase, basal metabolism, means the chemical activity of the organism, at rest; that is not doing work, but not asleep. It may be measured by calculating the amount of oxygen being inhaled and the amount of carbon dioxide being exhaled. Basal metabolism may be affected inherited characteristics, but it also depends on diet, weight and general health.

Migraine. Severe headache involving attacks of pain, usually in one side of the head, nausea and vomiting. The pain is caused by narrowing of the blood vessels inside and outside the skull, followed by dilation, for reasons which are either hormonal, allergic or unknown. Migraine can occur in childhood, but usually begins at puberty; it often runs in families. Attacks usually happen during rest periods (weekend holidays) or, in women, around the time of menstruation. Stress, smoking and alcohol also have an effect. Women often find that migraine attacks subside during pregnancy or after the menopause.

Narrowing of the blood vessels causes the attack to begin with a tight feeling on one side of the head. At the same time the blood supply to one half of the brain is disturbed, causing symptoms in the other side of the body, such as tingling in the arm or leg. In rare cases temporary paralysis or aphasia occurs. After about 20 minutes the constricted veins dilate, and a pounding headache begins rapidly, finally leading to nausea and vomiting. A substantial number of patients experience only the headache, and not the symptoms associated with constriction of the blood vessels. A regular regime is essential if attacks are to be prevented. Medical treatment is directed mainly at preventing attacks, but there are drugs which can be given during them.

Milia. Small creamy-white spots on the skin, usually on the nose and face, often seen in newborn babies. They are caused by an accumulation of sebum (grease) under the skin because the sebaceous glands are still closed. The condition is harmless, and the spots disappear spontaneously.

Milk excess. Milk production goes into full swing in the first few days after a baby's birth. The baby does not imtially take all the milk, however, and in consequence too much is left in the breast. Accumulation of milk can also occur later on during breast feeding. The woman experiences a full, tight, sometimes painful feeling in one or both breasts. Hard places in the breast indicate swellings of the lactiferous glands. The symptoms are usually reduced by beginning each feed with the breast containing more milk, and allowing the baby to suck from this breast until it is completely empty. Slight massage with extended fingers towards the nipple helps to empty the breast. Care must be taken over hygiene because there is a greater risk of mastitis when milk has accumulated there

Minimal brain dysfunction. Term used to describe poor educational performance. The name is controversial, because it suggests a brain disorder, which has not yet been shown to be so. In most cases there is no known cause.

There is no simple medical solution to the problem; parents, doctors, psychologists and teachers have to work together. The development of this pattern of behaviour is highly dependent on the attitude to the child, and the possibility of finding a suitable form of education. The prognosis is favourable in many cases; symptoms usually decline after puberty.

Miscarriage. Spontaneous abortion before the 16th week of pregnancy. The birth of an immature baby incapable of sustaining life after the 16th week is sometimes also inaccurately called a miscarriage; in a true miscarriage the foetus, the placenta (which is still forming) and associated membranes are all expelled at once. After the 16th week, foetus and placenta are usually expelled separately, as in a normal birth.

About 10 per cent of all pregnancies end in miscarriage. Even after several miscarriages the cause almost always lies with the foetus, very rarely with the mother. The notion that sexual intercourse during pregnancy can cause a miscarriage is unfounded for the same reason.

Mitral valve defects. The mitral valve is between the left atrium and left ventricle of the heart; it can become constricted (stenosis), or leak (insufficiency). Mitral stenosis is caused by inflammation of the valve in rheumatic fever; over the years scar tissue forms in the valve, causig constriction. As a result the left atrium has difficulty in pumping blood from the lungs into the left ventricle, so that the lungs become excessively full of blood, resulting in shortness of breath, coughing and cyanosis. Tension on the wall of the right atrium can cause atrial fibrillation. Mitral valve stenosis is treated by medication to stimulate correct heart function; in severe cases the valve can be replaced by an artificial one.

Molluscum contagiosum. Contagious virus infection of the skin, characterized by small blobs with a central indentation from which a porridge-like substance can be expressed. The condition sometimes occurs as small-scale epidemics among school-children. The skin abnormality is usually on the buttocks or arms, and can spread all over the body. It can occur in adults, usually on a lesser scale; if a single blob occurs in an adult it can be theateningly like a basilioma, a form of skin cancer. Molluscum contagiosum clears up spontaneously after a few months; if the parents are not prepared to wait, the spots can be removed by a dermatologist.

Morning sickness (hyperemesis gravidarum) Vomiting during pregnancy, sometimes preventing food being taken and causing acidosis. Morning sickness and vomiting occur in the first three months in 50 per cent of pregnancies. Nausea is experienced upon waking. After vomiting, the woman feels better remarkably quickly and is able to eat. As a rule the vomit consists only of gastric mucus and bile. Frequent meals, five or six a day, with large amounts of carbohydrates and only a little fat, often appear to help. A serious form of vomiting during pregnancy occurs if vomiting continues after three months and no fluid or food at all can be kept down. The woman grows thin and is in danger of dehydration. She should be admitted to hospital in order for the liquid deficiency to be made good.

Removing the woman from her familiar surroundings often also has a positive effect. This supports the idea that psychological influences play a part in causing excessive vomiting during pregnancy.

Motion sickness (travel sickness) Symptoms occur as a result of prolonged and perhaps violent movement of a kind to which one is unaccustomed, as in a bus, car, boat or aircraft. The cause is overstimulation of the organ of balance, and confusion because the organ receives unusual information from the other organs necessary in keeping one's balance: eyes joints and muscles. This results in dizziness, nausea, often vomiting and sweating. Not everybody suffers to the same extent: the symptoms can be increased by apprehension or fear. Habit usually causes the symptoms to diminish,. only two per cent of people never become accustomed to a particular unusual movement. Habituation diminishes after the movement stops, however, so that motion sickness can recur. Also becoming accustomed to one movement does not necessarily enable one to cope with others.

The best way to control motion sickness is by prevention. Many preparations are available from chemists; they can prevent nausea, but may make the patient sleepy, so they must not be used by car drivers. There are also plasters available containing a motion sickness remedy; wearing the plaster behind the ear gives protection against motion sickness for a few days.

Motor neurone disease. Fairly rare condition of unknown cause, although a hereditary influence can be detected in some cases. It revolves degeneration of motor nerves, affecting the nerve sheaths running from the cerebral cortex to the spinal cord grey matter and the anterior horn cells in the spinal cord.

Early symptoms are muscular weakness, wasting of the muscles in one of the limbs sometimes in the face or throat. This can end in paralysis. Irritation of the motor nerve cells in

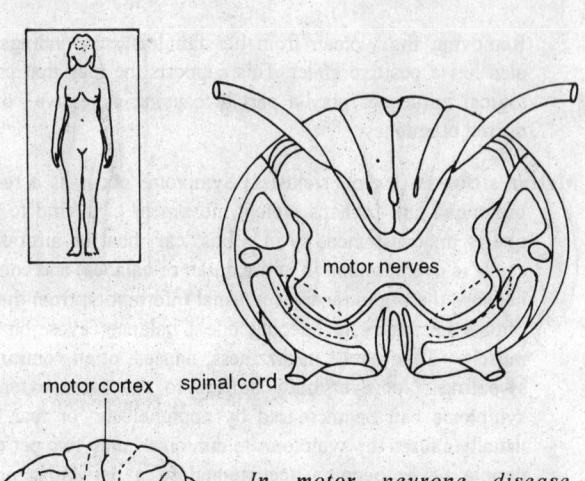

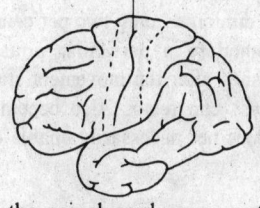

motor cortex   spinal cord

In motor neurone disease (amyotrophic lateral sclerosis) the motor neurones in the cerebral cortex and spinal cord fail, causing paralysis

the spinal cord grey matter causes small muscular convulsions, together with increasing clumsiness and difficulty in walking and then general paralysis of almost all muscles. The patient dies of paralysis of the respiratory muscles, or pneumonia caused by choking. There is no effective treatment. Physiotherapy may beneficial.

Mouth ulcers (aphthous ulcers) Small, superficial ulcers in the mucous membrane of the mouth, occurring above all on the inside of the lips and the tongue. They are yellowish-white, with a red, inflamed edge. Eating is difficult, because they can be very painful. They often clear up spontaneously after a time, but can unfortunately recur. The cause is not known, and no effective treatment has so far been developed. Easing the pain is a possibility. Stomatitis herpetica is a similar condition, common in children who have been in contact with the herpes simplex virus; as well as the usual cold sores on the lips, ulcers develop in the mouth, less obvious than the mouth ulcers under discussion, but spreading throughout the mouth.

Fever is often associated with this condition, and even though the cause is known, there is still no treatment. If the virus returns it produces cold sores but no ulcers.

Mucous. mucus. The former is an adjective referring to mucus, a noun. The most common use of mucous is to describe the membrane consisting in part of cells that secrete mucus.

Mucus is a clear, viscous fluid consisting of lipids, some minerals and dead cells from the membrane where it has been formed. It acts as a protective barrier, for example, in the lining of the nose, and as a lubricant as in the intestines.

Multiple sclerosis. Neurological disorder associated with the damage to nerve tissue in the brain and spinal column; the cause is unknown. Multiple sclerosis (MS) causes widespread foci of inflammation in the myelin sheath of a nerve; the insulating material around the nerve tracts is broken down, with the result that impulses can no longer be transmitted. Damaged material is replaced with scar tissue. The first symptoms often occur unannounced, and disappear completely within a few weeks or months. The situation is then repeated the symptoms are renewed, but on each occasion they leave residual symptoms behind. Tension and fatigue can worsen the condition.

Multiple sclerosis sometimes develops so slowly that the patient remains relatively active for several decades; on the other hand there are cases in which brain tissue breaks down so rapidly that death occurs within weeks.

Mumps (parotitis) Infectious disease of the salivary glands caused by a virus. The illness occurs worldwide, mainly in children in their fifth to ninth year, but also in young adults (in barracks, for example), and above all in the winter and spring. About a third of sufferers undergo no discomfort. By the age of 20 about 60 per cent of the population has had mumps.

Infection occurs through the air or direct contact with saliva.

A patient is infectious to those around him five days before symptoms appear until about nine days afterwards. The mumps virus causes infection of the air passages, where it multiplies, and is conveyed in the bloodstream to the salivary glands and organs such as the brain and reproductive organs.

Two to three weeks infection the illness begins with high fever and pain when chewing. The salivary glands on one side swell, and other glands swell a few days later. The swelling is painful, particularly when the mouth is opened. Sometimes the salivary glands on the other side of the face swell as well. Most patients suffer from headaches.

Swelling of the salivary glands subsides after about a week and disappears completely after three weeks. Mumps is usually harmless in children, and generally clears up without persisting symptoms. In young adult males there is an increased possibility of inflammation of the testicles (orchitis). One testicle swells painfully, and sometimes the other testicle can be affected as well. This complication is practically always completely cured, seldom resulting in sterility. The mumps virus sometimes also causes meningitis or pancreatitis.

Infection with mumps results in immunity to the virus; it is a disease which you have only once. It can be prevented by immunization, but this is rarely used. Treatment is by controlling the pain and a liquid diet. There is no medication effective against the mumps virus itself. In the case of orchitis, corticosteroids can be used to limit the possibility of irreparable damage.

Muscular disorders. Muscular dystrophy is a hereditary muscular disease characterized by the breakdown of muscular tissue. Myositis can be caused by abnmormalities of the body's defence system (polymyositis and dermatomyositis). Muscular disorders can also be caused by conditions of the nervous system. In myasthenia gravis the junction of nerve and muscle is affected. Myotonia is a muscular condition associated with delayed muscuclar relaxation. In congenital myotonia, usually menifesting itself in childhood, the eyes cannot be opened when they are tightly shut, and the hand is not released when grasped. Myatonia atrophicans begins between the ages of 20 and 30; as well as the above-mentioned characteristics muscular tissue decay also sets in, particularly in the lower arms, neck and face. Both forms of the disease are hereditary. The congenital form usually runs a favourable course, and may clear up spontaneously in later life; myatonia atrophicans progresses slowly and can cause invalidity. Certain metabolic disorders also cause symptoms of muscular disease, then known as metabolic muscular disease. For example muscular weakness or even muscular decay can result from an excess of thyroid hormone or crotricosteroids in the blood. Low blood potassium content is also associated with muscular weakness.

Muscular dystrophy. Condition in which muscular fibre gradually degenerates; the muscles weaken, and deposits of fat can cause them to swell. There are various forms of muscular dystrophy, all of which are hereditary and have no known treatment. There are three principal categories. In the pseudo-hypertrophic form (Duchenne type) calf and underarm muscles are enlarged, and there is weakness in upper and lower limb muscles; the disease begins before the age of three, and affects mainly boys. Patients have difficulty with walking and climbing steps. The disease causes a high degree of invalidity. The

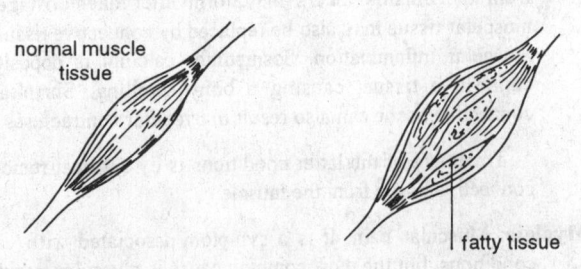

normal muscle tissue

fatty tissue

In muscular dystrophy a muscle looks well developed because of the presence of fatty tissue. In fact it is much weaker than normal.

limb girdle variety begins between the ages of 10 and 30, and is equally common in men and women. Muscles are seldom enlarged, but this form too causes severe invalidity in the course of years.The third group is the facioscapulohumeral variety (Landouzy-Dejerine type); it can begin at any age. Eyelids, droop and the upper lip may also protrurde: later shoulder muscles are affected and possibly limb-girdle muscles. This variety of the disease develops slowly, and most patients can lead normal life.

Muscular tumours. Abnormal growth of muscular tissue. The best-known is a uterine myoma (fibroid). Myoblastoma is also benign: this is a round tumour which can occur in the tongue or under the skin. Treatment, if desirable, is by surgical removal of the tumour.Rhabdomyosarcoma is a rare but highly malignant muscular tumour; it can occur in striated and cardiac muscle, but usually in the muscles of a limb or the buttocks. It grows extremely rapidly, and can achieve a size of 25 centimetres. The prognosis is bad, even under such drastic treatment as the amputation of limbs, because the tumour metartasizer rapidly especially, to the lungs and bones. Tumours originating in connective tissue also occur in muscles; they include the benign fibroma and the malignant fibrosarcoma. Swellings in muscle may have another cause, such as injury to or haemorrhage in the muscle, which may resemble a tumour from the outside. Scars may form after haemorrhage, and muscular tissue may also be replaced by connective tissue after muscular inflammation. Sosmetimes calcium is deposited in connective tissue, causing a bony swelling. Shrinkage of connective tissue can also result in irregular contractures.

Treatment of the latter conditions is by surgical removal of connective tissue from the muscle.

Myalgia. Muscular pain. It is a symptom associated with various conditions, but the most common cause is muscular strain. The immediate source is large quantities of waste products, such as lactic acid, which are produced by muscular activity, and by microscopic damage to muscular cells; it is produced in particularly large quantities when oxygen supply to the muscle is deficient. Pain of this kind can be prevented and treated by encouraging circulation in the muscle by warmth and massage, and by continuing to use it. Cramp is almost always associated with myalgia. A number of hereditary muscular disorders associated with increased muscular tension (myotonia) also cause muscular pain. Pain in the shoulder girdle or pelvic girdle muscles may be the result of polymyalgia rheumatica. Naturally muscular pain is also present in cases of tearing and inflammation of muscles, and is one of the symptoms of viral diseases such as influenza. Polyneuritis, the simultaneous inflammation of various nerves, which can occur in alcoholic poisoning and diabetes, often has myalgia as its first symptom.

Myasthenia gravis. Muscular disorder characterized by loss of strength and increasing proneness of the muscles to fatigue. The condition originates from an abnormality at the point where nerve stimuli are transferred to muscular tissue. Normally a nervous impulse liberates a chemical transmitter substance, acetylcholine, at the nerve ending; acetylcholine transmits a nerve impulse to the muscle. This process is disturbed in myasthenia gravis. The cause is unknown, but it is assumed to be an autoimmune disease in which antibodies are formed that work against the body's own protein and cell structures.

Myasthenia gravis occurs above all in women between the ages of 20 and 40. Symptoms often occur in the face first, in the form of drooping eyelids and double vision, especially in the evening. The muscular weakness can show in difficulties in speaking and swallowing. Other muscles in the body can be affected. Symptoms are not always present to the same extent, but can worsen rapidly in the event of tension or heightened emotion.

Myelin. A fatty substance enclosing the long processes or axons of some nerve cells. Major nerves visible to the naked eye are actually collections of cells wrapped in myelin. In the brain, the white matter also consists of neurons inside myelin, but the grey matter is nerve cells without this insulation. Myelin increases the separation between the cell and body fluid surrounding it. Nerve signals pass much more rapidly through myelinated nerve cells than through those which are not insulated.

In *multiple sclerosis,* the myelin sheath is lost by nerve cells regulating different parts of the body.

Myeloma, multiple. Form of cancer in which antibody-forming white blood cells grow unchecked. The body needs some antibodies to protect itself against infection; in multiple myeloma there is no shortage of the cells concerned, but the quality of the antibodies is insufficient, and resistance to disease is lowered.

White blood cells are produced in the bone marrow, and formation of tumours by these cells drives out other cells, such as red blood cells, causing anaemia, associated with fatigue and pallor. A characteristic feature of multiple myeloma is bone pain, and the bones also soften, so that fractures occur more readily.

The prognosis is unfavourably for this disease. Treatment with drugs to inhibit cell growh is sometimes prescribed.

Myocarditis. Inflammation of the muscular tissue of the heart, usually caused by viral or bacterial infection, or the effects of certain chemicals or radiation. The condition is associated with general inflammation following temporary injury of the heart muscle cells. Mild myocarditis is characterized by rapid heartbeat and possibly rhythmic disturbances. If the condition is severe so many cells may become damaged that the heart can no longer pump blood adequately, causing heart failure. Treatment is by avoiding physical exertion, and taking medication if necessary (antibiotics, corticosteroids).

Myopia (short sight) Abnormality of the eye in which it cannot focus on distant objects, because refraction is too great or the eyeball is too long, so that the image is focused in front of the retina. A normal eye focuses parallel beams precisely on the retina; close objects can be brought into focus by increasing the refractive power of the lens (accommodation).

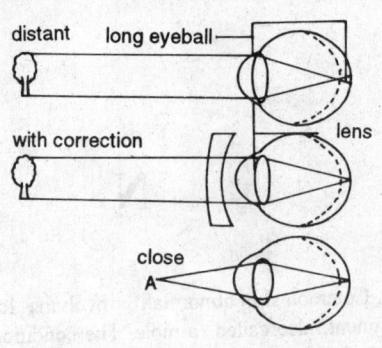

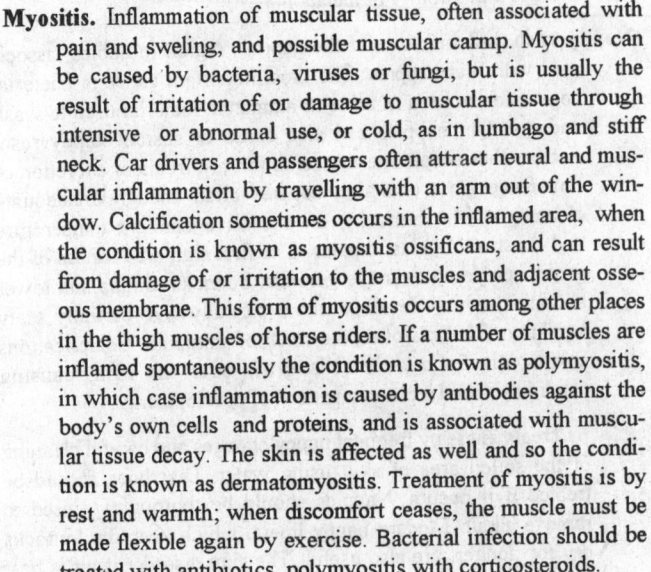

Myopia; the eyeball is too long, which means that the image is incorrectly focused on the retina, causing blurred vision. The problem is solved by corrective spectacle lenses. Close work causes no problems.

Myopia is corrected by negative lenses in spectacles or contact lenses.

Myositis. Inflammation of muscular tissue, often associated with pain and sweling, and possible muscular carmp. Myositis can be caused by bacteria, viruses or fungi, but is usually the result of irritation of or damage to muscular tissue through intensive or abnormal use, or cold, as in lumbago and stiff neck. Car drivers and passengers often attract neural and muscular inflammation by travelling with an arm out of the window. Calcification sometimes occurs in the inflamed area, when the condition is known as myositis ossifacans, and can result from damage of or irritation to the muscles and adjacent osseous membrane. This form of myositis occurs among other places in the thigh muscles of horse riders. If a number of muscles are inflamed spontaneously the condition is known as polymyositis, in which case inflammation is caused by antibodies against the body's own cells and proteins, and is associated with muscular tissue decay. The skin is affected as well and so the condition is known as dermatomyositis. Treatment of myositis is by rest and warmth; when discomfort ceases, the muscle must be made flexible again by exercise. Bacterial infection should be treated with antibiotics, polymyositis with corticosteroids.

N

Naevus. Common skin abnormality involving local accumulation of pigment, also called a mole. The condition is in fact so common that it can hardly be considered abnormal. It is a small brown to back patch, consisting of a dense accumulation of skin pigment, on which a few hairs may grow.

There are variants set deeper in the skin, which show through as blue. If a naevus increases in size, starts to itch, bleed or become ulcerated a doctor should be consulted immediately as there is a possibility of melanoma.

Nappy rash. Inflammation of the genital region in babies, associated with wet nappies. The most important cause is bacterial conversion of urea in urine to ammonia; material used to wash and disinfect nappies can also cause or sustain nappy rash. Factors that encourage the condition are frequent excretion of thin faeces, not changing nappies often enough, inadequate cleaning of the buttocks, an excessive ambient temperature and constricting plastic pants. The first sign are redness of the groin, spreading over the genitals, buttocks, thighs and lower abdomen, which develops into a partially wet, partially scaly condition. There is often the smell of ammonia. Complications can occur if *Candida* cells grow over the rash, causing candidiasis, and a chronic pattern of development.

Treatment is by frequent nappy changes and careful cleaning of the soiled area of skin using water. Diarrhoea should be treated if it occurs. Nappies should be thoroughly rinsed to remove alkali. Modern nappy liners, which keep the buttocks dry for longer, are also useful. The skin disorder itself is best treated with zinc ointment.

Nausea. Feeling of being sick closely associated with vomiting, often preceding or accompanying it, sometimes vomiting relieves nausea completely, or reduces the feeling. Causes, as with vomiting are stimulus of the stomach wall or the vomiting centre in the medulla oblongata of the brain. Some brain conditions, particularly tumours and high pressure in the brain, which sometimes cause vomiting are not unnaturally also associated with nausea. Well-known and frequent causes are motion sickness (including—carsickness and seasickness), overeating and excessive consumption of alcohol. Nausea is also often felt in the first month of pregnancy, particularly in the morning (morning sickness); this is caused by hormonal changes that occur in pregnancy.

Neonatal jaundice. Yellow colouring of the skin caused by accumulation of bile pigment, occurring when the liver cannot, or cannot adequately, convert bilirubin into a water-soluble form. This can cause jaundice in full-term babies on the 3rd or 4th day of life, but the condition occurs more rapidly and severely in premature babies, in whom blood bilirubin levels can reach dangerous heights, requiring treatment. The condition can be caused in a number of ways: blood group or rhesus incompatibility, infection, metabolic disorders, blockage of the bile ducts and so on.

Nephrotic syndrome. Increased porosity of the kidney filter system to protein, permitting heavy protein loss in the urine, and thus blood protein deficiency. This in turn leads to a decline in the blood's capacity to retain moisture, causing oedema in body tissue, principally in the face and legs. Fluid can also accumulate in the abdominal cavity (ascites). Blood fat content usually rises at the same time. A form of nephrotic syndrome occurs in children in which typical globules of fat are excreted in the urine (lipid nephrosis). The cause of this condition is unknown. In 75 per cent of adults with nephrotic syndrome the cause is a kidney disorder such as glomerulonephritis. The other 20 per cent are caused by general diseases such as diabetes mellitus, pre-eclampsia, amyloidosis in rheumatic conditions and malaria Diagnosis is by removal of a piece of kidney tissue with a hollow needle for tests (biopsy).

Nerve compression. Pinching of a nerve, with short-or long-term interruption of the nerve function.

Nerve damage mainly occurs because of an interruption of the blood supply. One well-known example is carpal tunnel syndrome, in which a nerve in the hand is pinched by wrist tendons that are too tight. Various nerves in the arm can be pinched by faulty posture, by the use of crutches under the armpits, or by carrying a heavy rucksack. Thus there are many examples of nerve compression. The first symptom is tingling in the area innervated by the nerve. Numbness and paralysis occur if the pressure is continuous.

This condition can often be remedied by correcting faulty posture. Sometimes an operation must be performed.

Nervous disorders. The various nerve conditions can be classified according to cause. Neuritis (inflammation) does not often occur. In nerve compression, a nerve is damaged by pressure resulting from a slipped disc carpal tunnel syndrome or Bell's palsy. Neuropathy is a neural damage resulting from e.g., vitamin B deficiency (Wernicke's disease), metabolic disturbances such as diabetes, poisoning, or disturbances in the blood supply. A neurinoma is a neural tumour that occurs mainly on the eighth cranial nerve. The primary symptoms of nerve conditions are pain, numbness and slack paralysis.

Neuritis. Inflammation of a nerve with a loss of function. This leads to slack paralysis and/or numbmess. The best-known form is inflammation of the optic nerve causing temporary blindness (neuritis retrobulbaris). In a third of cases, it is a precursor of multiple sclerosis.

Occasionally one or more nerves may become inflamed after excessive work, exposure to cold, or other causes. Sometimes such inflammation resembles an allergic inflammatory reaction. Although the inflammation may affect any nerve, the most frequent instance is shoulder neuritis in young adults.

This often affects only one side. Parts of the nerves in the shoulder are affected. The symptoms are sudden pain in the shoulder and upper arm, followed by slack paralysis of the local muscles. The disorder usually takes a benign course and the pain generally disappears after a few days. The paralysis, however, may take many months to disappear.

Bacterial inflammation of nerve ends occurs in leprosy, mostly with a reduced sensitivity to pain. There is no direct means of treating inflammation of the optic nerve. In the case of shoulder neuritis, remedies are administered to reduce inflammation and soothe the pain, and at the same time the condition may be treated with local heat and physiotherapy

Neurinoma. Benign tumour, originating in the connective tissue around a nerve, usually the auditory nerve. The first symptoms are daffiness in one ear, often with an associated whistling

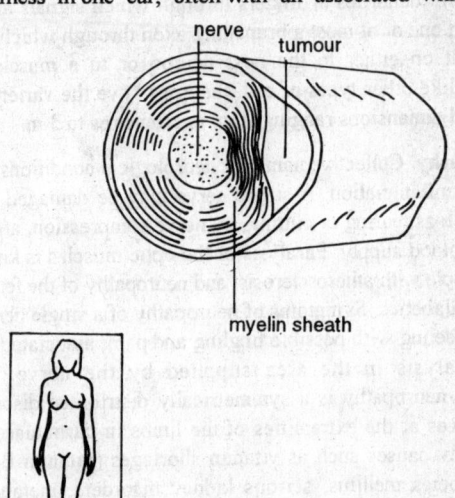

A neurinoma is a benign tumour originating in the myelin sheath if a nerve; it can exert pressure on a nerve.

sound. As the auditory nerve runs with the nerve from the organ of balance, it is possible that problems of balance may also occur (vertigo). Later, pressure on the nearby trigeminal nerve can cause loss of feeling in and paralysis of the face. Finally, the tumour can exert pressure on the brain stem, causing paralysis in the rest of the body. If the tumour has advanced to this extent the diagnosis is practically certain. It is usually possible to remove the entire tumour by surgery, but loss of hearing in one ear can probably not be avoided because the tumour has usually grown rigidly together with the auditory nerve. Loss of feeling in or paralysis of one-half of the face is usually completely cured by removal of the tumour.

Neuron. A nerve cell. It consists of a body containing the genetic material and most of the energy conversion and synthesizing machinery of the cell plus two kinds of processes or extension: dendrites or fingers through which signals are received, and one or at most a branching axon through which signals are sent on either to the next neuron or to a muscle or gland. Unlike other types of cell, neurons have the variety of shapes and dimensions ranging from micrometres to 3 m.

Neuropathy. Collective name for neurological conditions not caused by inflammation. A single nerve may be damaged by injuries such as tearing or cutting, by nerve compression, and disorders in blood supply. Paralysis of the optic muscles is known in old people with atherosclerosis, and neuropathy of the femoral nerve in diabetics. Symptoms of neuropathy of a single nerve are loss of feeling with possible tingling and pain, associated with slack paralysis in the area supplied by the nerve. So called polyneuropathy is a symmetrically distributed disorder of the nerves at the extremities of the limbs in particular. There are many causes such as vitamin shortages (vitamin B_1 and B_{12}), diabetes mellitus, serious kidney disorders, metabolic disorders, poisoning with various medicines and heavy metals and widespread disturbances in blood supply to the nerves of the kind that occur in rheumatic conditions, lupus erythematosus and other socalled systemic diseases. Polyneuropathy can also occur in cancer patients, for no known reason. The condition usually develops over several weeks, often beginning with loss of feeling, pain and tingling in the feet and lower parts of the legs, possibly resulting in muscular decay and slack paralysis. Later the same problems occur in the hands and forearms.

Treatment is aimed at the underlying cause. Damage to a nerve can be repaired by surgery, pressure should be released on a compressed nerve, vitamin shortages are corrected and diabetes and other metabolic disorders should receive appropriate treatment. In the early stages bed rest, warmth and physiotherapy are also important.

Neurosis. Habits, qualities and psychological symptoms that cause the patient severe difficulty, associated with unsuccessful attempts to change. Almost everybody has 'neurotic' traits to a certain extent. The symptoms of genuine neurosis are anxiety compulsive neurosis, phobias inferiority complex conversions insomnia and depersonalization. There may also be physical symptoms and causes or psychosomatic disorders. A neurosis can also show as a character disturbance as in hysteria. The cause of a neurosis is usually in the patient's youth; congenital traits, the situation in which someone was brought up and education are all factors affecting personality development from birth. Each phase of growing up has its own problems; ideally a child comes to terms with these before passing to the next phase but almost everyone has some problems not entirely solved from an earlier stage. Defence mechanisms are used to exclude problems from the patient's consciousness. This is often successful, but the problems then come indirectly to light in symptoms and character traits which the patient himself does not understand. Psychotherapy can clarify the unconscious background of the neurotic symptoms and problems from the past, so that the patient can learn to deal in a different way with residual difficulties.

Night blindness. Condition in which the patient sees badly in poor light, caused by inadequate retinal rod function. Some time is always needed for accommodation when passing from light to

darkness; the rods may need an hour to achieve maximum
night vision. The rods may be absent congenitally, but the
condition can also be caused by vitamin A deficiency, the
vitamin from which chemicals in the rods are formed. Night
blindness also occurs as a complication of other conditions,
and as a precursor of some retinal disorders.

Poor nutrition can also cause night-blindness. If night-
blindness is a complication of another condition, that condition
must be treated. Only if vitamin A deficiency is the cause is
treatment with that vitamin effective.

Nipple disorders. Problems that affect the nipple, the site on the
breast into which the ducts on the 15-20 separate breast glands
discharge. A normal variant is a nipple which has been retracted since birth; this may occur on one or on both sides. The
same is also true of the additional nipples which can occur in
the line from the armpit to the groin. If a nipple suddenly
retracts, this may indicate that the milk passages or the breast
tissue are affected. A biopsy is usually necessary in order to
determine the nature of the condition. Cracks in the nipple are
rare except in breast feeding mothers. Redness and scales on
the nipple and the surrounding area can indicate an allergic
reaction in the skin. This usually occurs on both sides; when it
is present only on one side it may be a sign of a malignant
growth in the milk ducts under the nipple.

Secretions from the nipple of varying colour and occurring
in one or both nipples may arise. A milk-like secretion occurring with women of child-bearing age is usually bilateral. It
may be caused by a disturbance in the hormonal balance of the
hypothalamus and the pituitary. Taking certain medicines, no-
tably antidepressants and the contraceptive pill, can also give
rise to a milk like secretion.

Abnormal secretions from the breast, such as bloody, flesh-
coloured or yellowish-green secretion, are a sign of a disorder
in the milk passages or lactiferous glands and further examinations (mammography, contrast X-rays or biopsy) are usually

required in order to determine whether the condition is benign or malignant.

Nosebleed. There are many possible causes. The commonest is damage to a blood vessel in the nasal mucous membrane caused by an injury, picking the nose, or blowing it too vigorously. It sometimes occurs with no clear cause, particular in patients with blood clotting problems or those who use anticoagulants. A nosebleed should be stopped as follows: blow the nose well once (to remove blood clots that may inhibit sealing of the affected vessel). Sit upright and hold the nose closed for at least ten minutes. If bleeding has not stopped after half an hour, a doctor should be consulted. If necessary the affected vessel can be sealed by cauterization.

Nymphomania and satyriasis. The first term was originally used for women who have several orgasms within a short time, but is now reserved for a practically insatiable sexual desire which the patient herself usually finds irksome. Inability to reach orgasm, even by masturbation, is an important feature; the condition can be long standing or occur in attacks. The rarely mentioned male equivalent is satyriasis. Social norms and values establish the point at which sexual behaviour becomes abnormal; levels of sexual desire and expression vary, and there are no rules about the frequency of sexual contact. Very frequent sex creates problems only if one partner is keener than the other. Hypersexuality can be physical or psychological, origin: therapy is according to the cause, and sometimes involves the use of sex hormones.

Nystagmus. Involuntary rhythmic movement of the eyeball, which may be continuous or spasmodic. According to the direction of movement it is designated horizontal, vertical, rotary or pendulum (to and fro). The condition is by no means abnormal: it occurs in anyone looking through the window of a moving train, for example. The same occurs in reading. Eye movements of this kind are abnormal only if they occur when looking at stationary objects. Nystagmus can also be caused by irritation of the organ of balance in the inner or by the entry of warm water into one ear. Nystagmus can be caused by an illness; a long period spent in the dark (as with miners, for example) causes temporary nystagmus, and the condition also occurs in disorders of the organ of balance such as Meniere's disease and in disorders of the central nervous system, such as multiple sclerosis and cerebral tumours or haemorrhage. Specialist examination is necessary to establish the cause: treatment is not always necessary or possible. Sometimes surgery is needed to remove the source of irritation to the organ of balance.

O

Obesity. Exceeding the normal weight by more than 20 per cent. The normal weight is calculated on a basis of height, age and sex. The Quetelet index is also often used as a measure of overweight. For this purpose the weight in kilograms is divided by the square of the height in metres. If this calculation results in a figure between 20 and 24, the weight is within the norm, whereas if the figure is higher than 27 it is possible to speak of obesity.

Obesity is always the result of food intake larger than the body requires. The excessive amount of energy which has been absorbed is stored by the body in the form of fat. Food which is rich in calories (with much fat and many carbohydrates or sugars) assists the production of body fat. The same applies to alcohol, which also contains a large number of calories. The excessive storage of body fat is hardly ever caused by disease, and it is therefore not generally useful to carry out an extensive examination in order to detect particular metabolic disturbances such as a thyroid gland which is urderfunctioning. Obesity should be distinguished from conditions in which the amount of liquid in the body is increased (oedema). Body weight also increases in oedema, but this is usually only temporary. When the cause is treated (it may be cardiac weakness or nephritis), surplus body fluid is lost by urination and the weight can decrease by several kilograms in a few days.

Obsession. Can be a compulsive urge to do something (compulsion neurosis), but also certain fears (phobia) can become an obsession. Also certain thoughts, words or fantasies may recur persistently in the consciousness; the patient may not wish to think the thought, but still it comes. A harmless example is a song which keeps repeating itself in the mind. Less harmless are obsessive thoughts which the patient finds a torment.

Occipito posterior presentation. Abnormal position of the baby's head during birth. With a normal presentation the head has to turn during passage through the birth canal, and as a result the baby ends up with its head against the mother's pubic bone. This is necessary, because the head cannot pass through the pelvic aperture in an oblique or transverse position, unless the head is very small or the pelvis very large. If this turn is not made, or if the back of the head is turned in the direction of the mother's sacrum, the position is known as occipito posterior presentation. A narrow pelvis or weak contractions can cause the problem. A decision on what action to take is made on the basis of the cause, the progress of the birth and the condition of the child at the given moment.

Oedema. Increase in the quantity of fluid in the space between tissue cells, caused by leakage from blood vessel walls. It usually occurs first in the lower parts of the body; if the patient is standing, in the ankles and if the patient is lying down, in the back. A soft, usually painless swelling appears; the skin is tight and shiny. Firm pressure on the skin causes an indentation which remains when the pressure is removed. Oedema can occur for very many reasons. The most important are raised blood pressure in the veins, altered blood composition, and reduced lymph removal (lymphatic oedema). Pressure in the veins is raised by standing for a long period, varicose veins, thrombosis or heart failure.

Oedema, lymphatic. Swelling caused by insufficient drainage of lymph. The swelling is not painful and the skin is not discoloured; in the early stages it yields easily to pressure, and hardens later. The condition can be present at birth and is a result of an abnormality in the lymph ducts. In most cases lymphatic oedema occurs after inflammation, surgery or exposure to radiation; radiation in particular can cause shrivelling of lymph ducts and nodes, thus restricting lymphatic flow. Usually the cause cannot be removed, so treatment is directed at the swelling (for example by wearing elasticated stockings).

Oedema, pulmonary. Accumulation of fluid in the lungs, which restricts oxygen and carbon dioxide exchange and causes shortness of breath and cyanosis. The condition is associated with gurgling respiration, the coughing up of pink, foaming fluid, chest pain and fever. The condition occurs when the small blood vessels in the lungs fail to retain fluid, which is then as it were sweated out into the lungs. It can be caused by the inhalation of poisonous gases (such as chlorine if toilet cleaners are used incorrectly). In can also be the result of heart and blood vessel diseases associated with lung congestion such as heart failure and some abnormalities of the heart valves. Diagnosis is by means of the above symptoms and X-rays.

Oesophagitis. Inflammation of the mucous membrane of the oesophagus, often caused by chronic gastric acid irritation; the stomach is not affected by this acid, but the oesophagal mucous membrane is. Normally there is no gastric juice in the oesophagus, but if the valve mechanism at the entrance to the stomach is not functioning properly, some acid may flow back (so-called reflux), when the condition is known as reflux inflammation of the oesophagus. Inflammation also occurs as a result of tumours or stricture, and after accidentally drinking corrosive liquids. Gastric acid reflux causes heartburn and pain behind the breastbone, sometimes associated with regurgitation of food. Discomfort increases with lying, bending straining and lifting, and also in cases of overweight, pregnancy, and excessive smoking.

Oesophagus, disorders of. The oesophagus (or gullet) is a hollow pipe consisting of a thick layer of muscle lined with mucous membrane; its function is the transportation of food from the mouth to the stomach. The swallowing phase of this transport is voluntary; then food moves down the oesophagus without conscious intervention, under the influence of the involuntary nervous system. Disorders of the oesophagus usually cause difficulties in swallowing and pain behind the breast-bone,

sometimes associated with regurgitation of food, and heartburn.

Oesophagus, diverticulum of. Protusion of the oesophagal wall as
a result of localized weakness in the muscular layer, occurring
almost anywhere in the oesophagus, but usually in the upper
section, causing the most discomfort. A so-called Zenker's diverticulum forms a pear-shaped swelling just above the entrance to the oesophagus; the swelling can become so large
that it can be felt from the outside at the left of the neck.
Pieces of food accumulate in the sac. Diverticulum of the
oesophagus causes problems in swallowing because of the pressure of the sac on the oesophagus. Immediately after a meal
food can be regurgitated from the sac, enter the air passages,
and cause coughing fits. Another symptom is mouth odour
because of the presence of half-digested food near the throat.
The diverticulum shows on a contrast X-ray.

Treatment is by surgical removal.

Oesophagus, Spasm of. Contraction of muscular fibre in the wall
of the oesophagus, occurring in the form of rings, or on several
levels at once, when they are known as ladder spasms. They
are usually caused by a nervous condition, sometimes by a
disorder of the muscular fibre. Symptoms depend on the site of
the disorder; in the upper part of the oesophagus it feels like
something stuck in the throat; lower down the passage of food
can be blocked. Treatment is by rest; drinking water can help,
and valium is a possible drug treatment.

Oesophagus, stricture of. Localized constriction of the oesophagus,
making it less easy for food to pass, and occurring as a result
of a benign or malignant tumour. Benign strictures usually
consist of connective tissue which has formed in the wall in
the course of time, usually as a reaction to irritants, as in
inflammation of the oesophagus caused by gastric acid reflux,
or the accidental drinking of corrosives (ammonia, strong acids). An unusual form occurs particularly in women over the
age of 40, often associated with iron deficiency and inflammation of the tongue (Plummer Vinson syndrome). Malignant

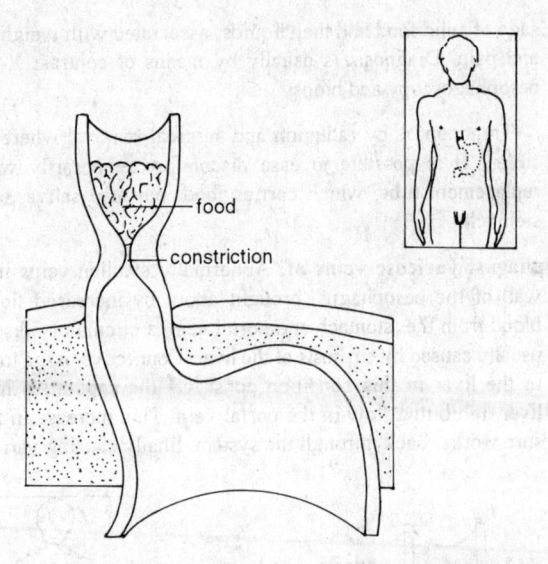

food

constriction

If the oesophagus is constricted food gets stuck, causing pain and tightness of the chest.

strictures are the result of cancer of the oesophagus. Particular symptoms of benign structure are difficulties in swallowing and, in the case of gastric acid reflux, heartburn and smarting behind the breastbone. If the stricture is malignant it is associated with increasingly severe problems in swallowing, loss of weight and reduced appetite. Pain is rare in such cases. Oesophagoscopy and possibly biopsy are the best instruments of diagnosis. Treatment of benign stricture is by stretching; malignant strictures are treated in the same way as other cancers of the oesophagus.

Oesophagus, tumour of. Usually malignant; benign tumours are rare, and usually unproblematical. Cancer of the oesophagus occurs principally in men between the ages of 50 and 80. Risk factors are excessive consumption of strong alcoholic drink and stricture of the oesophagus. Characteristic symptoms are increasing difficulty in swallowing, and finally, restricted passage of solid food and then liquids, associated with weight loss and pain. Diagnosis is usually by means of contrast X-rays, oesophagoscopy and biopsy.

Treatment is by radiation and surgical removal where possible. It is possible to ease discomfort temporarily with a replacement tube, which carries food, but also saliva, to the stomach.

Oesophagus, varicose veins of. Abnormally swollen veins in the wall of the oesophagus, brought about by increased flow of blood from the stomach and portal vein, a circulatory disorder usually caused by cirrhosis of the liver. Connective tissue formed in the liver in this condition constricts the capillaries in the liver, inhibiting flow in the portal vein. This increase in pressure works back through the system, finally causing varicose

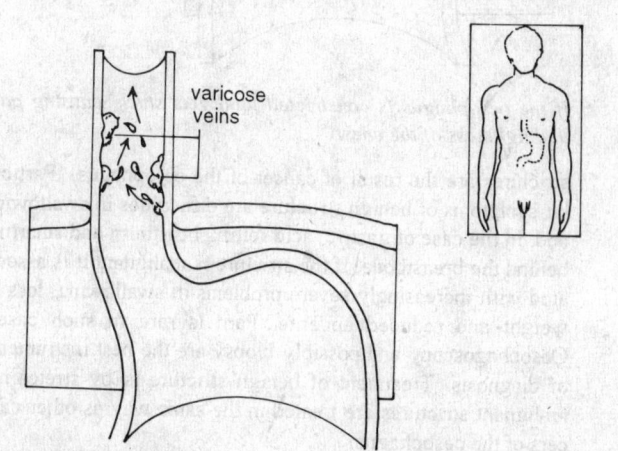

varicose
veins

Varicose veins of the oesophagus can cause dangerous haemorrhage because there is no counter pressure to stem the bleeding.

veins in the oesophagus. Such varicose veins can cause haemorrhage without warning: food moving along the oesophagus bursts one of the protruding veins, causing violent haemorrhage and the vomiting of blood (haematemesis). Such haemorrhage is potentially fatal. Treatment is by medication to close the blood vessels or the introduction of a balloon to seal them by physical pressure. When the haemorrhage is staunched it is possible to make a connection (shunt) between the portal vein and another major vein, thus taking intestinal blood past the liver, reducing pressure in the portal vein and shrinking the varicose veins.

Ophthalmoplegia. Whole or partial failure of one or more of the muscles responsible for moving the eye in its socket, caused either by a disorder in the associated nerve or the muscle itself; the former is more common. The condition usually affects one eye. The eye is normally moved in its socket by six muscles, provided with impulses by three nerves. If a muscle is paralyzed the eye cannot move in certain directions, and is dragged adrift by the unaffected muscles. This causes double vision (diplopia), because the images presented to the brain by the two eyes no longer correspond. The commonest failure is of the sixth cranial nerve, which controls the muscles that turn the eye outward. This nerve has a long run round the skull, and is thus susceptible to crushing if the skull is injured. Ophthalmoplegia is difficult to treat; surgery is sometimes possible.

Paralysis of the muscles can occur as a result of disorders of one of the associated cerebral nerves.

Orchitis. Inflammation of one or both testicles, the organs lying in the scrotum which produce sperm. Testicular inflammation usually occurs in combination with epididymitis.

A rapid onset of testicular inflammation may be caused by an infection of the urinary tract, prostatitis, epididymitis, during an attack of mumps, as a result of the venereal disease gonorrhoea and other infectious diseases in which bacteria can reach the testicles via the blood, and as a result of accidents in which the testicle is damaged.

Testicular inflammation causes the scrotum to swell, and is very painful. The same symptoms also occur with torsion of the testicle, and here surgical treatment is necessary.

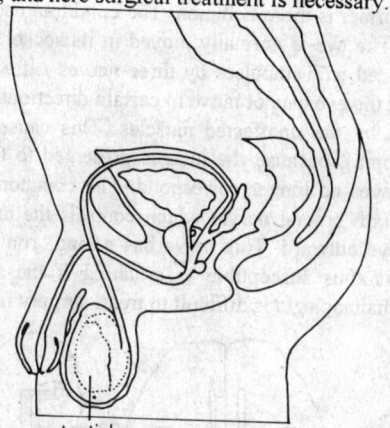

testicle

Inflammation of the testicle (orchitis) can be a cause of reduced fertility in later life.

With children, inflammation occurs mainly during mumps, and mumps can cause testicular inflammation in adults too. Treatment consists of complete rest, pain relief and the administration of antibiotics. Sometimes the inflammation becomes chronic and antibiotics are again of considerable assistance. Such disorders usually damage the tissues and infertility may be a consequence of testicular inflammation.

Orgasm, lack of. Orgasm is the moment of passage from the climax of sexual tension to complete relaxation, associated with intensely pleasant sensations. Inability to reach this climax occurs in both men and women, but is commoner in women. There are numerous causes, such as inexperience in dealing with one's own or partner's body, fear or guilt feelings about sex and the enjoyment of it, hostile feelings towards a partner, or failure to find satisfaction oneself. Painful sexual intercourse (dyspareunia) as a result of physical disorder can also inhibit orgasm.

In general the cause is faulty sexual technique. Often men (and women) are under the impression that the penis alone can bring sexual satisfaction, and there are indeed women who experience orgasm during intercourse, but most women reach orgasm by stimulation of the clitoris. Men rarely suffer from lack of orgasm; if they do it is usually because of impotence or physical or psychological problems. The difficulty can usually be obviated by education, love and patience; sometimes therapy by discussion and exploration of one's own and one's partner's body can solve the problem.

Osis. The word-ending denotes a disease process, usually one in which something increases abnormally. Thus *toxoplasmosis* is an infection characterized by growth in the number of the toxoplasma protozoon such that signs and symptoms of disease develop.

Osmosis. Passage of a pure solvent, for example, water, from a compartment containing a lesser concentration of a solvent or solvents to a compartment containing a greater concentration when the two compartments are divided by a membrane which allows the passage of the solvent but not the solutes. This physical process occurs in inorganic as well as organic situations, but it is very important in the latter. Thus, the relative volumes of blood and other body fluids is strongly influenced by osmosis.

Osteoarthrosis. Chronic condition of one or more joints in which the cartilage wears and the adjacent bone produces a knobbly growth in reaction.

The cartilage of the joint is first roughened, then gradually disappears, and this and the bone growth cause deformity of the joints, such as Heberden's nodes on the fingers.

Osteoarthrosis is largely associated with old age, affecting almost everyone in their lifetime. The condition is as frequent in men as women, and begins around the age of 40. A patient may be more susceptible because of heredity. Osteoarthrosis can occur in younger people through undue strain on a joint, or through abnormalities of the joints caused by injury, growth disturbances, tumours or inflammation.

Usually the joints of the leg, such as the hips and knees, are affected, but the condition can also occur in the spinal column (particularly the neck) and in the feet, toes, hands and fingers, Early symptoms of osteoarthrosis are usually stiffness of the joint, followed by pain which increases under pressure and decreases when the joint is not being used. A grating sensation can occur with movement.

Osteochondritis. Inflammation of bone and associated cartilage. It thus occurs only in parts of the body where these two tissue occur, such as joints and the cartilaginous growth plates in bones. Such inflammation occurs in children with congenital syphilis, but can also be the result of inflammation of the bone marrow. Generally the term is used to include disorders, usually in young people, in which bone and tissue decay occur as a result of deficient blood supply. Sometimes a piece of dead bone is lodged in the joint, causing pain and difficulty in movement. This can occur in various joints but the commonest site is the head of the thigh (Perthes' disease) the lower part of the shin (Osgood-Schalatter's disease) and the spinal column (Scheuermann's disease). The cause of these condition is unknown.

Treatment is by rest, possibly with the limb in plaster, after which the condition heals spontaneously.

Osteogenesis imperfecta. Congenital disorder that causes bones to fracture easily, resulting from a hereditary abnormality. It often affects several children in a family, and is commoner in girls than boys; arm and leg bones in particular are thin and brittle, leading to fractures. Other characteristic symptoms are a bluish tinge to the white of the eye and deafness caused by ingrowing bone in the middle ear. Ligaments are often slack, allowing extreme movement of joints; it may be possible to push the fingers back on to the wrist, for example. Teeth may be missing. A striking feature is that fractures heal less well than fractures in healthy bone. As the childgets older the bones become less brittle, and after puberty the high degree of fragility has almost disappeared. If the frequent fractures in childhood are properly treated, to avoid invalidity, the prognosis is good; no other treatment is possible.

Osteomalacia. Metabolic bone disorder in adults, related to rickets. Both conditions involve characteristic incomplete calcifition, resulting from vitamin D deficiency, lack of calcium in food or reduced calcium absorption by the intestine. Vitamin D is important in calcium absorption and calcification of bones; it is formed in the skin by sunlight from substances containing cholesterol. Lack of vitamin D can be the result of dietary deficiencies or lack of sunlight, and its absorption can be impaired by disorders of the alimentary canal. Osteomalacia can also occur in pregnant women, who pass a great deal of their calcium to the growing foetus. Characteristic features of the disorder are deformed bones, pain and muscular weakness (because calcium also affects muscular function, explaining the extreme fatigue also associated with the condition). Most forms of osteomalacia and rickets react well to large doses of vitamin D and calcium, but existing deformities cannot be corrected.

Osteomyelitis. Inflammation of the bone marrow, usually combined with inflammation of the surrounding bone, caused by bacteria, viruses or fungi, but in 90 per cent of cases by staphylococci.

Osteomyelitis occurs predominantly in children. Bacteria

from an inflamed tonsil or boil reach the bone marrow via the bloodstream; usually the shin or thigh is affected, often near the knee. The first sign is often pain in the knee, associated with fever and nausea.

Bacteria can also reach the bone from outside through injury at any age and in any bone. If bone marrow inflammation is not quickly recognized and treated it will spread and there is danger that an abscess may form which, by increasing pressure and damaging the blood vessels of the bone, can limit blood supply, causing bone death. The dead bone floats loose (sequestered) in the abscess. As the process of inflammation proceeds, the abscess can break through the bone to lie under the periosteum, then break through this, and possibly form a fistula to the surface of the body. In such a case bacteria in the encapsulated abscess die, stopping the inflammation, but the encapsulation prevents the body from clearing away the abscess. Diagnosis is by symptoms, a blood test which may show the cause of inflammation, and bone examination by X-rays or possibly bone scan, in which radioactive material is injected which accumulates in the affected bone. A special photograph makes this visible. It may also be advisable to look for inflammation elsewhere in the body, which could be a source of the bone inflammation. Bone tumours give similar symptoms to bone marrow inflammation, and checks should be made for these too.

Osteoporosis. Condition in which bone breaks down more rapidly than it is produced; in contrast with osteomalacia, calcification of the bone is normal. The various structures in the bone are thinner, and therefore weaker, and fractures easily occur; vertebrae can collapse, causing lack of height, kyphosis and backache. Osteoporosis has many causes, the commonest of which is lack of load on the bone, for example in patients bedridden for a long time or older people with restricted movement. The condition is encouraged in older women by decreased female sex hormone production after the menopause. Osteoporosis is one of the most important causes of hip fractures in older people. In modern times weightlessness can cause deficient bone loading: astronauts who spend long periods in space find that osteoporosis can be a problem. The condition is also associated with certain disorders such as osteogenesis imperfecta, and excessive thyroid hormone and corticosteroid levels; the latter are used in the treatment of various illnesses, but can also be produced in excess by the body (Cushing's syndrome). Treatment of osteoporosis can consist of increased activity, such as exercises for the elderly; avoiding long-term confinement to bed; a diet high in vitamins D and C calcium, phosphate and protein; and the administration of sex hormones or anabolic steroids. The latter are hormonal preparations that encourage tissue (and thus also bone) formation. Certain resultant bone conditions, such as collapsed vertebrae, cannot be cured; painkillers may be prescribed.

Otitis media (middle ear infection) The middle ear is the cavity behind the eardrum containing the auditory ossicles, small bones that transmit sound from the eardrum to the inner ear and the auditory nerves. Middle ear inflammation frequently occurs in children, usually affecting both ears. In adults generally only one ear is affected. Inflammation often begins as the result of a cold or other infectious illness such as measles, scarlet fever or a sore throat. The mucous membrane of the nasal cavity and the pharynx swells up. The same occurs in the Eustachian tube, which connects the pharynx with the middle ear. The tube becomes blocked, mucus can no longer pass to the pharynx and accumulates in the middle ear, where inflammation can occur, causing pus to form from the bacteria and dead cells.

Blockage of the Eustachian tube by an enlarged adehoid can also cause inflammation. The child snores, sleeps with its mouth open, and is subject to frequent colds and inflammation of the middle ear. If the complaint persists the adenoid can be removed.

Another cause of inflammation of the middle ear in children is swimming in chlorinated water, which causes swelling of the mucous membranes, blocking the Eustachian tube. Swimming should be cut down inflammation of the middle ear occurs regularly.

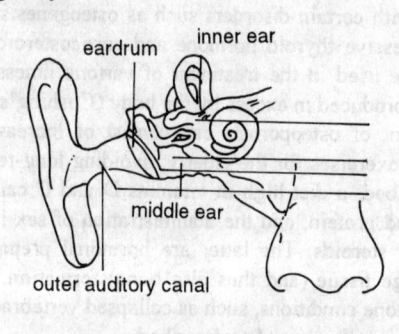

Otitis media causes pain, loss of hearing and a distended eardrum.

Middle ear inflammation causes earache, possibly severe. In infants the symptoms are not so clear. There is usually fever, but sometimes the child simply has difficulties in taking nourishment. When pus forms in the middle ear the pain is more severe, the patient feels extremely ill and hearing is badly affected. Inflammation of the middle ear can persist for a long time-more than six weeks-and the ear will discharge matter throughout this period.

Otorrhoea. Discharge of pus from the ear as a result of perforation of the eardrum in otitis media (inflammation of the middle ear). Under normal circumstances inflammation of the middle ear clears up after spontaneous or induced perforation of the eardrum or after treatment with antibiotics; the discharge of pus and blood from the ear stops and the eardrum closes again. Sometimes inflammation persists, the eardrum remains open, and the discharge continues. The inflammation has then usually become chronic. The cause can be undetected mastoiditis or a source of infection in the nose or throat such as an enlarged and inflamed adenoid, sinusitis or bronchitis. Chronic otitis media is sometimes also associated with cholesteatoma.

Otosclerosis. Hardening of bone in the inner ear, limiting movement
of one of the ossicles which transmit sound vibrations to the
inner ear and resulting in hearing difficulties. This disorder
often occurs shortly after puberty, is now more common in
women than men, and is sometimes worse during pregnancy.
Sound enters the ear through the auditory canal, and is then
transmitted to the tympanic cavity, which contains the three
auditory ossicles: the hammer, the anvil and the stapes. The
ossicles transmit sound to the inner ear, where the vibrations
stimulate nerves. In otosclerosis hardening of the bone in the
inner ear prevents the stapes from moving, thus hindering the
passage of sound to the inner ear. The patient becomes hard of
hearing, usually in both ears; the condition is sometimes stable
for a period, and then suddenly deteriorated, frequently followed by another stable period. Total deafness caused by
otosclerosis is rare. Ringing in the ears (particularly a fluting
tone) frequently occurs, and the patient sometimes complains
of slight dizziness and an unsteady feeling similar to drunken-
ness, because the balancing mechanism of the inner ear is
affected. Women are more troubled by ostosclerotic dizziness
during menstruation.

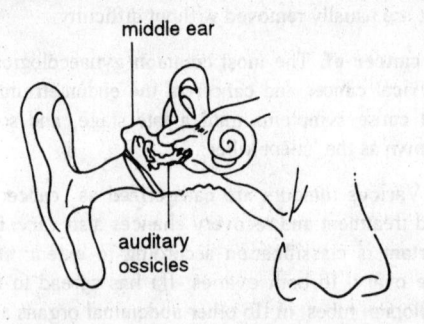

middle ear

auditary
ossicles

*Otoselerosis is stiffening of the auditory ossicles, the small
bones in the middle ear, causing hearing loss.*

Many other disorders can cause hearing difficulties including congenital deformation of the ossicles and adhesions and
malformation caused by inflammation of the middle ear. In

otosclerosis hearing difficulties occur gradually and it often runs in families.

Ovarian cyst. A cyst is a cavity containing fluid or a semi-fluid mass. Ovarian cysts usually occur in sexually mature women, and seldom become malignant. Some are small and of little significance; others can reach the size of footballs. The various types of cyst require various treatments. A possible complication of cyst is that it can twist on its axis and cut off the blood supply to the ovary, causing severe pain, and potentially the death of the ovary. An emergency operation is essential. A corpus luteum cyst often occurs during a hydatdiform pregnancy; it is 6 to 7 cm in size and disappears of its own accord. A follicle cyst is 1 to 10 cm across and contains light-coloured liquid; it too disappears or bursts spontaneously, although it may be removed if persistent or painful. Endometrial cysts contain blood, and are often painful at menstruation or when they burst, and surgery can be necessary. Dermoid cysts are benign tumours, and can occur in the ovaries; they contain skin structures such as hair, sebum, nails and teeth. They can easily twist on their stem and do not disappear spontaneously, but are usually removed without difficulty.

Ovary, cancer of. The most common gynaecological cancer after cervical cancer and cancer of the endometrium; it often does not cause symptoms until a late stage, and so is sometimes known as the 'silent killer'.

Various tumours are categorized as cancer of the ovary, and treatment and recovery chances also vary. Even more important is classification according to extent: stage Ia affects one ovary, Ib both ovaries, IIa has spread to the uterus and Fallopian tubes, in IIb other abdominal organs are affected , in III there is extensive metastasis in the abdominal cavity and in IV metastasis to other parts of the body.

Treatment is usually by surgery (removal of the ovary and, where necessary, the entire internal reproductive apparatus) and medication to prevent cell division. These cytostatic drugs have many side-effects, and are more effective in proportion to the amount of cancerous tissue removed.

Cancer of ovaries occurs most frequently between the ages of 40 and 60.

Ovulation, lack of (Anovulation). This can be deliberate, as in women using the contraceptive pill; a normal physiological phenomenon, as in pregnancy and often in breast feeding; or an illness or symptom of a disorder. There are various more or less serious causes of anovulation, and it can occur occasionally or persist for years. Ovulation can be missed for several consecutive months through stress or fatigue, in cases of rapid loss of weight or an underweight condition (such as anorexia nervosa), or in women who take part in endurance sports such as marathon running. In these cases anovulation is probably a natural protection against having a pregnancy in unfavourable conditions. Various disorders of the ovaries prevent ovulation, such as ovarian cysts, diseases or tumours of the thyroid or it may be the result of high levels of corticosteroid hormones. Gynaecological and endocrinological tests over a long period may be necessary to establish the cause; treatment and the possibility of treatment depend on the cause.

P

Paget's disease. Bone disorder in which the normal process of bone formation and resorption is accelerated, with the formation process dominating. Bones form freakishly, however. The disease occurs principally in older people; about 3 per cent of people over 50 are sufferers, but in very different ways. The cause is unknown; the disorder sometimes occurs in several members of the same family. Characteristic symptoms are thickening of the bones of the skull, increasing its circumference, and deformity of the lower and upper legs. The patient's that may become too small, and his trousers too long. Thickening of the skull can cause headache, and possibly also deafness through narrowing of the ear canal. The led deformities often cause the patient to waddle.

Usually there is little real discomfort. The disease is uncurable, but sometimes its advance can be prevented by medication with calcitonin, a thyroid hormone which reduces bone resorption white at the same time inhibiting bone formation (which is normally a reaction to the resorption). Further treatment is by physiotherapy and painkillers, if needed.

Pancreas, tumour of. Tumours of the pancreas can be benign or malignant (cancer of the pancreas). Benign tumours are rare, and usually affect the islets of Langerthans, which then overproduce insulin, leading to a sharp drop in blood sugar levels (hypoglycaemia).

Cancers of the pancreas are also uncommon, although they have appeared increasingly in the last few years. They are commoner in men than women, usually in later life (from roughly age 40 to 50). The tumour is usually close to the entrance of the tube leading from the pancreas to the intestine.

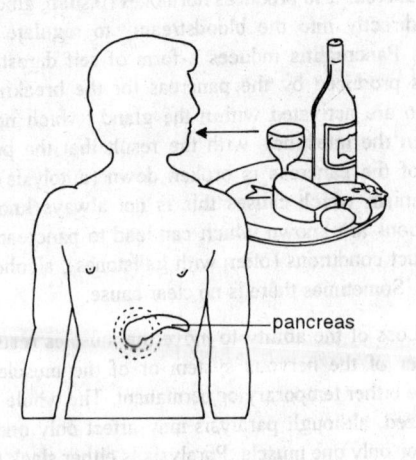

—pancreas

Acute pancreatitis can often occur after a heavy meal and high alcohol consumption.

The symptoms are initially vague and not necessarily typical. Cancer of the head of the pancreas is usually accompanied by persistent pain in the abdomen, loss of weight and jaundice the latter as a result of pressure on the bile duct. If the tumour is in the tail of the pancreas it produces piercing pain, often radiating to the back, and alleviated by bending and associated with weight loss and vomiting, but no jaundice. Cancer of the head of the pancreas can also cause narrowing or even closure of the duodenum by obstructing the bile duct (ileus). Because the symptoms of cancer of the pancreas are atypical it is often diagnosed at a late stage, usually after the occurrence of jaundice.

Pancreatitis. Inflammation of the pancreas, a serious abdominal condition. The pancreas is the gland opening into the duodenum. The bile duct flows into the exit from the pancreas, which produces digestive enzymes to break down protein, fat and carbohydrate in the intestine so that they can be absorbed.

The pancreas also produces hormones (insulin, glucagon) which pass directly into the bloodstream to regulate blood sugar levels. Pancreatitis induces a form of self digestion. The enzymes produced by the pancreas for the breaking down of protein are activated within the gland (which normally happens in the intestine), with the result that the protein in the cells of the pancreas is broken down (autolysis). The direct mechanism which causes this is not always known. Several conditions are known which can lead to pancreatitis: mumps, bile duct conditions (often with gallstones), alcohol abuse and injury. Sometimes there is no clear cause.

Paralysis. Loss of the ability to move the muscles resulting from a disorder of the nervous system or of the muscles. Paralysis may be either temporary or permanent. The whole body can be paralyzed, although paralysis may affect only one part of the body, or only one muscle. Paralysis is either slack (chiefly as a result of neural conditions) or spastic (conditions of the spinal cord or brain), depending on the cause.

In slack paralysis the muscles are limp and eventually atrophy. The motor, nerves are affected, and in consequence the relevant muscles receive little or no stimulus. The causes are conditions such as spinal muscular atrophy or poliomyelitis. Disorders of the nerve roots of the spinal cord include slipped disc and the Guillain-Barre syndrome. Nerves can also be affected in the course of a disease, as in certain forms of neuritis or in the carpal tunnel syndrome. Slack paralysis can also occur in serious muscular disorders such as muscular dystrophy.

Paranoia. Paranoia, or persecution mania, is the conviction that one or more people are tying to injure, kill or in some other way harm the person concerned. Everybody misinterprets other people's behaviour on occasion, and feels himself unjustly treated or cheated. An idea of this kind can take on the nature of a delusion in certain mental illnesses such as schizophrenia, psychosis and dementia. Paranoia occurs principally when the sense of reality is reduced or lost. The delusion is a means by which the patient explains fears, ideas and events which he does not understand. For someone who does not think himself ill a psychiatric investigation can seem like proof that he is being held prisoner. Someone who cannot or will not see that he is demented will not ascribe the fact that he keeps losing things to his own forgetfulness, but will think that someone is stealing from him. Any delusion is a part of a more general syndrome; thus treatment depends on the particular illness. In general it is necessary to enlist medical assistance.

Paraphimosis. Condition which occurs when a tight foreskin (phimosis) cannot be pulled back over the glans penis; the narrow front end of the foreskin lodges in the groove behind the glans. Obstruction of blood flow then causes the glans and the foreskin to swell, and the foreskin cannot be pulled back into its normal position. The tighter the foreskin the greater the obstruction and swelling. If consulted quickly a doctor can gently squeeze out the swelling and pull back the foreskin; if this is not possible, a small cut in the foreskin can help. To avoid repetition the foreskin may be widened or removed by surgery (circumcision).

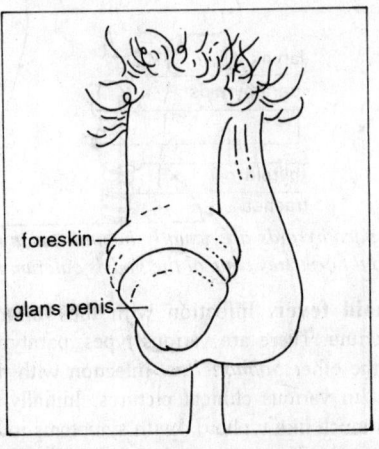

In paraphimosis the foreskin can be pulled back over the glans penis, but gets stuck behind it, causing the glans to swell painfully.

Parathyroid glands, disorders of. Conditions in which the mineral content of the body is not properly regulated. There are two forms, hyper-and hypoparathyroidism, over-and underactivity of the glands respectively. The parathyroids are hormone-producing glands, usually four in number, hidden on either side of the thyroid in the neck; their function is to control the level of calcium and phosphates in the body. Underactivity can be caused by the accidental removal of the parathyroids during a thyroid operation. In new-born babies the function of the parathyroids can be inhibited by excessive phosphate content in food (cows' milk) but in most cases the cause is unknown.

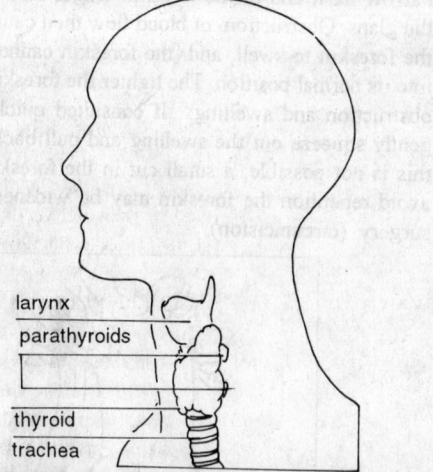

larynx
parathyroids
thyroid
trachea

The parathyroids are usually behind the thyroid gland. Parathyroid hormones control the body's calcium levels.

Paratyphoid fever. Infection with the *Salmonella paratyphi* bacterium. There are various types: paratyphoid A, B and C and the other *Salmonellas*. Infection with these bacteria can result in various clinical pictures. Initially the infection can seem much like typhoid, with symptoms in organs other than the bowels. This is particularly so with paratyphoid B, but it occurs rarely. There is a form confined to the intestines, with symptoms akin to gastroenteritis, sometimes caused by paratyphoid B or C, but more often by other salmonellae. There is a short incubation period of 8 to 48 hours, followed by sudden nausea, vomiting, colic fever and diarrhoea, sometimes with blood and mucus. Usually the bacteria are carried in contaminated food (such as pork, poultry and salads). The patient usually recovers spontaneously in 2 to 5 days; young children may suffer from dehydration. The bacteria remain in some patients, who are designated carriers if there are still bacteria in the faeces after 6 months. Carriers can contaminate large quantities of food, particularly if they are kitchen workers, for example. Diagnosis is by faeces culture.

Parkinson's disease. Common chronic disorder of the part of the nervous system responsible for muscular co-ordination (the so-called extrapyramidal system), causing disturbed posture and movement usually starting in middle age. The cause is low dopamine (a brain protein) levels because of a decay of certain cells in the deeper parts of the brain, with no clear cause; it may be encephalitis or a series of small strokes. Lowered dopamine content causes domination by the cholinergic cerebral proteins and affects brain cells causing stiffness, reduced mobility and tremor. The first feature to attract attention is reduced swinging of the arms when walking . Because automatic movements are affected the patient notices that he has to think consciously before he can perform certain movements. Walking becomes slower and more difficult, with an increasingly bent posture; sudden turning or stopping is difficult. One the other hand the patient may be able to move very rapidly in situations involving stress. Hand movements also become slower and more difficult: handwriting may become smaller and indistinct. The face is mask-like, and speech monotonous and indistinct. The tremor is most marked in the hands, which look as though they are counting money or rolling pills. Head and feet may also tremble. The tremer is most pronounced when the patient is at rest, and declines when purposeful movements have to be carried out. It is worsened by emotion. In the later stages the mind can be affected, and dementia may occur, together with psychological disturbances such as depression, confusion and sometimes even psychosis.

Paronychia. Infection of the cuticle of a nail, which swells up and becomes red and painful. Sometimes pus can be seen through the skin. The disorder can be caused by various bacteria, most commonly by staphylococci and streptococci; they usually reach the cuticle through a small cut or splinter. A small quantity of pus accumulates under the skin, and cannot find an outlet. Pressure increases; it is felt as a throbbing pain. A doctor can release the pus through a small incision in the cuticle, and the condition heals rapidly. If the inflammation is not treated, it will spread, and even lead to the formation of a whitlow. Nail-forming tissue can also be affected, causing the nail to fall off; it will not grow again. A particularly stubborn form of paronychia is caused by the fungus *Candida*. If this form is not treated rapidly, the nail can be permanently malformed.

Pathy. Gr. Pathos-suffering. A suffix designating a disease or abnormal process.

Pellagra. Skin disorder caused by niacin (vitamin B group) deficiency. The skin abnormality is associated with diarrhoea. The skin of the entire body is covered with sharply defined, scaly, red patches, followed by inflammation of the skin. The vitamin occurs in numerous foodstuffs, including green vegetables, cereals, fruit and meat. The condition is rare in the West. Treatment is with B-complex vitamin tablets or by injections if there is intestinal disturbance.

Pelvis, Inflammation of (*adnexitis*). Inflammation of the female pelvic organs, usually but not always caused by infection. The condition can be very painful, particularly in menstruation, when all the pelvic organs have an increased supply of blood and the menstruating uterus pulls on surrounding organs.

A non-gynaecological cause is untreated appendicitis which causes adhesions in the pelvis. Non-infectious causes are endometritis and trapped retroverted uterus, when irritation, swelling and adhesion are the cause of the inflammation.

Most pelvic inflammation is caused by infections originating in the cervix and oviducts, as in gonorrhoea. The chance of inflammation is increased by a tampon or intra-uterine device (coil) kept in position for too long.

Pelvic inflammation is fairly often the cause of infertility in women, but can sometimes be corrected by microsurgery.

Thorough treatment of all infection of the female genital organs is the only way to reduce the incidence of pelvic inflammation.

Pelvis, narrow. Relatively narrow pelvic passage making chidlbirth difficult or impossible.

The ends of the pelvic bones form an almost circular opening through which the child must pass at birth, and the possibility of this is governed by the size of the pelvis and of the child (particularly the head). There are various forms of female pelvis. Women with slightly masculine body structure-broad shoulders and narrow hips-may have a very narrow pelvis. Another cause of narrow pelvis may be rickets, poliomyelitis or tuberculosis of the vertebrae. A pelvis broken in an accident may also be narrowed.

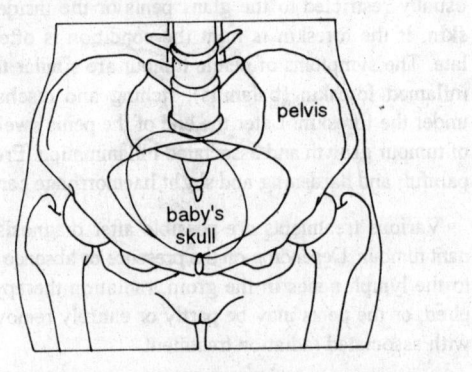

A narrow pelvis can cause difficulty in the birth of the baby's skull.

The width of the pelvis is usually checked in a test between the 36th and 38th week of pregnancy and a decision may be made to deliver the baby by Caesarean section. In doubtful cases the birth should always be in hospital so that an operation is possible if the need arises.

Pemphigus. Serious skin disorder involving the formation of blisters all over the body. Symptoms are large blisters and abrasions on all skin surfaces. The blisters are displaced if pressure is applied to an edge. The disorder continues to spreed, so that after a period of years so much of the body is affected that the patient dies, but with modern medication this rarely occurs.

The cause of pemphigus is the formation of immune substances against the material that normally holds together the cells of the skin. This weakens the skin to the extent that blisters can arise spontaneously. The illness can occur in young patients.

Pemphigus is treated with a substance derived from hydrocortisone. Very high dosages are needed, which can have serious side-effects.

Penis, tumour of. Tumour rarely occur in the penis itself; they are usually restricted to the glans penis or the inside of the foreskin. If the foreskin is tight the condition is often discovered late. The symptoms of penile tumour are similar to those of an inflamed foreskin (balanitis); itching and discharge of fluid under the foreskin. Later the end of the penis swells as a result of tumour growth and associated inflammation. Erection is then painful, and hardening and slight haemorrhage can occur.

Various treatments are possible after diagnosis of a malignant tumour. Depending on the presence or absence of metastasis to the lymph nodes in the groin, radiation therapy can be applied, or the penis may be partly or entirely removed, possibly with associated radiation treatment.

It is known that cancer of the penis rarely occurs in men who practise good genital hygiene, i.e. thorough washing of the penis with the foreskin fully retracted . Circumcized men run the least risk of late detection of cancer of the glans penis.

Pericarditis. Inflammation of the membrane that encloses the heart, resulting from viral or bacterial infection, or as the expression of a disorder elsewhere in the body (rheumatic fever, kidney failure, malignant tumours etc.).

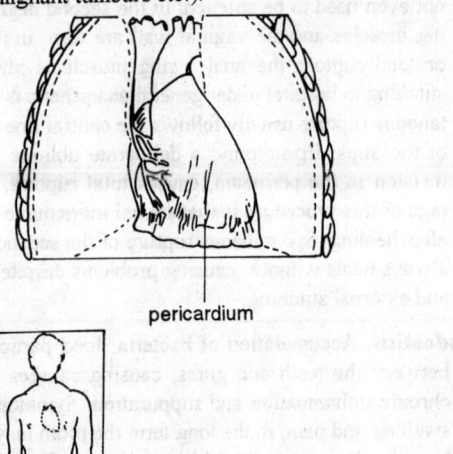

pericardium

In pericarditis the heart rubs painfully against the pericardium at every beat.

Pericarditis from an infection causes symptoms such as chest pain, fever and rapid heartbeat. Treatment depends on the cause of the infection: bacteria are controlled with antibiotics; with viruses only pain killers are needed. If the condition is part of another disorder there is usually considerable accumulation of fluid in the pericardium, which presses on the heart and reduces its efficiency. If so much fluid accumulates as to be dangerous the condition is known as cardiac tamponade. The fluid must be drained using a hollow needle. Treatment is directed at the disorder causing the inflammation.

Perineum, rupture of. Tearing of the tissue between vagina and
anus usually during the birth of the head, or less often the
shoulders, of a baby during labour. The most important factors
are a large baby, a narrow vagina or a baby driven out with
great force at the last minute. The injury is assigned a degree
of severity. In the first degree only the skin is torn, and may
not even need to be stitched: in the second degree the underlying muscles and the vaginal wall are torn; in the third degree
or total rupture the anal   ring muscle is affected and then
stitching in hospital under general anaesthetic is required. Spontaneous rupture usually follows the central line in the direction
of the anus. Episiotomy, a deliberate oblique lateral surgical
incision in the perineum, causes total rupture. The disadvan-
tage of this procedure is that sexual intercourse is often painful
after healing. Spontaneous rupture of the second degree almost
always heals without causing problems despite heavy internal
and external stitching.

Periodontitis. Accumulation of bacteria, food particles and plaque
between the teeth and gums, causing cavities (pockets) with
chronic inflammation and suppuration. Symptoms are redness,
swelling and pain; in the long term the tooth may become loose
because the surrounding bone tissue is affected. The cause is
not always clear. It is often poor oral hygiene, but the condition also occurs when oral hygiene is good. A general disease
such as diabetes mellitus can be a factor.

Treatment is by rinsing, removal of plaque, possibly supplemented with antibiotics or the lancing of abscesses and removal of excess gum.

Periostitis. Inflammation of the periosteum, the firm mucous connective tissue that lines the outer surface of a bone. As well as
capillaries which supply it with food, the periosteum contains
bone-building cells and is therefore important in bone formation particularly after a fracture. Periostitis can be caused by
local irritation, such as tennis elbow, by osteitis by tuberculosis bacilli and by a wound which allows bacteria (usually
staphylococci) to penetrate. During dental treatment of the roots

of teeth, injury to the jaw's periosteum can cause inflammation, which is responsible for the subsequent painful swelling. The symptoms of periostitis are pain and localized redness of the skin. If pus or moisture accumulates between the bone and periosteum, the membrane is lifted, and because of its bone-building function forms an extra layer of bone. Treatment of periostitis depends on the cause. Bacteria relating to a particular disorder are destroyed with antibiotics. If pus forms the infected area must be opened and drained.

Peritonitis. Inflammation of the peritoneum, the membrane that lines the abdomen and encloses the abdominal organs. Peritonitis is not an independent disorder, but a complication of various abdominal conditions. It can be caused by bacteria, by infection of perforation of various abdominal organs, and by chemical irritation. Causes can include appendicitis, salpingitis or ectopic pregnancy, Pancreatitis perforation of the stomach cholecystitis, or inflammation of the large intestine (diverticulitis, ulcerative colitis).

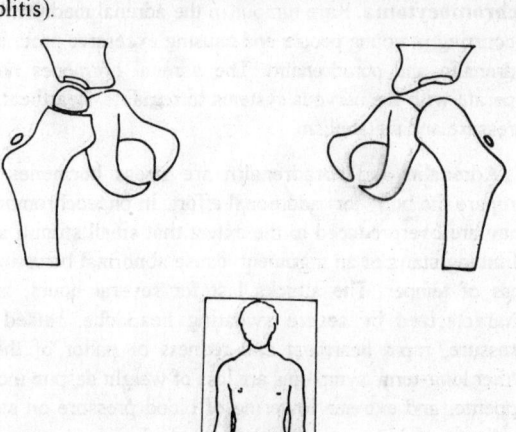

In Perthe's disease the head of the hip joint is destroyed by a local disturbance in the blood supply.

Perthes' disease. Growth disturbance in the head of the femur at hip level, one of the forms of osteochondritis. It occurs in children between the ages of 5 and 12 and is associated with hip pain and lameness. For as yet unknown reasons the growth of the femur head and the growth plate (epiphyseal cartilage) is disturbed, and these parts of the bone die. Decay of the epiphysis can cause the head of the bone to slip away (epiphysiolisis): the head is also completely destroyed and replaced by spontaneous new growth, which is soft and easily deformed at first. If weight is placed on the leg at this phase, the new head can be deformed, possibly causing permanent invalidity. It is important that the disorder is recognized at an early stage and other possibilities, such as arthritis, excluded. Diagnosis is by hip X-ray. Treatment is by taking the weight off the hip for long periods, so that the head of the femur can form as normally as possible. Prognosis is good if the disorder is recognized and treated early enough.

Phaeochromocytoma. Rare tumour in the adrenal medulla, usually occurring in young people and causing excessive production of adrenalin and noradrenalin. The adrenal hormones normally operate with the nervous systems to regulate heartbeat, blood pressure and metabolism.

Adrenalin and noradrenalin are stress hormones which prepare the body for additional effort. In phaeochromocytoma they are overproduced to the extent that small stimuli such as climbing stairs or an argument cause abnormal behaviour like loss of temper. The attacks last for several hours, and are characterized by severe sweating headache, raised blood pressure, rapid heartbeat and redness or pallor of the face. Other long-term symptoms are loss of weight despite increased appetite, and extreme lowering of blood pressure on standing up from a dying or sitting position, which can cause vertigo or fainting. Examination should be made of the level of the hormones concerned in the blood, and the possibility of a tumour in the adrenal glands should be investigated. Treatment is by removal of the (usually benign) tumour and by careful regulation of blood pressure by medication.

Pharyngitis. Inflammation of the mucous membrane of the throat and the surrounding lymph nodes. Acute Pharyngitis is a short-lived infection, caused by a virus or bacteria. Most people have at least one attack of pharyngitis a year. The symptoms are a dry, tickling throat, smarting and pain when swallowing, and generally also fever and nausea. The throat is red and swollen with a coating. Recovery occurs within a few days.

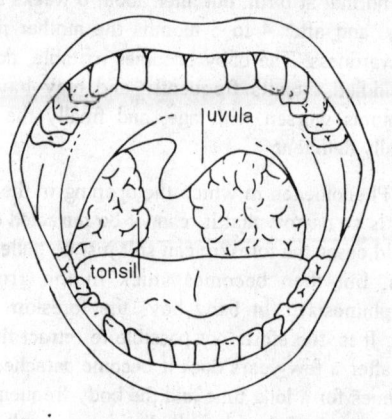

If an abscess forms behind a tonsil the uvula is displaced towards the healthy tonsil.

A complication of bacterial pharyngitis can be the formation of throat abscesses. With viral infection complications rarely occur, meningitis being a rare exception. Acute pharyngitis can also accompany another illness, such as measles, German measles or glandular fever, and the doctor should always be aware of this. If the patient is very ill, the disorder is probably acute tonsillitis, or it could be a streptococcal infection. This is a serious condition, with possible, though rare, complications such as scarlet fever, glomerulonephritis or rheumatic fever.

Pharynx. The throat; more accurately, the space linking the air passages through the nose, the entrance to the oesophagus, and the mouth.

Phenylketonuria. Serious congenital metabolic abnormality that occurs in 1 in 15,000 births, caused by lack of the liver enzyme that converts the amino acid phenylalanine (which occurs in all protein) and which thus accumulates in excessive quantities in the blood. The brain is affected, and the child becomes backward; normal nutrition is thus poisonous. Such children seem normal at birth, but after about 6 weeks the urine smells musty, and after 4 to 6 months the mother notices signs of backwardness. The baby becomes irritable, does not want to be cuddled, vomits frequently and may have convulsions. Symptoms worsen with age, and finally the child becomes mentally deficient.

Phimosis. Phenomenon in which the opening in the foreskin of the penis is so narrow that it cannot be retracted over the glans. In mild cases the foreskin can still just be pulled back over the glans, but then becomes stuck in the groove behind it (paraphimosis). In baby boys the foreskin is stuck to the glans. It is, therefore, not possible to retract the foreskin, and only after a few years does it become detached. If adherence continues for a long time and the body frequently suffers from inflammation of the glans (balanitis), a small surgical operation can release the foreskin. Such boys do not usually have a genuine phimosis; good penis hygiene prevents adherence from recurring. Genuine phimosis should be treated by surgery to widen or remove the foreskin. Regular stretching of the foreskin is not an appropriate way of remedying the condition and apart from this it is also very painful. Phimosis later in life is usually the result of foreskin shrinkage caused by inflammation. Treatment is also by removal of the foreskin.

Phobia. Severe anxiety about a certain object or situation, despite simultaneous awareness that the anxiety is unfounded. Directed anxiety is known as fear; there is a vague dividing line between exaggerated caution and fear. If someone is afraid of walking along the top of a wall, that is normal; but if a patient will not take more than two steps up a ladder, he is afraid of heights. Many other people are afraid of spiders or mice. Phobia is a state of severe anxiety, or an obsessive concern that a spider or mouse might appear. The best-known phobias are fear of stains, often associated with compulsive washing, agoraphobia, claustrophobia and fear of heights. It may be that the object of the phobia symbolizes something important in subconscious conflicts (defence mechanism), as in children who develop school phobia through fear of being deserted by their parents. In such cases treatment is by psychotherapy to make the conflict conscious and to allow the patient to come to terms with it. Phobia can also result from a bad experience: if a child is bitten by a dog he is likely to be afraid of all dogs; in such cases behavioural therapy is often effective. Phobia usually leads to avoidance behaviour, and is self-reinforcing. The patient does not allow himself to see that he can cope with the situation. Also the fact that there is genuine fear when confronted with the feared situation is seen by the patient as proof that the situation is alarming.

Pigeon chest. Chest deformity in which the breast bone seems to protrude, although in fact caused by sunken cartilage on each side. The condition is generally congenital, runs in families, and is sometimes associated with congenital heart conditions; it can also be a consequence of rickets.

A pigeon chest restricts the movement of lungs and heart, and can sometimes cause partial shrivelling of the lung (atelectasis). The opposite condition is funnel chest, characterized by severe inward slanting of the lower part of the breast bone; this condition too is probably caused by misplaced cartilage. If they cause problems both conditions can be treated by surgery.

Pituitary disorders. The pituitary gland is about the size of a pea, situated in a bony cavity at the base of the brain. Its function is to produce a number of hormones which regulate metabolic processes. Thus the pituitary gland controls growth, the quantity of water in the body, the formation of milk in the breasts, contraction of the womb during labour and the function of the thyroid, adrenal and sex glands. Disorders cause over-or under-production of one or more of these hormones, and can result from a pituitary tumour or brain damage, although often the cause is unknown. Excess growth hormone production can cause gigantism or acromegaly, excess sex hormone (FSH and LH) early puberty and too little fluid-regulating hormone (ADH) can lead to diabetes insipidus in which the kidneys excrete to much water with the urine. If the pituitary gland fails completely, all the hormones are underproduced. Some of the symptoms are listlessness, fatigue, muscular weakness, weight loss, loss of libido, loss of armpit and pubic hair, and lack of menstruation in women. In children growth slows down. Treatment is aimed at restoring normal hormone levels in the blood. Excess production can be controlled by surgical removal of (part of) the pituitary gland, by radiation therapy or by drugs to suppress hormone production. If the pituitary gland fails, synthetic hormones can be supplied, by injection, tablets or nasal spray. In the last case the active substances reach the bloodstream via the nasal mucous membrane. Such treatment usually restores normal bodily function almost completely.

Pituitary Gland. A small clump of cells about the size of a pea. The gland is buried in the bone that forms the base of the skull and roof of the mouth and is connected by the pituitary stalk consisting of neurons and local blood vessels to the part of the brain called the hypothalamus. The pituitary has a scientific name, hypophysis.

In humans, the glands is divided into two segments, the posterior or neurohypophysis and the anterior or adenohypophysis. The former secretes two hormones antidiuretic hormones, also called vasopressin, and oxytocin, both of which may be formed in the hypothalamus. The anterior pituitary secretes five hormones, growth hormone or somatotraphin, adrenocorticotrophic hormone (ACTH), thyroid-stimulating hormone, and three sex-related hormones, follicle-stimulating hormone, luteinizing hormones (female) or interstitial-cell stimulating hormone (male) and prolactin. All five are secreted in response to factors released into the local circulation by neurons in the hypothalamus, and their secretion is probably always stopped when hypothalamic neurons release a chemical with an opposite effect.

Pituitary tumour. Usually benign growth of certain cells in the pituitary gland. Symptoms are related to the function and site within the pituitary gland, which is about the size of a pea. Its function is to produce various hormones: a tumour can stop this process or the cells of which the tumour consists can become hyperactive and produce a particular hormone in excessive quantities, usually with associated under-production of others. Excess growth hormone production can cause gigantism or acromegaly and excess sex hormone (FSH and LH) can lead to early puberty; other effects depend on the site and size of the tumour. The pituitary gland is in a cavity at the base of the brain, near the intersection of the left and right optic nerves. A larger tumour can exert pressure on these nerves, possibly causing blindesss and persistent, increasingly severe headache. A pituitary tumour is diagnosed by measurement of certain blood-hormone levels; an X-ray of the skull shows enlargement of the pituitary cavity. Treatment is by surgery to remove the tumour, or radiation therapy. It is sometimes sufficient to check cells which are producing excess hormone using drugs.

Pityriasis Rosea. Harmless and common skin condition with characteristic 'medallions', yellow on the inside with a red edge, usually scally. A few days after the first patch appears smaller patches occur all over the rump, usually less distinct, but probably also with the 'medallion' effect. The cause is unknown; viral origin is suspected by unproven. The condition heals spontaneously after 6 to 8 weeks, and causes no difficulty other than skin abnormalities, thus ho treatment is necessary.

Pityriasis versicolor. Slightly itchy, superficial fungus infection of the skin, with characteristic brown patches, caused by *Malassezia furfur*, which can be detected in the patches by microscopic examination. The patches form on chest, back and shoulders; they are usually pale pink to brown. In dark-skinned people the patches are lighter than the surrounding skin, darker if the skin is fair, hence the name 'versicolor'.

Pacenta, detached. Detachement of the palcenta from the wall of the womb during pregnancy. It is caused by bursting of an artery at the point where the plancenta joins the uterus; the increasing discharge of blood wholly or partially detaches the placenta from the uterine wall. Detachment of the placenta is associated with sudden, continuous and often severe pain in the lower abdodmen. The uterus hardens as a result of the violent contraction, and does not relax. The baby can no longer be felt, and its heartbeat cannot be heard. With a major detachment, blood supply to the baby ceases, causing its death within a short time.

Placenta, disorders of. Inadequate placental function can have serious consequences for the unborn baby in the womb. The function of the placenta is the transport of nutrients and waste products, and exchange of blood and gases between the mother and baby. The placenta also produces hormones which are responsible for, among other things, sustaining the pregnancy. Sudden detachment of the placenta terminates blood supply abruptly (acute insufficiency), and usually causes the death of the foetus. Insufficiency can also arise gradually (chronic insufficiency), leading to under-development of the pregnancy. The child's growth is backward, and it can show oxygen deficiency. Abnormalities of placental structure or position in the womb can impair optimal blood supply, but usually it is abnormalities of the blood vessels in the mother's part of the placenta or the womb that are responsible for the deficiency. High blood pressure and diabetes mellitus can be factors in bringing about these abnormalities, which lead to minor haemorrhages and infarctions which impair the function of the placenta. The weight of the placenta is also a measure of its capacity, although it must also be seen in the context of the weight of the child. After birth it is also important to weigh the afterbirth and to check it for abnormalities, which could indicate or explain deficient growth in the child.

Placenta, retained. Failure of the placenta (afterbirth) to be ejected within an hour of the birth of the baby. After the birth of the baby the placenta detaches itself from the wall of the contracting uterus, but may not always be expelled immediately. If little blood is being lost, there is no harm in waiting, but after an hour the chance of serious post-natal haemorrhage is increased. Then usually attempts are made to expel the afterbirth by abdominal manipulation; this is also necessary if severe haemorrhage sets in immediately after the birth. If the placenta, or part of it, is still retained after manipulation, it is removed under general anaesthetic.

Placenta praevia. Placenta that overlies the cervical canal, so that the baby's head pressing against it can cause haemorrhage from the placenta. Painless loss of blood without contractions

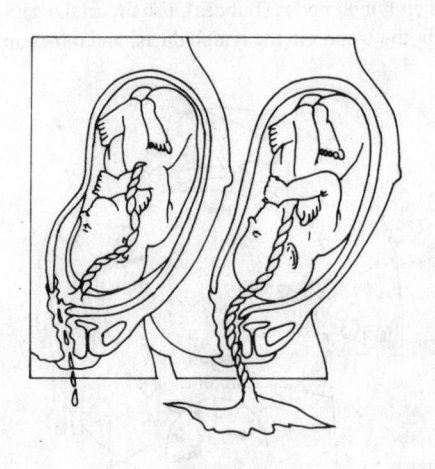

If delivery is normal and the placenta is born first the baby could suffer from orxygen shortage; for this reason a Caesarean delivery is customary if the placenta is presented at the entrance to the womb.

and hardening of the uterus in the second half of pregnancy can be a sign of placenta praevia. The first haemorrhage usually stops spontaneously, but subsequent ones can be so severe that there is danger to the mother of shock. Another sign of placenta praevia is malpresentation: low placental positioning prevents stable head presentation. The position of the placenta can be established by sonography; if placenta praevia is discovered the delivery must be by Caesarean section. The problem is unlikely to recur in a subsequent pregnancy.

Plague. Infection with the bacterium *Yersinia pestis,* transmitted to man by rat-fleabite. Plague still occurs in India, Pakistan, China, Indonesia and Africa, but is now rare in Western Europe. Many rodents are infected with plague bacteria, but only the rat can transmit it to man. The rat flea can only jump short distances, so infection can only be caused by rats living close to man (house or ship rats). There are two forms of plague in man: bubonic and pneumonic. Bubonic plague is characterized by swollen lymph nodes (buboes), usually in the groin. Bacteria reach the blood via the lymph ducts, and infection can then

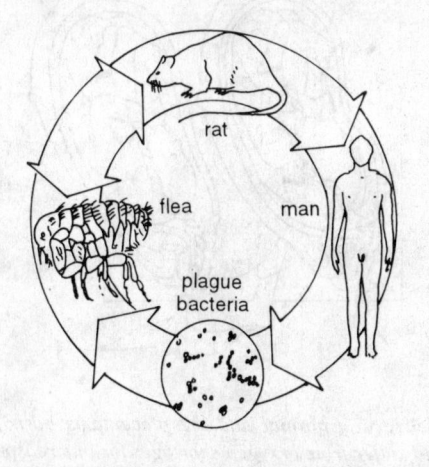

Cycle of infection with plague bacteria.

spread to many organs, including the lungs. Two to ten days after biting by the rat flea the patient has high fever, small skin haemorrhages and swelling of the luymph nodes. Pneumonic plague can be passed from person to person by coughing; this condition can also occur in connection with bubonic plague. After 2 to 3 days the patient is short of breath, and vomits watery mucus, later containing blood. Formerly few people recovered from this form of plague.

The most important measure against the disease is rat control and destruction of rat fleas. Infection can be prevented by vaccination, and is practised in areas in which plague occurs and for travellers to such areas. The disease itself is treated with antibiotics.

Plasma. A sticky, yellowish fluid smelling sweet when it is fresh. It consists of water, proteins, salt, glucose and other dissolved substances being transported around the body such as hormones. Plasma may also be looked upon as blood minus all cells and formed elements, platelets, found in whole blood.

Platelet. A piece of a large cell found in bone marrow and perhaps the lungs from which other blood cells are formed. Platelets lack nuclei and cannot reproduce themselves, but the same is true of red blood cells. Platelets are also called thrombocytes (Gr. *thrombo*=lump, clot) because they are required for the clotting process. They collect in a damaged place in a blood vessel and both secrete proteins that assist clotting and themselves form a matrix around which the clot forms. Not all of the functions of these small cells are understood; for example they contain the hormone adrenaline, and two other hormones which also act as chemical transmitters of signals between neurons, but the roles of these substances in the blood are unclear.

Plegia. (Gr. *plege* = a blow, stroke) A suffix which means the *paralysis* of the part, or a *stroke*.

Pleurisy. Inflammation of the mucous membrane surrounding the outer lung membranes (pleura), which consist of two layers separated from each other by a thin film of fluid. The inner layer is in contact with the lung, the outer layer with the wall of the chest; the film of fluid allows them to slide freely against each other. The space between the layers of membrane, the pleural cavity, is a vacuum, so they cannot drag on each other. Dry pleurisy is a condition in which the two layers adhere to each other because of the formation of fine threads of protein; this is almost always caused by a process in the lung directly under the pleura. This can be inflammation, as in tuberculosis, or lung cancer or a blood clot in the pulmonary artery. The adhesion occurs only at the site of the disorder. The condition can also occur in association with a general disease such as chronic rheumatoid arthritis. The adhesion prevents the pleura from sliding smoothly against one another, causing pain on breathing and coughing. Breathing is more shallow than usual.

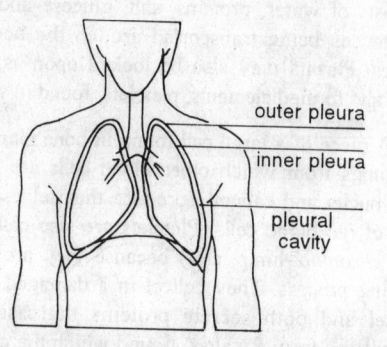

outer pleura

inner pleura

pleural cavity

In cases of pneumonia or pleurisy breathing is painful because of friction of the inflamed tissue.

The further development of the condition is uncertain. There are three possibilities: usually fluid is formed, so that the dry pleurisy changes to the wet form; the threads can disappear spontaneously; or they can develop into a definitive (no longer painful) adhesion of the pleural layers. In wet pleurisy an abnormal quantity of fluid accumulates in the pleural cavity; the condition tends to be preceded by dry pleurisy. The pain disappears with the fluid. The condition is most usually caused by pneumonia or lung tumours. A small quantity of inflammation fluid causes little discomfort; larger quantities cause shortness of breath through pressure on lung tissue. The symptoms of the primary disease predominate; coughing, fever and expectoration of sputum for pneumonia; loss of weight, general malaise and coughing for malignant tumours. Pleurisy is detected by knocking and listening to the chest.

Plummer-vinson syndrome. Rare combination of oesophagal stricture and iron-deficiency anaemia, with reduced gastric juice production. Other symptoms may include inflammation of the tongue (glossitis), nail abnormalities (spoon-shaped nails) and an enlarged spleen. The syndrome occurs particularly in middle-aged women. The principal difficulty is in swallowing solid food, which sometimes lodges in the air passages.

Pneumoconiosis. Malfunction of the lungs caused by inhalation of dust. The condition is infrequent, and associated with certain occupations—it is an occupational disorder.

The function of the lung deteriorates according to the quantity of substance inhaled, and the disorder is classified according to the nature of substance. The most common varieties are: silicosis (accumulation of silica or sand particles), and asbestosis) accumulation of asbestos fibres). Silicosis occurs in jobs such as quarrying, sand-blasting and grinding. The sand particles cause the formation of knots in the alveoli, resulting from the clustering of layers of connective tissue cells. As the disorder develops the knots of tissue form masses, a condition known as interstitial fibrosis, which gives a characteristic image on a chest X-ray. The knots show up as denser patches on the film, and the area around is brighter because of excess air in the lungs, the result of ephysema, wastage of the lung with expansion of the alveoli. Lung function tests show decrease in lung capacity and in the ability to breathe out quickly and powerfully. The disorder can be prevented by wearing good quality masks.

Asbestosis, the accumulation of asbestos fibres, occurs in the asbestos industry and in the manufacture of insulation material. The condition is characterized by the large-scale formation of connective tissue, particularly in the lower part of the lung (an effect of gravity). Scar tissue forms, and there is deformation of the alveoli. Shortness of breath is the most important symptoms of this condition, at first when the patient is active, and subsequently at rest as well. A chest X-ray shows slight, non-specific deviations, and an increased stripe pattern. Sometimes asbestos particles are found in the sputum. Lung function is restricted.

Pneumonia. Inflammation of the lung, the terminal sections of the air passages, and the tissue in between, usually caused by bacteria or viruses, sometimes by a fungus. In the alveoli, oxygen is removed from inhaled air and replaced with carbon dioxide. In pneumonia inflammation cells and fluid accumulate, with the result that the alveoli cannot fill properly with air, making the process of breathing difficult. The cause of the disease reaches lung tissue in inhaled air, or via the blood from an inflamed area elsewhere in the body. In the presence of factors that increase the risk of pneumonia it can be advisable to vaccinate the patient against influenza; this is particularly important for older people or chronic bronchitis and asthma sufferers. Inflammation can also occur (obstruction pneumonia) if a branch of the air passages is constricted by a tumour, inflammation or a foreign body (a peanut, for example). Aspiration or swallowing pneumonia can occur through the inhalation of pus or a piece of inflamed tissue, after a tonsillectomy for example. Disorders in the swallowing process can also cause this form of pneumonia.

The first signs of pneumonia are often cold shivers and a rapid rise in body temperature. If the source of infection is a virus, pneumonia is usually preceded by a cold or influenza. A mixture of pus and mucus forms in the lungs as a result of the inflammation reaction, and this is coughed up as sputum which is clear, yellowish-green or rust-brown according to the cause of the illness; it can also contain pus or blood. Local irritation of lung tissue can occur, causing pain in the side or chest, particularly when the patient breathes deeply or coughs. In cases of infection with certain bacteria, cold sores often occur at the same time.

Pneumonia is treated with antibiotics, and the patient usually recovers within two to three weeks. Regular knocking on the chest helps in coughing up the sputum; sometimes excess pus has to be removed by suction. A rise in the patient's temperature during treatment suggests a complication such as pleurisy, empyema or sepsis (blood poisoning).

Pneumothorax. Trapping of air between the lung and the chest wall. This space, the pleural cavity, normally contains no air at all, so that the lung is held firmly against the thoracic wall. If air gets in, the negative pressure responsible for holding the lung against the throax is removed, and the lung collapses partly or wholly. Air can penetrate from the inside (through a hole in the lung) or from outside (through a wound in the chest wall). If air leaks from the lung the condition is known as 'spontaneous pneumothorax', and is quite common among

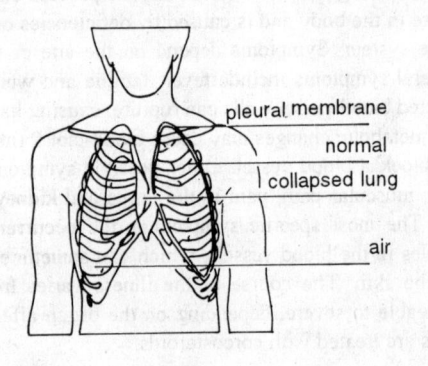

In pneamothorax air penetrates the membranes of the chest, thus raising the air pressure in the thoracic cavity and causing collapse of the lung tissue.

young men between the ages of 15 and 35. Older people with disorders such as emphysema run a greater than normal risk of pneumothorax, because large thin-walled blisters form in lung tissue, and can burst easily. Pneumothorax can also be the result of an accident : if a rib breaks it can damage the lung and release air into the pleural cavity. Finally, air can enter from the outside via an opening in the chest (a stab wound, for example).

Poliomyelitis (infantile paralysis; polio) Viral infection that affects mainly young people. Its symptoms resemble those of influenza. Polio also sometimes results in paralysis. The cause is the polio virus, which can affect the anterior horn cells of the spinal column—those that provide the muscles with impulses. Damage to these cells causes slack paralysis. The symptoms initially are fever, possibly followed by a similar feeling to influenza, diarrhoea and a stiff neck, and this is all most patients experience. About 1 per cent of patients then have sudden muscular pain, and paralysis of one or more nerve groups in the trunk and/or limbs.

Polyarteritis nodosa. Inflammation of large and medium-sized arteries, leading to tissue alteration. The process can occur anywhere in the body and is caused by deficiencies of the autoimmune system. Symptoms depend on the site of the disorder. General symptoms include fever, fatigue and weight loss; the affected blood vessel walls can rupture, causing haemnorrhage; also metabolic changes may cause blood-clot formation, which can block a blood vessel. Other possible symptoms are headache, muscular pain, pain in the joints and kidney abnormalities. The most specific symptom is the occurrence of small nodules in the blood vessels, which can sometimes be felt under the skin. The course of the illness varies from scarcely noticeable to severe, depending on the organ affected. Severe forms are treated with corcosteroids.

Polymyalgia. Muscular disorder that occurs particularly in older women. The first sign is usually severe pain in the muscles around the shoulders and hips, often associated with muscular stiffness and limited movement in the shoulder and hip joints. This joints themselves show no abnormality. The disorder is usually associated with loss of weight, fever and anaemia. Tests on affected muscle tissue reveal no abnormalities, but blood tests show a significant increase in red blood cell sedimentation rate (ESR). Polymyalgia is often associated with arteritis temporalis, inflammation of the small arteries at the temple. Probably these two disorders are components of the same disease, of which the cause is unknown. Because arteritis can lead to blindness, polymyalgia patients should be examined for abnormalities in the arteries of the temple. Both conditions are treated with corticosteroids Physiotherapy and heat treatment can be important in maintaining and restoring mobility to muscles and joints.

Polyp, intestinal. Initially benign intestinal tumour. Polyps may occur throughout the larger intestine, and sporadically in the small intestine, increasing with the age of the patient. In later life about 10 per cent of the population has one or more polyps, particularly in the last section of the large intestine. They

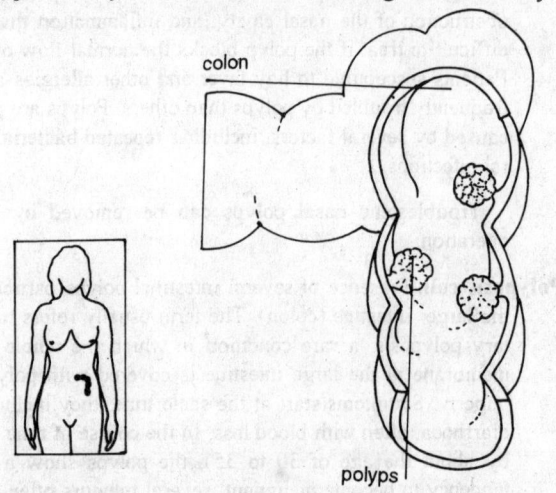

colon

polyps

Polyps in the colon are extrusions of mucous membrane on a stalk; they can become malignant.

can also be hereditary, so-called polyposis coli, but this is rare. Intestinal polyps usually cause no symptoms but there can be slight blood loss or even significant haemorrhage with bright blood in the faeces, or black faeces (melaena, when the blood is partly digested). Large polyps can cause sporadic intestinal obstruction. Certain polyps (so-called villous adenoma) are more likely to become malignant (intestinal cancer); in others the likelihood is slight. Most malign intestinal tumours do not originate from polyps. If the above symptoms occur the possibility of a malignant tumour must always be investigated, by contrast X-rays or by rectoscopy. The polyp may possibly be removed at the same time. As a rule any polyp larger than 1 cm, or a rapidly-growing polyp, must be removed and examined in a laboratory (biopsy).

Polyp, nasal. Soft protusion of mucous membrane that occurs in the nose and elsewhere. Nasal polyps can occur inside the nose or on the mucous membrane of the sinuses. The glassy, bluish-grey polyps are benign, but can cause difficulties in breathing through the nose, problems with smell and speech through obstruction of the nasal cavity, and inflammation that can be difficult to treat if the polyp blocks the normal flow of mucus. Patients susceptible to hay fever and other allergies are more frequently troubled by polyps than others. Polyps are probably caused by several factors, including repeated bacterial and viral infections.

   Troublesome nasal polyps can be removed by a minor operation.

Polyposis coli. Presence of several intestinal polyps particularly in the large intestine (colon). The term usually refers to hereditary polyposis, a rare condition in which the whole mucous membrane of the large intestine is covered with polyps from puberty. Symptoms start at the same time; they include slight diarrhoea, often with blood loss. In the course of time (usually by about the age of 30 to 35), the polyps show a marked tendency to become malignant; several tumours often occur at the same time. After diagnosis by coloscopy the only treatment is the whole or partial removal of the colon, possibly supplemented with colostomy. If a decision is made to join the small intestine to the rectum, thus allowing faeces to be passed in the normal manner, regular checks are necessary to find any new polyps in the rectum, which must be cauterized.

Pons, tumour of. Benign tumour (acoustic neuroma) that originates in either the nerve responsible for hearing or that responsible for balance, which leave the inner ear together and enter the brain as the eighth cranial nerve.

As the tumour grows it exerts increasing pressure on its surroundings, causing gradual deafness, often with tinnitus (ringing in the ears). Possible failure of the inner ear can also lead to slight problems of balance, but adaptation usually means that these are not severe. The development of microsurgery has meant that it is often possible, if the tumour is discovered early, to remove it in its entirety, without damaging other nerves or brain tissue.

Porphyria. Collective name for a number of disorders involving overproduction in the body of substances called porphyrins. Symptoms vary according to the porphyrin concerned, varying from slight to potentially fatal. Most forms are hereditary.

The condition can affect the skin (a brown discoloration); large blisters often form after exposure to sunlight, warmth or certain medicines. The liver may be affected; accumulation of porphyrins can cause jaundice and in the long term cirrhosis of the liver. Other symptoms are epileptic attacks and convulsive abdominal pain. The disorder is diagnosed by the presence of certain substances in the urine, which may turn bright red. Treatment is by avoiding circumstances which can worsen the condition (walking in the sun, drinking alcohol, taking certain medicines and eating certain foods).

Post-partum Haemorrhage. Loss of more than half a litre of blood before and after expulsion of the placenta (afterbirth), which is always associated with loss of blood, normally stopped by pinching of the blood vessels in the contracted uterus. This process can be disturbed if the placenta is retained, or because part of it has remained in the womb. Post-partum haemorrhage can also be the result of extreme stretching of the womb during pregnancy because of a multiple pregnancy or an excess of amniotic fluid. Because of the danger of shock the woman must be taken immediately to hospital. Treatment is in the first place for shock, followed by scraping the uterus under anaesthetic and the administration of drugs to induce uterine contractions.

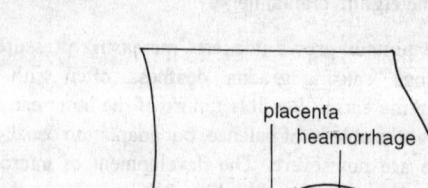

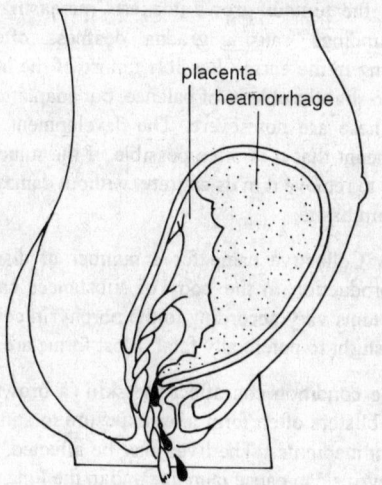

Post-partum haemorrhage usually occurs because the plancenta has not been completely released and thus the womb cannot contract properly.

Pre-eclampsia. Term for a number of symptoms that can affect a woman during pregnancy and which threaten both the baby's development and the mother's life. The most significant is high blood pressure, which develops in the last three months of pregnancy. The body often retains liquid at this stage, and this is reflected in weight gains of more than 500 grams per week on average.

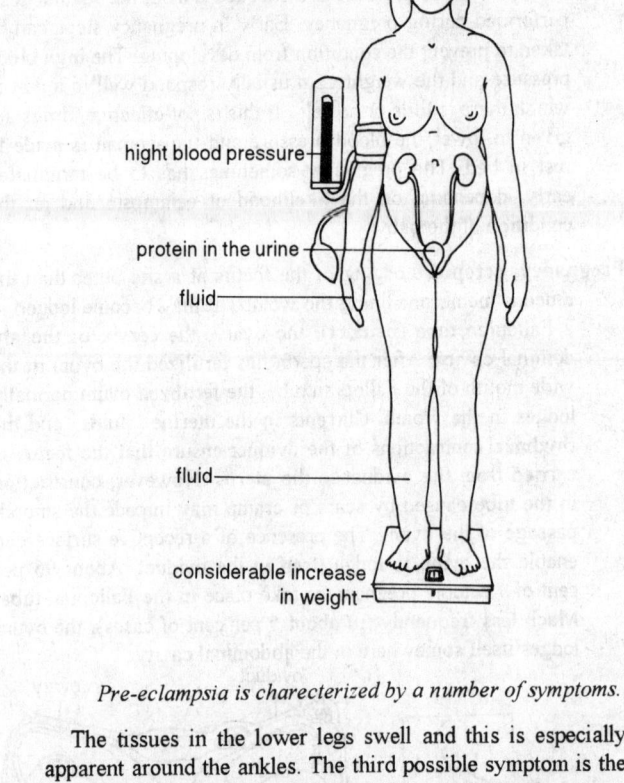

fluid

hight blood pressure

protein in the urine

fluid

fluid

considerable increase
in weight

Pre-eclampsia is charecterized by a number of symptoms.

The tissues in the lower legs swell and this is especially apparent around the ankles. The third possible symptom is the elimination of protein in the urine. This indicates damage to the kidneys. Women who, before becoming pregnant, had high blood pressure, kidney conditions or who are diabetics, are most at risk. The danger of these complications during pregnancy is that they increase the risk of the placenta malfunctioning. This retards the baby's growth and the baby is underdeveloped. At a late stage in pregnancy, the woman can suffer symptoms such as headache, nausea, vomiting, drowsiness, and seeing spots and stars. The woman may suffer a fit of eclampsia at any time; fortunately this is rare. Weight, urine and blood pressure are checked during the regular tests performed during pregnancy. Early in pregnancy steps can be taken to prevent the condition from developing. The high blood pressure and the weight gain usually respond well to a diet in which there is little or no salt. If this is not effective, drugs are given to lower the blood pressure and the woman is made to rest in bed. The pregnancy sometimes has to be terminated early, depending on the likelihood of eclampsia and on the condition of the baby.

Pregnancy, ectopic. Lodging of the foetus at a site other than the mucous membrane lining the womb. It may become lodged in a Fallopian tube (oviduct), the ovary, the cervix or the abdominal cavity. After the sperm has fertilized the ovum in the wide mouth of the Fallopian tube, the fertilized ovum normally lodges in the womb. Currents in the uterine fluids and the rhythmic contractions of the oviduct ensure that the foetus is carried from the oviduct to the uterus. However, constriction in the tube caused by scars or cramp may impede the smooth passage of the ovum. The presence of a receptive surface can enable the ovum to lodge itself in the oviduct. About 95 per cent of ectopic pregnancies take place in the Fallopian tube. Much less frequently (in about 5 per cent of cases), the ovum lodges itself somewhere in the abdominal cavity.

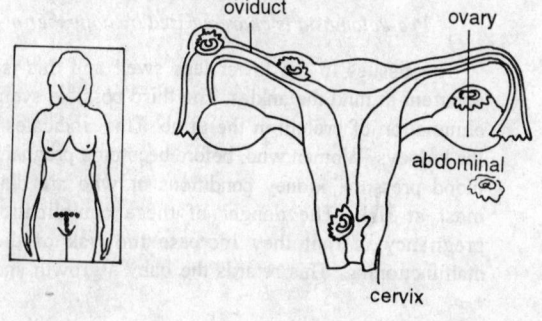

Pregnancy, multiple. Pregnancy in which more than one baby is
present.

Twins occur in about one of eighty pregnancies. Triplets or
a larger number of foetuses are extremely rare, and occur almost exclusively after treatment to stimulate ovulation. The
chance of complications is somewhat higher in multiple pregnancy. The placentas, which are too small in proportion to the
size of the babies, can sometimes be insufficient for the baby's
needs at an early stage. Malfunction of the placenta is increased by the regular incidence of high blood pressure and
the increased tendency to retain fluid. These last-mentioned
factors roughly quadruple the likelihood of pre-eclampsia. For
these reasons, rest and a salt free diet are usually precribed
from early on the pregnancy. A pregnancy in which there are
twins normally lasts for less than 37 weeks and birth is premature. One complications of labour is that one of the babies is
often a breech delivery. This in the case of prematurely born,
immature babies, is an additional strain which threatens survival. A woman with a multiple pregnancy is usually kept
under observation; delivery almost always takes place in hospital.

Pregnancy, underdeveloped. Slower growth than normal of a pregnant woman's womb at a given stage of the pregnancy. This
often reflects retarded growth in the baby. Slow growth is
usually detected during a pregnancy check, because the uterns
is either not growing at all or is not growing enough. The
growth is measured by the rise in the roof of the uterus as
measured against the mother's pubis and naval and the curve
of her ribs. For example, when the pregnancy reaches 20
weeks, the uterus is normally at the level of the navel. If it is
found that the uterus is too low, this does not in itself mean
that the pregnancy is underdeveloped. The first question is
whether the supposed duration of pregnancy is correct. The
pregnancy may have begun later because of menstrual cycle of
more than four weeks, and in such cases a low uterus is in
fact entirely normal. A pregnancy can be confirmed as underdeveloped only after repeated measurements.

The diagnosis can be made with greater certainty with the aid of an ultrasound examination (echography). In this technique, a picture of the baby is formed by the reflection of sound waves. The dimensions of the head and other parts of the body are compared with standard values or with the results of measurements taken in previous examinations.

Premenstrual syndrome. Group of symptoms caused by the monthly cycle of sex hormone production, occurring in women who are not on the pill or using other sex hormones. Many women experience the syndrome to a mild degree; the only consolation

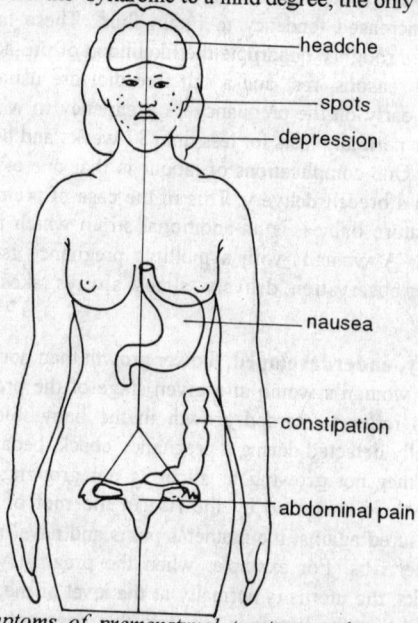

The symptoms of premenstrual tension syndrome (PMS) are caused by a strong reaction to monthly hormonal changes in the pituitary gland and ovaries.

that can be offered is that a normal cycle is an essential prerequisite, and thus the syndrome is a sign that all is well for the woman concerned. Possible symptoms include fatigue, irritability, hypersensivity, painful breasts,(sometimes with painful benign tumours in the breasts), a distended feeling in the abdomen, constipation, flatulence, retention of a few litres of fluid and headache or migraine. The symptoms usually disappear when menstruation begins. They are caused by sex hormones and their natural fluctuations. Symptoms do not always occur, and the necessity for treatment is viewed in various ways. There are experts and also women patients who blame the premenstrual syndrome for every misfortune and every squabble. This can be taken to excess. A woman once submitted a defence for murder on the grounds of diminished responsibility as a result of premenstrual tension. At the other end of the scale there are doctors and women who trivialize the problem completely. Naturally discomfort and pain are difficult to measure, and any genuine complaint should be taken seriously.

Presbyopia. Worsening near vision caused by the normal decrease in accommodation in older people.

Accommodation is the ability to make the lens of the eye bulge in order to focus on closer objects. The older a person gets, the less elastic the lens becomes, and the closest point at which the eye can focus becomes increasingly far away; this is illustrated by the fact that an older person has to hold a book or newspaper farther and farther away in order to be able to read it.

Priapism. Sudden and persistent penile erection, without previous sexual stimulation, and not resulting in ejaculation. The erection is painful, and persists because blood cannot flow out of the erectile tissue. Priapism can occur in patients with bone-marrow conditions, inflammation of the genitals, diabetes mellitus, leukaemia and some infectious diseases, and as a result of coagulation of blood in the erectile tissue. Hospital treatment is necessary, and often difficult. Sometimes gentle massage under anaesthetic helps, or the administration of female sex hormones. In some cases the only possible therapy is the surgical removal of erectile tissue.

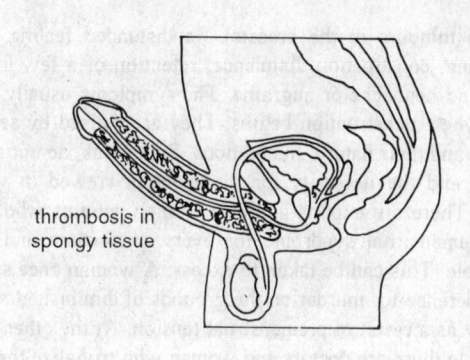

thrombosis in
spongy tissue

Priapism is a painful erection caused because the blood vessels in the spongy tissue of the penis are blocked, with the result that the blood cannot flow out.

Prickly heat. Skin condition which develops as a result of exposure to excessive heat and is characterized by large red pimpled spots.

This condition occurs mainly on the skin of the trunk or on those parts of the skin which are kept warm by clothing. It is an abnormal reaction of the skin to heat, and there is a cogenital predisposition to it. Such heat rashes occur in reveral members of certain families, while other families remain entirely free of the condition.

Proctitis. Inflammation of the rectum, the last section of the intestine before the anus. The condition is often part of more general inflammation, for example of the whole large intestine, as in ulcerative colitis, or the result of infection with gonorrhoea.

Symptoms are directly dependent upon the cause and include diarrhoea and loss of mucus and blood. Gonorrhoea is associated with pain and a burning sensation, and a white or yellow discharge.

Diagnosis can be rectoscopy with a bacterial culture to confirm gonorrhoea or other bacterial infections. Treatment is according to the particular condition.

Prostate, cancer of. Malignant tumour of the gland under the bladder which partly encloses the urethra in males. This form of cancer is very common in men over 60. As in the case with an enlarged prostate caused by a benign tumour, there are problems with urination. But the major symptom is pain, usually localized around the anus and penis, and sometimes in the region of the stomach. The pain is not relieved by urinating, which is made difficult because of pressure on the urethra by the tumour. There is no force behind the stream, and urine dribbles out in small quantities, meaning more frequent visits to the toilet (at night as well).

Prostate, enlargement of. The prostate gland, which is set beneath the bladder and partly encloses the urethra in men and boys, can become enlarged in various ways. The commonest is a benign tumour (adenoma). The tumour grows slowly, and replaces normal prostate tissue. Because the urethra runs through the prostate the first noticeable symptoms occur when urinating. The urethra is constricted by the tumour, making urination more difficult; there is no force behind the stream, and urine often dribbles out. The patient can thus pass only a little urine at a time, and often has to get up in the night for the purpose. Because the condition develops slowly, many men do not consult a doctor. The disorder is said to be an old man's disease, but it can have serious consequences in the long run. The bladder can no longer be fully emptied, which can cause infection of the urethra and even damage to the kidneys.

Prostate gland. A male sex organ which secretes much of the seminal fluid in which sperm are suspended during ejaculation. It is actually a group of glands and muscle fibres forming a ring of tissue around the urethra or tube connecting the bladder to the exterior. It lies just below the bladder.

Prostatitis. Inflammation of the prostate gland, which is set beneath the bladder and partially encloses the urethra in men and boys. If the condition develops quickly, it is usually caused by an infection elsewhere in the body which reaches the prostate via the blood. For example, bacteria originating in the urethra can be associated with the venereal disease gonorrhoea. Prostatitis causes severe pain in the area between anus and penis; the pain can be such that the patient is unable to urinate. Treatment with antibiotics is necessary to control the infection, which can also be chronic, with vague back pain, pain between anus and penis and the need to visit the toilet increasingly frequently.

Protein. With carbohydrate (for example, sugar) and fat, protein is a major constituent of all organishes and therefore of food. It is made up of carbon, hydrogen and oxygen, like the other constituents, plus nitrogen and to a lesser degree, sulphur. These elements form small molecules called amino acids. About twenty different amino acids are joined together in long, often branching chains to form thousands of proteins each of which has its unique structure and function. The major functional classes of proteins are structural, like the molecules that form the working parts of muscle cells; transport, like haemoglobin in red blood cells; defence, like antibodies, and enzymes. Structural protein is constantly needed during growth and for maintenance and repair.

The normal body can synthesize all the proteins it requires. Indeed, the role of the gene is to direct the synthesis of a protein. Body cells can also synthesize the amino acids out of the basic elements, but eight of them may be made too slowly or in quantities too small to satisfy need. These essential amino acids ought to be supplemented from the food we eat.

Only meat products and certain plants, for example, peas and beans, can provide the nitrogen required for amino acid synthesis. Although nitrogen is part of the air, it exists in a chemically-inert state which makes it unusable by body cells. We acquire nitrogen by eating amino acids. As far as protein is concerned, food digestion consists of the breakdown of animal or vegetable protein to its constituent amino acids. All essential amino acids can be obtained from meat, eggs, fish and milk products, but no single plant food contains all of them.

Prusitus vulvae (Vulvar itching) Itching of the external female sex organs. It can have many causes. The itching can be the consequence of vaginitis; the accompanying discharge irritates the vulva. A venereal disease such as syphilis or gonorrhoea often causes itching; crab louse and scabies on the vulva can also cause it. Some general disorders such as diabetes are associated with itching because regular infections occur. Skin diseases often also affect the vulva.

Pseudo-arthrosis. Incomplete calcification of the first tissue (soft callus) that forms between two parts of a bone after a fracture with the result that the two parts of the bone can still move relatively to each other. If a fracture heals normally the

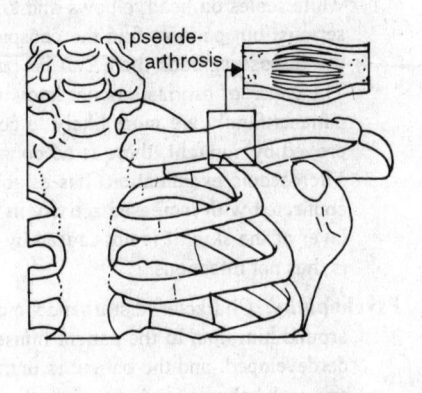

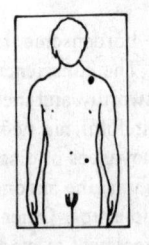

Pseudo-arthrosis can occur in various parts of the body if a fracture is badly set and immobilized.

two parts of the bone are joined together by the soft callus, then growth takes place from the internal and external bone membranes to form bone and cartilage, and finally the joint is completed with bone tissue.

Pseudo-croup. Inflammation and swelling of the mucous membrane under the vocal cords in children, with hoarseness, a yelping cough and difficult, noisy breathing. The condition occurs almost exclusively in children between the ages of one and five, and begins in the early evening; the condition is usually allergic.

Psittacosis. Respiratory infection with pneumonia caused by *Chlalmydia psittacosi,* a micro-organism that occurs in parrots, but also in parakeets, pigeons chickens and other birds; the birds themselves are sometimes merely carriers. The disease is transmitted to human beings by inhalation of substances contained in the feathers or excrement of infected birds.

Psoriasis. Skin disorder characterized by red patches and silvery white scales on head, elbows and knees. The condition is not serious, but patients find the conspicuous patches irksome. If the disease spreads there can be patches all over the body. The cause of psoriasis is not known exactly. Members of the patients family are more likely to contract it; it is usually improved by sunlight; there is no connection with certain foods. Microscopic examination has established that the disorder is connected with increased activity in the cells forming the base layer of the skin; it is not caused by a virus or bacterium, and is thus not infectious.

Psychopathy. Character disturbance more burdensome to those around him than to the patient himself. The conscience is underdeveloped, and the patient is untrustworthy and inclined to criminal behaviour. A psychopath must fulfil his needs. His tolerance of frustration is low: small annoyances or disappointments make him ill. Psychopaths cannot imagine anyone else's situation, or enter into long, deep relationships. Other people are objects used for his satisfaction. Treatment is made difficult by the fact that everything that goes wrong in the patient's life is ascribed to others, and never to himself. One cause of psychopathy can be lack of affection or teaching in early life. A certain amount of trust in other people is needed to form a conscience and the ability to place oneself in other people's shoes; love security and a structured life in early childhood are essential for this.

Psychosis. Mental disorder in which perceptions and ideas cannot be related to reality. Many people form mistaken ideas, but correct them when the true situation is pointed out. Psychotics cannot make this correction. They perceive things which do not exist (hallucinations) or are convinced of something which is not so (delusions). Consciousness may or may not be lowered (as in delirium), but this does not help. Short-term psychotic conditions occur in association with serious and devastating events in a person's life, and as a result of intoxication with alcohol, LSD and other drugs. Psychoses can also be caused by brain disorders and physical illnesses. This can be the result of serious neurosis and can occur at certain periods in life (childbirth and pubertal psychosis). Periods of psychosis can also be part of general psychiatric illness: schizophrenia and manic-depressive psychosis. Treatment is by medication (neuroleptics) to suppress the psychotic symptoms; if psychosis is itself a symptom of another disorder, that disorder should be treated.

Psychosocial problems. Generally caused by a particular situation in which the individual finds himself; these circumstances or society are always part of the cause. Psychosocial problems in the narrower sense are characterized by the fact that they disappear when the cause is identified and assistance directed at the circumstances. Social work is extremely important in helping the patient to come to terms with and solve problems in this category, which can be caused by loneliness divorce, educational problems,. bereavement, and so on.

Psychosomatic. A symptom or disease with a mental as well as a physical component or cause. It focuses attention on the supposed duality of the human being, part matter and part mind or soul. Increasingly with the development of the brain sciences in the second half of this century, mind has been recognized as a function of brain. No matter that mind remains a poorly understood function, it does not exist without brain and is wholly embodied in that physical entity. If that hypothesis is more correct than the old notion of duality, then a psychic origin is no less physical than an infection or a broken leg, for example, but it may be unidentified. This being the case, psychosomatic takes on the meaning of multifactorial; that is, the symptom or disease is caused by a number of factors, some of which may be identifiable while others, especially those associated with emotions and states of mind, are not yet identifiable.

Emotions for example, can certainly produce physical effects ranging from *diarrhoea* to loss of consciousness in fainting. Equally obviously, physical disorders like *heart disease* can produce *anxiety, depression* and *fear*. Emotions can be shown to be associated with the signals in groups of brain cells which are also involved with the release of powerful hormones, both physical events with psychic aspects.

Asthma is a classic case of a psychosomatic disease. It is caused in part by *allergy*, a fairly well understood physical sequence of events, and in part by fear, tension or stress, words without precise, measurable meanings. The contemporary view is that the lack of precision arises out of ignorance of the relevant physical events rather than because these phenomena have a different kind of reality called psychic.

Because of arguments like these, the word psychosomatic has tended to be much less frequently heard, but the duality behind it has not disappeared. Today, people talk instead about holistic medicine which takes into account the whole person. The notion implies, if it does not openly assert, that there is a non-holistic medicine: the traditional Western medicine that focuses on measurable physical relationships   while playing down or ignoring the powerful and no less real emotions and similar psychic phenomena. It is of course a nonsensical formulation. Doctors ignore what they cannot explain only at the greatest risk to themselves and their patients and all but the most ignorant and blinkered know it. No school of medicine could have existed for five minutes let alone 500 years which failed to recognize patients worries, fears and stresses—or the observable physical causes of their ills. "Holism", indeed, may be the most important if not the only quality that Chinese, Hindu, Bantu and Western medicine have in common.

Psychosomatic disorders. Disorders with physical symptoms, but having a psychological cause. It is known that psychological factors can to a large extent affect the course of an illness, any complications and the speed of recovery. Hereditary factors are significant: some people react excessively with part of the autonomic nervous system to emotional pressure. The patient's circumstances also play an important part, as does the structure of his personality. It is not known for certain how body and mind interact. The most important psychosomatic disorders, or disorders with a psychosomatic component, include stomach ulcer, ulcerative colitis, and other intestinal inflammation, asthma, essential high blood pressure rheumatoid arthritis anmd migraine. People with a psychosomatic illness often make use of defence mechanirms to suppress conflicts and aggression. It is possible that psychosomatic disorders are themselves such a mechanism, and related to a conversion symptom. The physical aspect of the illness must of course be treated, and a change in lifestyle or psychotherapy can be helpful. It is usually necessary for the patient to accept psychological treatment.

Puberty, delayed. Lack of sexual maturity in girls of 13 to 14 and boys of 15 to 16. The cause can be hereditary abnormalities such as hypothyroidism, Turner's and Klinefelter's syndromes chronic malnutrition and chronic illness (of the heart, lung or kidneys) or inadequate sex hormone production because of an abnormality in the brain or the genitals. Such children seem more childish than their age would suggest which can have a harmful effect on psychological development. In girls the breasts do not increase in size, pubic hair does not grow, and menstruation does not begin. Boys have no pubic hair, the penis does not grow, the testicles are absent or remain small, and the voice does not break. The children may or may not grow to the correct height, depending on the cause of the abnormality. Diagnosis is by taking the family history and making external, laboratory and X-ray examinations.

Puberty, early. Sexual maturity before the age of eight in girls and ten in boys. Both show an early development of secondary sexual characteristics. Girls' breasts increase in size and menstruation is usually early. In boys the penis, testicles, pubic hair and underarm hair grow, the beard begins to grow, and somewhat later the larynx increases in size and the voice breaks. As a growth spurt is usually associated with puberty, such children are often tall for their age, but this in itself need not cause anxiety because an early growth spurt is often shorter than usual. The cause of early puberty is not always known; this is the case in 40 per cent of boys and 85 per cent of girls. The cause can be a pituitary tumour, which causes overproduction of sex hormones (FSH and LH); this can also occur because of hyperactivity of the sex cells themselves (in the testicles, ovaries or adrenal cortex). If the adrenal cortex is overproducing at birth, in a girl this can give rise to male external genitals, while the internal genital organs are female (pseudohemaphroditism). The abnormality is caused by excess male sex hormones, which can make it difficult to establish the child's sex at birth. Diagnosis is by family history, physical appearance and extensive laboratory tests.

Puerperal fever (childbed fever) Infection of a woman's internal genital organs, usually in the first week after having a baby, associated with fever and a foul-smelling discharge. Such infection can easily occur immediately after childbirth, because the woman's resistance is low. The interior of the womb is still accessible and the wound at the site of the placenta with residual blood clots is an ideal breeding-ground for bacteria. During birth this area is almost always affected, and in some cases true inflammation occurs, which can spread in various ways to other organs in the abdominal cavity. leading to danger of the once dreaded peritonitis. Puerpetal fever is an alarming condition; as well as general symptoms such as headache, dullness and loss of appetite a foul-smelling discharge indicates the presence of inflammation. Treatment is by bed rest and drugs to stimulate the womb to expel dead matter. Antibiotics may also be prescribed. Good hygiene before, during and after childbirth are essential to reduce the chance of infection.

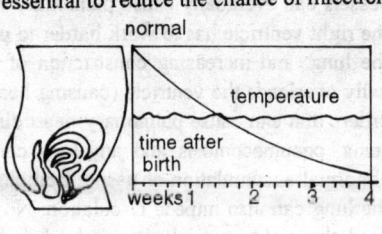

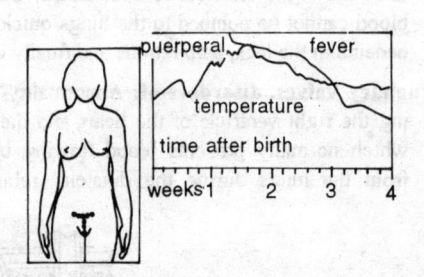

In puerperal fever there is fever after the first week, and a foul-smelling discharge from the vagina.

Pulled muscle. Tearing of muscular fibre, which usually also damages blood vessels in the muscle because muscles have large numbers of blood vessels which provide oxygen and remove waste products. Tearing a muscle thus also causes haemorrhage, known as haematoma. Other symptoms are pain, particularly when using the damaged muscle, and resultant restricted movement. As muscular fibre on both sides of the damaged area contracts, and indentation may be felt at the point of the tear. Muscles can also be torn by injury from the outside, which may also damage other tissue. This is particularly common in sports such as wrestling. Sudden convulsive muscular contraction can also cause tearing; damage of this kind occurs in badly-trained muscle and those affected by muscular conditions.

Pulmonary heart disease (cor pulmonare) Failure of the right-hand side of the heart caused by lung abnormalities; any lung condition associated with narrowing of the pulmonary blood vessels can eventually cause pulmonary heart disease because the right ventricle has to work harder to pump enough blood to the lung, and increasing constriction of the blood vessels finally overloads the ventricle (causing heart failure). Lung disorders that can cause pulmonary heart disease include emphysema, pneumoconiosis and any lung condition involving the abnormal accumulation of tissue. Embolisms in the arteries of the lung can also impede circulation. No discomfort is caused until the right ventricle is overloaded, but as soon as it is, blood cannot be pumped to the lungs quickly enough, causing oedema in the legs, palpitations and finally cyanosis.

Pulmonary valves, disorders of. Abnormality of the valve dividing the right ventricle of the heart and the pulmonary artery, which normally prevents blood flowing back into the heart from the lungs during the diastole (relaxed) phase in the

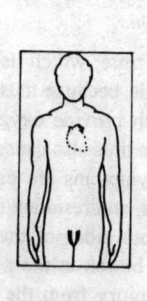

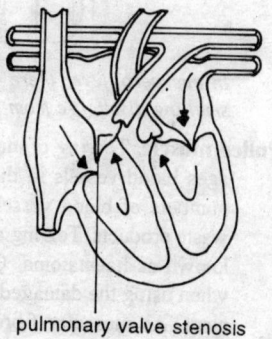

pulmonary valve stenosis

Disorders of the pulmonary valve are insufficiency or stenosis of the valve. In stenosis the blood can pass through the valve only with difficulty.

hearbeat. A valve can be constricted (stenosis) or leak (insufficiency), but the latter is rare in the pulmonary valve. Pulmonary stenosis is almost always congenital. The consequence is that the right ventricle can pump too little blood to the lungs, causing symptoms such as cyanosis and shortness of breath. Medication is pointless; the only effective treatment is surgery to widen the valve.

Purpura. Purplish-red haemorrhages, a symptom of capillary inflammation, whcih destroys the blood vessels and causes multiple small haemorrhages just below the surface of the skin. They show through as purple patches and sometimes form blisters. The commonest cause is an allergic inflammation of the blood vessels : the body reacts to the presence of a foreign substance in the blood vessels by forming antibodies . In some cases the condition is not confined to the skin, but affects internal organs and can damage the kidneys (among others). Another cause of purpura is the presence of too few platelets in the blood, possibly because too many blood platelets are being broken down in the spleen or because too few platelets are being manufactured, as in leukaemia. If the cause of purpura is treated the symptoms should disappear spontaneously, in which case no treatment is necessary for the skin condition itself.

Pyelitis. Inflammation of the renal pelvis and often also of kidney tissue, usually subsequent to inflammation of the urinary tract, such as inflammation of the bladder (cystitis). Pyelitis occurs particularly as a result of restriction of the flow of urine, by kidney stones for example, tumours of the renal pelvis or pregnancy. Inflammation of the bladder can also lead to pyelitis in conditions such as urine retention resulting from an enlarged prostate or nerve failure. Chronic pyelitis is usually caused by an anatomical abnormality of the uninary tract and/or restricted urinary flow. In severe cases the kidneys can be damaged to the extent of causing kidney failure, associated with uraemia. The symptoms of pyelitis include fever, back pain and pain associated with urination. In chronic cases the predominant symptoms are exhaustion and loss of appetite. Treatment is by high fluid intake and antibiotics. The root cause of the inflammation should also be sought. Contrast X-rays and sonographic examination of the kidneys are also possible.

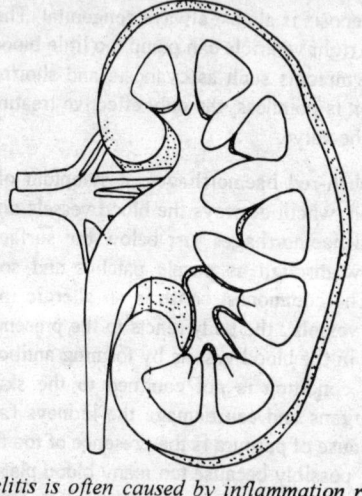

Acute pyelitis is often caused by inflammation rising from the urinary tract.

Pyloric Stenosis. Constriction of the exit from the stomach caused by convulsive contraction (spasm) or constriction of the pyloric muscle. The condition occurs particularly in boy babies two to six weeks old, and sometimes in adults as a complication of stomach ulcers. It prevents the passage of food from the stomach to the duodenum. In infants the symptoms develop gradually in 1 to 2 weeks, but sometimes begin suddenly. The most important symptom is vomiting with great force, so-called projectile vomiting, which can project vomit over several metres. The vomiting is worst in the mornings and evenings. All other symptoms are the direct result of the vomiting: loss of weight small quantities of faeces, relatively dry nappies and possibly dehydration. Treatment is by surgery to cut open part of the constricted muscle; only in mild cases can medicine be given and developments awaited. If pyloric stenosis occurs as a result of a stomach or duodenal ulcer the symptoms are less drastic, consisting of vomiting and a full feeling in the stomach.

R

Rabies (hydrophobia). Viral disease that occurs in man and other mammals; foxes and bats are the principal carriers in the wild. The virus is present in infected animals' saliva, and human beings are infected by biting, scratching or licking. The virus cannot be transmitted through undamaged skin, but could pass through the mucous membrane of mouth or eyes, for example. The virus lives and multiplies in the nerves and brain. First symptoms may occur between ten days and two years after infection with the disease.

In man the symptoms are fever, pain and tingling at the site of the wound. Saliva is thick and viscous and contains the virus. Restless, excited behaviour, linked with uninhibited screaming, ends in a genuine fit.

Radiation sickness. Symptoms that occur after exposure to an overdose of radioactivity or X-rays. The severity of the condition is detrermined by the intensity and duration of radiation. The total radiation does is calculated from the number of separate occasions on which the patient has been exposed to radiation. Thus frequent short exposure is as dangerous as one large dose. Children are more sensitive to radiation than adults, because it has a particular effect on growing and dividing cells.

Raynaud's Disease (dead fingers). Condition of the blood vessels in the fingers in which they occasionally become constricted so that circulation to the fingertips is temporarily restricted. The condition affects mainly young women. The blood vessels are hypersensitive to stimuli that cause constriction (including cold and emotion). An attack begins with one or more fingers of both hands turning pale and 'dead'. After a few minutes or hours the narrowed vessels dilate spontaneously, circulation is restored and the fingers become red and painful. Treatment consists of protecting the hands from cold (by wearing gloves, for example) and giving up smoking. Medication and surgery usually have no effect.

Rectum, Prolapse of. Protrusion of rectal mucous membrane (incomplete prolapse) or mucous membrane and rectal wall (complete prolapse) through the anus. Incomplete prolapse occurs quite often in children, in whom it can be caused by problems in defecation. In adults with complete prolapse weakening of the pelvic muscles and loose suspension of the rectum can be factors.

Symptoms consist of difficulties with defecation, including an increase of the prolapse during defecation, and possibly swelling, haemorrhage and irritation of the mucous membrane and even tissue death. With complete prolapse diagnosis can easily be made by inspection. Treatment is by surgery to suspend the rectum more securely. In mild cases the diet should be adjusted so that less pressure is needed for defecation.

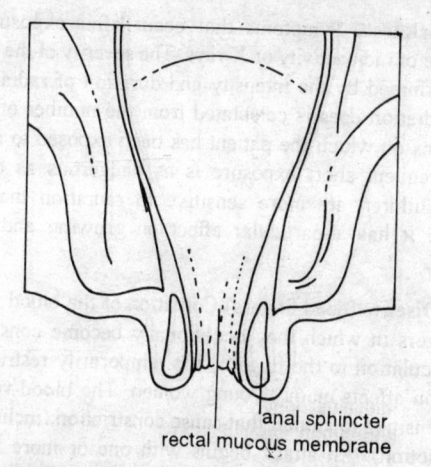

anal sphincter
rectal mucous membrane

In prolapse of the rectum the mucous membrane protrudes through the anal sphincter.

Reflex Action. Inborn, involuntary response to a stimulus which is determined by a preset nervous pathway. Many reflex actions involve muscles normally under voluntary control but override any willed action. Starting a reflex action by an act of will is even more difficult than stopping one.

There are dozens of reflex actions, most of them concerned with movement and balance. Thus, muscles resist contraction and tend toward a relaxed state. In order for any movement to be carried out smoothly, muscles with opposite actions like the large muscle in the front of the upper arm and the less prominent muscle at the back of the arm work against each other. I wish to bring the spoon in my hand to my mouth, but the balanced interplay of muscles required to complete the action is largely reflex. Various brain centres are involved in the control of these reflex actions, but malfunction in one of them can severely impair a movement if not completely destroy it, as happens in *Parkinson's disease,* for example.

One of the simplest and most familiar reflex actions is the knee-jerk. You acoss your legs, and the doctor strikes your knee just below the cap with a sharp blow. The blow slightly stretches the ligament and pulls the large leg muscle. Sensors signal the change to the spinal cord, but in the knee-jerk, the message goes to the brain only afterwards; the signal is transmitted on a second neuron through the spinal cord and to a third reuron running back down the leg to effectors which tighten the opposing muscle while the first muscle relaxes. The result is the characteristic, slightly overcompensated kick. You can mimic the knee-jerk by thinking about it, and you can also prevent it happening if you try. But otherwise, the reflax action follows its normal course unless there is damage or mulfunction somewhere in the pathway.

Breathing and heartbeat have strong reflex controls which are much more complex. Release of wastes, temperature regulation, eye movement, tears and of course salivation in the presence of food are all examples of reflex actions. As in the case of Pavlov's dog, they can be used as the foundation for a kind of learning called conditioned reflex. Thus, the great Russian physiologist rang a bell before giving dogs food. The salivation in the presence of food became associated with the sound of the bell, though it is interesting that the chemical content of the saliva produced by the conditioned response differed from that of the normal saliva mixed with food.

The Harvard psychologist, B.F. Skinner, took the study of conditioned reflexes one step further. He allowed the animal to change its environment in some desirable way, usually by producing food, in response to the conditioning stimulus. He called this operant conditioning. The animal learned faster because, according to behaviourist psychology, the learner was in control of the reward. Skinner argued that all learning is operant conditioning, but this theory remains highly controversial. Perhaps the contention will be finally resolved only when more is known about the physical basis of learning and memory; that is, how brain neurons are modified in the process.

Reflex disorders. Externally visible expression of a disorder of the nervous system. A reflex is a muscular contraction caused by a certain stimulus. Absence of a reflex or even a particularly strong reflex can provide information about neurological conditions or disorders of the spinal cord and brain. Reflexes used to test the nervous system include the knee tendon reflex, pupil reflex (narrowing of the pupil when a light is shone in the eye) or foot reflex (crooking of the toes when the sole of the foot is tickled). A reflex abnormality can appear on both sides of the body, or just on one. A certain stimulus (such as striking the tendon below the kneecap) directs a signal to the spinal cord by means of a sensory nerve; from there the signal is passed to the nerve which finally stimulates the muscle concerned to move. This so-called reflex pathway is limited by the brain to prevent overactivity of certain muscles. If this moderating influence fails-as a result of a brain disorder, for example-then the reflex is unduly strong, often associated with spastic paralysis.

Respiratory distress syndrome. Covering of the alveoli and the finest branches of the air passages with a deposit of fluid and protein which impairs oxygen absorption and carbon dioxide removal. The abnormality is linked with shortage of surfactant, which normally reduces surface tension in the mucous layer of the lung and makes respiration possible. The condition occurs principally in premature babies of mothers suffering from diabetes mellitus, and in infants delivered by Caesarean section.

Retention, urinary. Urine remaining in the bladder after urination. In acute retention, this arises suddenly; in the chronic condition, a little urine remains in the bladder each time urine is passed.

Urine retention is usually caused by constriction either at the neck of the bladder or in the urethra, as a result of sclerosis of the neck of the bladder, swollen bladder, bladder stones, a stone in the urethra or a narrowing of the urethra. In middle-aged men, the cause is frequently an enlarged prostate. One reason why retention can occur in women is pressure on the urethra as a result of prolapse of the bladder during pregnancy or in swelling of the uterus. Spinal cord disorders can also cause urine retention. Acute retention with stretching of the bladder is accompanied by pain, but in chronic retention this is usually not the case. Cystitis can early occur because some urine always remains in the bladder.

Retina. The light-sensitive hemicircle of tissue inside the eyeball at the back of the eye. It consists of a regular array of cells, no more than two or three layers thick. The outermost are farthest from the front of the eye and receive light which is in part reflected off the back inner surface of the eyeball. These cells are shaped like rods or like cones. The cones are concentrated near the visual centre of the retina and are the source of colour vision. Different groups of cone cells respond most actively to the red, blue and yellow wavelengths of light respectively. The rod cells are much more evenly distributed through the retina but occur alone around its outer margins. They respond

to lower light levels than are required to activate cone cells.
Towards the centre of the eye from these light-sensitive cells
are others which begin to process light even before it enters
the brain. The innermost cells are the neurons whose combined axons form the optic nerve linking the retina to the
brain. The retina is actually formed during foetal development
as a part of brain tissue and the eyeball grows around it from
connective tissue.

Retina, detached. Detachment of part of the retina at the back of
the eye from the vascular membrane beneath it. Usually a tear
occurs in the retina, through which aqueous humour can pass
between retina and vascular membrane. Detached retina causes
spontaneous, partial and painless loss of field of vision
(hemianopia). A retinal tear usually occurs in later life in people
with severe myopia (60 per cent of cases). In 35 per cent of
the cases, old age alone is the cause.

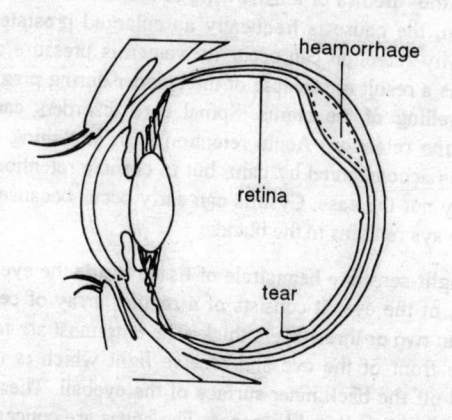

*Detached retina can occur as a result of haemorrhage behind
the retina or a tear in it.*

In cases of severe short-sightedness the eyeball is malformed,
and this slight stretching means that part of the retina is less
well supplied with blood, and terms more easily. Old age brings

abnormalities of the blood vessels, which can reduce blood supply to the retina; it becomes thinner, and can tear more easily. Sometimes the condition is caused by eye injury or a blow to the head, but in such cases too the retina is likely to have already been prone to damage in the first place.

Retina, disorders of. Usually caused by an illness affecting the whole body; both eyes are usually involved. The symptoms are generally the same for all conditions, but they vary in degree. They include declining sharpness of vision, (partial) loss of field of vision, lack of sensitivity to light possibly to the extent of night blindness, and sometimes oversensitivity to light stimuli. Sometimes objects are perceived incorrectly. Pain is rare. The conditions can usually be detected by examination of the eye with a special instrument (ophthalmoscope). The commonest source of difficulty is a disorder of the blood vessels in or of the blood supply to the retina. Other possibilities are inflammation, degenerative disorders, detachment of the retina, and tumours. Disorders occur in the wall of the small arteries in high blood pressure, diabetes mellitus, and severe cases of pre-eclampsia.

Retinoblastoma. Rare cancer of the retina of the eye that occurs in children under the age of three. The tumour causes blindness in one eye and if it grows further it appears as a greyish-yellow glowing mass behind the pupil. In 75 per cent of cases retinoblastoma occurs on one side only, in the other 25 per cent on both. The cancer may spread by metastasis to the brain. The retinal tumour can be discovered by examining the eye with a lamp. Treatment is by surgical removal of the whole eye. If both eyes are affected the eye with the more developed tumour is removed, and the other eye treated by radiation or by laser beams. Tests must also be made for metastasis. If other cancers are found, further treatment must follow; if treatment is executed speedily, recovery is possible.

Retrobulbar Neuritis. Acute inflammation of the optic nerve behind the eyeball in the eye socket, usually affecting only one eye causing loss of vision, and sometimes complete blindness.

Another symptom is headache, which is worsened by eyeball movement. The pupil reacts less well to light. The condition is usually caused by multiple sclerosis (in 60 to 70 per cent of cases), of which it is sometimes the first symptom. Another possible cause is an infectious disease elsewhere in the body, or sinusitis which has penetrated the eye socket; other less common sources are meningitis or an abscess in the vicinity of the optic nerve.

Rhea (Gr. *rhein* = to flow, run, gush.) Suffix designating something that flows. Thus, *diarrhoea* means to flow through.

Rhesus incompatibility. Reaction from contact between rhesus negative blood in a pregnant woman and rhesus positive blood in her unborn baby, causing breakdown of the child's blood. Rhesus positive blood contains a factor in the red blood cells which is absent in rhesus negative blood. The factor causes the defence system of people with rhesus negative blood to form antibodies on contact with rhesus positive blood cells, which they attack and kill. This situation arises when the mother is rhesus negative and the child rhsus positive (which can occur only if the father is rhesus positive). During a first pregnancy some of the baby's blood enters the mother's circulatory system, which begins to form antibodies. The child does not sufer from this, but a subsequent child (second and later pregnancies) with rhesus positive blood can get into difficulties because the mother's blood now contains antibodies. Severe anaemia occurs, accompanied by an excess of the waste product bilirubin, which the child cannot dispose of fully. The child becomes yellow (jaundice), and the bilirubin, which accumulates in the brain in particular, causes severe neurological disorders. If the child is to survive, birth must be induced. Blood transfusions are given to combat the anaemia, possibly even before birth.

Rheumatic disorders. Conditions that involve disorders of movement, associated with pain and limitation of movement, usually caused by inflammation processes in and around a joint. A large number of such inflammation are caused by disturbances of the body's defence system, so-called autoimmune diseases, in which the body produces antibodies against its own cell structures and proteins. This group includes disorders such as rheumatoid arthritis, polymyositis and dermatomyositis scleroderma lupus erythematosus, Bechterew's disease and Reiter's syndrome. Autoimmune disease primarily affecting other organs (such as ulcerative colitis and Crohn's disease) are often associated with arthritis. In rheumatic fever the inflammation is caused as reaction to infection with certain bacteria (streptococci, after tonsillitis or scarlet fever). Arthrosis is caused by wear and tear on cartilage in joints, and the reaction of the bones to this. It is thus not an inflammation reaction of the kind characteristic of the above rheumatic disorders. In gout, uric acid crystals are deposited in the tissue of the joints, causing irritation and consequential inflammation. Polymyalgia rheumatic is associated with restricted movement not caused by inflamed joints but by as yet not understood disease processes in the muscles.

Rheumatic fever. The characteristics of rheumatic fever are inflammation reactions around the joints and heart. The disease can occur in association with streprtococcal pharyngitis; in about 1 per cent of patients with a streptococcal infection the reaction between the bacteria and the body's defence mechanism is abnormally violent, and symptoms of rheumatic fever occur within 1 to 3 weeks. The most important symptom is a shifting inflammation of the joints: a number of large joints such as the knees, ankles and shoulders become inflamed successively, with associated pain, swelling and redness. Each joint remains inflamed for three to seven days, then the symptoms mvoe on. Small, painless bumps occur around the joints under the skin, and there is usually high fever. In roughly half the cases the heart also becomes inflamed (carditis) affecting the inner lining and the cardiac muscles. Cardiac inflammation causes rapid and/or irregular heartbeat, abnormalities in the electrocardiogram and in serious cases heart failure.

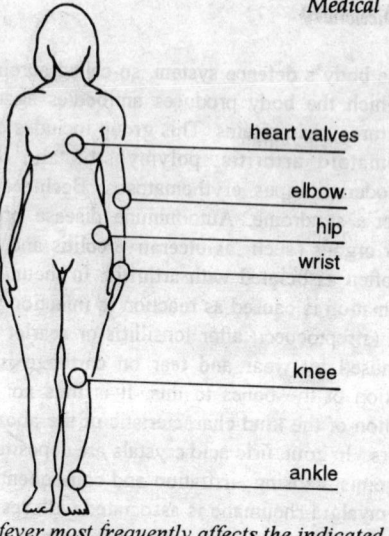

heart valves

elbow

hip

wrist

knee

ankle

Rheumatic fever most frequently affects the indicated areas.

Rheumatic heart disease. Heart condition that occurs during rheumatic fever, a disorder caused by streptococci and associated

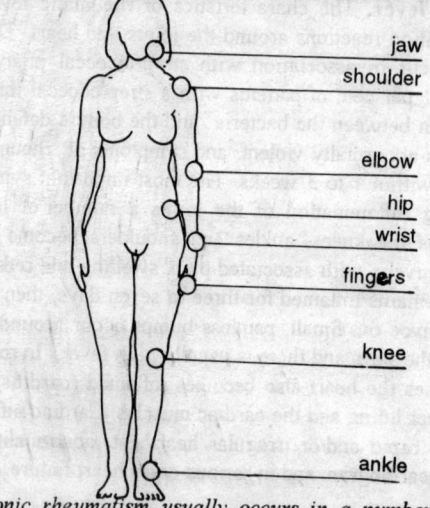

jaw

shoulder

elbow

hip

wrist

fingers

knee

ankle

Chronic rheumatism usually occurs in a number of specific joints.

with inflammation of the joints and cardiac muscle, together with the endo-and pericardium. The former condition causes swelling and leakage of the heart valves. The inflammation can lead to heart rhythm disorders, and valve leakage to heart failure. The severe inflammation is associated with fever and general malaise. Rheumatic fever is a serious condition which must be rapidly and thoroughly treated with long-term bed rest and the administration of antibiotics and corticosteroids.

Rheumatoid Arthritis. Common rheumatic disorder, characterized by inflammation of the mucous membrane of the joint, affecting the cartilage. Before the ago of 60 the disease is four times more common in women than men; after 60 the frequency is the same for each sex. It often affects more than one person in the same family, and occurs between the ages of 20 and 35, with a second peak between 50 and 55. It is probably an autoimmune disease, antibodies against the body's own protein, so-called rhematic factors, are often found in sufferers. Stiffnes, pain and swelling of the small joints of both hands are the first symptoms; other joints are affected at a later stage, again usually on both sides of the body. First the inflamed sinovial membrane swells, affecting cartilage and the bone underneath, which are gradually destroyed. The affected limbs stiffen at a later stage, which can be disabling. The condition can occur in any joint with a sinovial membrane, but it is not just a condition of the joints; abnormalities may also occur in tendons, mucous glands and blood capillaries. Subcutaneous lumps and nodules often form above the protruding joints of hands and elbows; other possible symptoms are fatigue, weight loss, fever and anaemia.

Rhinophyma. Abnormality of the skin of the nose, causing it to become enlarged, reddishpurple and bumpy. The symptoms are often incorrectly attributed to excessive drinking ('whisky nose'). Rhinophyma is caused by enlargement of the sebaceous glands in the nose, together with an increase in tissue, and as such is a particular form of rosacea.

Rhinophyma can be treated with antibiotics which reduce

the redness and some of the swelling. If this does not give satisfactory   results a skin specialist or plastic surgeon can reshape the nose by cutting out little strips, or by scaraping the skin.

Rib, cervical. Extra rib connected with the lowest vertebra of the neck and fused with the uppermost normal rib (or connected to it by a septum of tissue, often not completely). The condition occurs on one or both sides in 1 per cent of the population. It causes problems in only a very few cases, namely, when blood vessels and nerves of the arm, which normally run over the uppermost rib, are trapped because they have to run over the extra rib. Thr foremost oblique muscle of the neck, which is attached to the first rib, can cause further constriction.

Rickets. Disturbed metabolism of bone tissue in young children characterized by delayed bone formation and deficiency of vitamin D and calcium, the latter resulting from inadequate diet or reduced calcium absorption from the intestines. Vitamin D is important in calcium absorption and calcification of bones. It

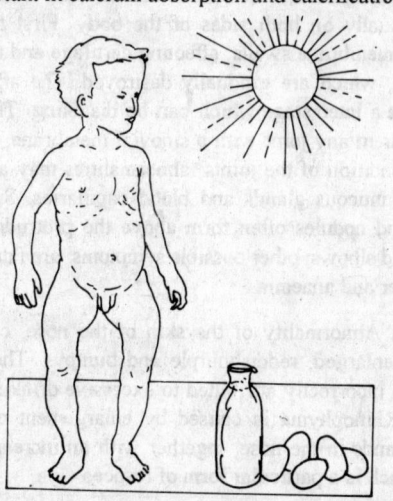

Rickets is caused by a shortage of sunlight and foodstuffs rich in vitamin D.

is formed in the skin from cholesterol substances under the effect of sunlight, and the deficiency is either dietary or caused by lack of sunlight. The condition was formerly prevalent in the West through lack of sun; now vitamin D is added to margarines and cooking oils, which has reduced the frequency of the condition. In developing countries it still occurs through lack of dietary calcium and fats, from which the vitamin can be formed. Characteristic signs are malformed bones, lumps on the cartilagenous outer ends of bones and delayed growth, bow legs or knock knees, and deformities of the spinal column (kyphosis, scoliosis).

Ringworm. General term for a fungus infection of the skin. Its name is derived from the particular form of the skin abnormality, which takes the form of a ring, with normal skin in the centre, occurring almost exclusively on the trunk and upper arms and legs. Fungus infections can affect hands and feet, but these take a different form. When a fungus penetrates the skin a small area appears in which the skin becomes red, somewhat swollen, and scaly. The area spreads gradually, from the edges. At the same time the centre heals, hence the impression of a gradually growing ring. Fungus can grow only if the skin is slightly alkaline, and slightly moist. The simplest way to prevent ringworm is to keep the skin as dry as possible, and restrict the use of soap to a minimum (because it tends to make the skin alkaline). Acid soap can be obtained. Once ringworm is present, these measures are not sufficient to clear up the condition; fungicidal ointment is also needed, and in some cases a fungicide must also be taken internally.

River blindness (onchocerciasis) Infestation with the nematode worm *Onchocerca volvulus*. The larvae have as an intermediate host a mosquito which lives near rivers, hence the name of the disease.

Blindness occurs only in those who have been infested for many years. Slight infestation by adult worms in subcutaneous connective tissue causes itchy skin abnormalities. The larvae can cause inflammation of the eye, resulting in blindness after a number of years as a result of corneal inflammation and iritis. Slight infestation needs no treatment; blindness can be prevented by medication for patients likely to be repeatedly infested.

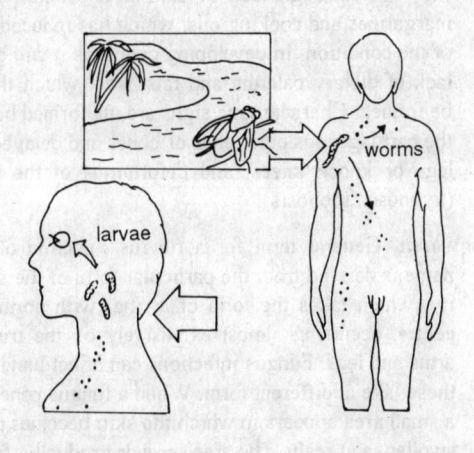

Cycle of the threadworm, which causes river blindness.

Rodent ulcer. Most common form of skin cancer, and also the least malignant, forming a glassy, greyish patch often with a rim, reminiscent of mother-of-pearl. As it grows it becomes indented in the middle, and ulceration is a possible complication. It occurs most frequently on the face and arms, but there is a form known as carcinoma of the trunk, which looks quite different, usually consisting of large red scaly patches not unlike those produced by psoriasis. The tomour can affect a much greater area than is apparent on the surface, and grows by means of feeler-like excrescences. Metastasis-spread to other parts of the body-can only occur at a very late stage. If an ulcer occurs spontaneously on the skin and does not disappear after the usual treatment, it may well be a rodent ulcer, and the surgeon should remove it in its entirety. To confirm diagnosis tissue removed should be examined in a laboratory, which will also confirm whether or not it has been completely removed, which is essential.

Rosacea. Disorder of the skin of the face involving red pimples and small suppurating blisters, occurring particularly in women over the age of 45. It affects the centre of the forehead, both cheeks, the bridge of the nose and the chin. Some experts hold that rosacea is caused by dilation of skin capillaries and consequent slowing of the blood flow. In severe cases abtibiotics are prescribed, not because of their ability to destroy bacteria, bu' because of a suspected side-effect.

Roseola. Harmless viral disease contracted exclusively by children between the ages of six months and three years. The disease begins with a mild cold in the nose, a slight temperature and reduced appetite. These symptoms often pass unnoticed, so that it is only when the skin rash appears that parents realize what is wrong. Small red spots form on the trunk and spread to the nape of the neck and the limbs. The spots fade away after two days and the body temperature then drops to normal.

Roundworms. There are a number of different roundworms, which can cause various diseases. Roundworm infection occurs throughout the world, affecting large population groups in the tropics and subtropics. Male and female worms exist; some, like the tapeworm, are hermaphrodite. Larvae develop from eggs, generally in the soil (*strongyloides,* hookworm, eelworm). People become infested by eating contaminated food, by larval penetration of skin, or by eating eggs or larvae in vegetables or meat (including trichomoniasis); wireworms have a mosquito as intermediate host, and the disease is transmitted by its bite. The threadworm is also a roundworm, and can be transmitted by eggs that remain on the hands or by inhaling air in which the eggs are suspended

Good hygiene (sanitary provision, handwashing, etc.) is the best way of preventing infection. Treatment by medication is possible.

S

Sadomasochism. Mental abnormality involving sexual satisfaction derived from hurting and being hurt. Sadism is the derivation of satisfaction from inflicting pain, humiliation or threat of violence. Masochism is the derivation of satisfaction from being hurt or humiliated. A situation in which both partners find satisfaction does not depend only on the presence of pain or threat. Erotic incidents involving pain, humiliation and threat are purposefully set up in consultation between the partners, according to personal preference. Roles (master and slave) may be assigned from the beginning. It is quite common for costume and 'props' such as whips and chains to be used in sadomasochistic play. The word play is apt in the context, because the partners respect and are usually very fond of each other, and both find the experience pleasurable and enjoyable.

Salivary duct stones. Formed in the salivary glands, usually the submandibular glands. The stone may be in the gland itself, or in the salivary duct. It consists of deposits of calcium salts from the saliva around a core formed by bacterial activity. Stones may block the duct wholly or partly, checking the flow of saliva. Symptoms are pain (sometimes severe) and swelling, particularly when eating, when the glands are activated. If such symptoms occur, a doctor should be consulted, who may be able to feel the stone in the duct. In cases of doubt diagnosis can be confirmed by X-ray. Complications include rapid infection of both mouth and gland; there is also a somewhat greater likelihood of caries (tooth decay) as a result of lowered saliva production. Treatment is by surgical removal of the stone; if it is in the gland itself, part of this may have to be removed as well.

Salivary glands, inflammation of. Usually in the parotid (under and in front of the ear) or submandibular (under the jaw) glands. The cause is usually viral or bacterial, sometimes blockage of a salivary duct (by a stone for example). The best-known inflammation of the salivary glands is probably mumps (parotitis), a viral infection of the parotid gland. Salivary gland inflammation is characterized by swelling and tenderness of the affected gland; with the parotid gland it is in the check, in front of the ear and down to the edge of the lower jaw, in the case of the submandibular gland under the edge of the lower jaw and at the corner of the jaw. Saliva production may decrease, with a dry mouth as symptom. Examination is directed at establishing the presence of a stone which may be causing a blockage, and distinguishing inflammation from a salivary gland tumour, which would also cause swelling. In children with a clear case of mumps such examination is usually superfluous.

Salivary gland tumours. Rare tumour of one of the salivary glands in the mouth, usually found in the parotid gland, below and in front of the ears (90 per cent of cases), and very rarely in the glands beneath the jaw or tongue. Tumours of the parotid gland are usually benign, but in rare cases they can become malignant; in the other two glands roughly half the cases are benign. With a tumour of the parotid gland there is swelling directly in front of and/or under the ear; the tumour is painless, and grows steadily. Possible complications include paralysis of one side of the face, facial pain or painful tic, all caused by pressure on a nerve. Malignant tumours are more likely to grow through into the surrounding area and can metastasize. Tumours of the other salivary glands behave in the same way, with swelling on the edge of the lower jaw or the bottom of the mouth. They do not exert pressure on important nerves.

Salpingitis. Inflammation of the Fallopian tubes, usually affecting both sides of the body and the surrounding abdominal tissue.

It is caused by gonococci, which cause gonorrhoea, or by bacteria. The condition occurs more frequently with the use of intra-uterine devices and in patients with numerous sexual partners. There is a greater chance of infection during menstrua-

tion and labour, because the mouth of the womb is wider open.
Salpingitis is usually associated with backache and high fever,
and sometimes with a pus-like discharge from the vagina. Pain
is felt if the mouth of the womb is moved during internal
examination, and the doctor can sometimes feel thickening of
the Fallopian tubes.

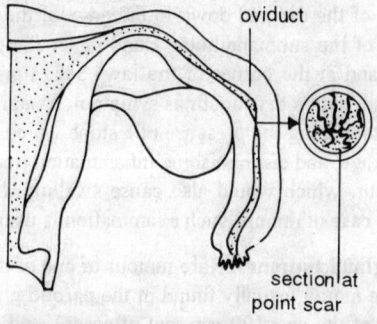

Salt. 1. Sodium chloride (NaCl) or table salt. 2. A chemical compound consisting of an acid and a base that neutralizes its
electrical charge. In the formation of a salt, water is usually a
by-product. In the body, potassium forms a second important
salt, again in combination with chloride.

Sarcoidosis. Granulomatous disorder characterized by the presence
of granulomas (accumulations of granular tissue), often in lymph
nodes or the lungs. Sometimes the disease is serious, and
hospitalization is necessary, but roughly 70 per cent of patients have no painful symptoms, and the disease is discovered
by chance at a medical examination. If the granules are in the
lung they cause coughing and shortness of breath, and there
can be a slight fever and fatigue as a result of the inflammation
reaction. In sarcoidosis of the skin it becomes reddish-purple,
tight and painful, with granules under the skin.

Scabies. Skin infestation with the itch mite, a small spider-like organism (0.2-0.5 mm long) which lives in the horn layer. The
mite makes channels up to 3 cm long, particularly in the skin
of hand and wrist, but also elsewhere in the body. The female

lays 2 to 4 eggs per day at the end of the channel; they hatch after a few days, and the larvae spread over the skin, permitting transmission of the disorder by intimate contact. The larvae are adult within 14 days, and live 1 to 2 months. An infested patient usually carries no more than 12 female mites. Scabies shows characteristic skin abnormalities consisting of small lumps, pimples and scaly lines which are very itchy,

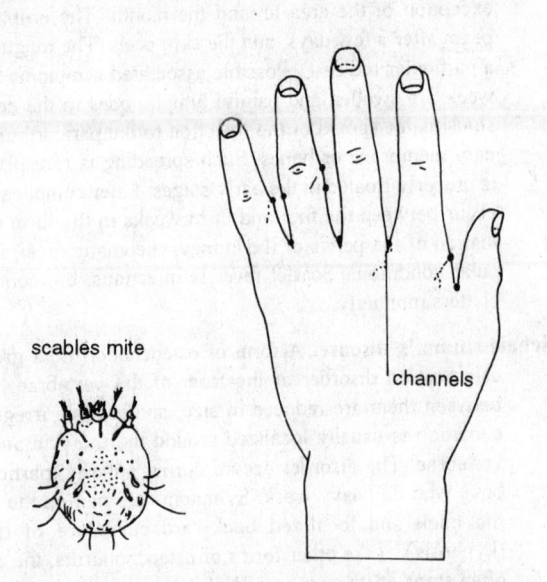

scabies mite

channels

The scabies mite digs small channels between the fingers. They itch, and scratching spreads the infection.

particularly at night. The symptoms are essentially allergic, and do not occur until after one month, but after 24 hours in the case of repeated infestation. Infection is caused only by female mites, and the larvae can be transmitted only by intimate contact with an infested person. Patients who wash regularly are unlikely to have mites under the skin. Treatment is with an ointment, repeated on the next day. Bedding and clothes must also be cleaned, and the patient should wash thoroughly in the evening. Although the itch may persist for some weeks, the above treatment should have killed the mites.

Scarlet fever. Acute streptococcal infection that occurs above all in childhood. The incubation period is one to seven days. The early stages of the disease include a severe cold in the nose, high fever and throat inflammation. Then a skin eruption in the form of small red spots covers the whole body, with the exception of the area around the mouth. The eruption disappears after a few days, and the skin peels. The tongue takes on a particular red cast. Possible associated symptoms in the first week are swollen and painful lymph nodes in the neck, otitis, sinusitis, or spread of the infection to the paricardium, pulmonary membrane or bones. Such spreading is rare if the illness is properly treated in the early stages. Later complications may occur between the first and third weeks in the form of inflammation of the pelvis of the kidney, rheumatic fever and a vascular condition. Scarlet fever is infectious, but contracting it confers immunity.

Scheuermann's disease. A form of osteochondritis, a growth and calcification disorder at the front of the vertebrae; the discs between them are reduced in size, and become irregular. The condition is usually localized around the thoracic and lumbar vertebrae. The disorder occurs during puberty, particularly in boys who do heavy work. Symptoms are pain in the centre of the back and localized backward curvature of the spine (kyphosis). Like other forms of osteochondritis, the condition often stops of its own accord; if it is recognized and treated at an early stage it is usually possible to prevent distortion of the vertebrae and resultant severe kyphosis. Diagnosis is from the characteristic changes in the vertebrae and discs as revealed by spinal X-rays.

Schizophrenia. Psychotic disorder in which symptoms occur in episodes, with intervening periods in which the mental powers are also in decline.

The patient's train of thought is difficult to follow, particularly because non-existent words are sometimes used as if they were common currency ('neologisms'). Consciousness is undisturbed, and the mood is not strikingly impaired, but certain ideas and delusions exert excessive influence: the patient is under the influence of other human beings, 'rays', poisons, and so on. Behaviour can be bizarre, with loss of decorum, hallucinations, and ceaseless, pointless, pseudo-scientific rumination on large and all-embracing topics.

Sciatica. Severe stabbing and radiating pain in one leg caused by irritation of or pressure on the sciatic nerve, the large nerve that runs from the base of the spine and down the back of the leg. The pain radiates from the buttock to the upper rear section of the leg, the back of the knee, the outer side of the

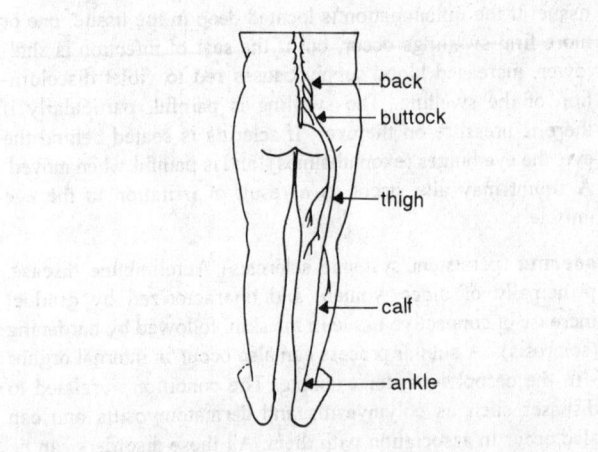

— back
— buttock
— thigh
— calf
— ankle

In sciatica the sciatic nerve is trapped, causing pain and irritation along a particular nerve pathway.

lower leg and the foot. Pain increases if the leg is bent or the hip flexed. The most usual cause is a slipped disc, in which part of the nerve is trapped. In older patients arthrosis of the vertebrae can reduce the nerve apertures in the spinal column, which also causes sciatica. Less common causes are pressure on the nerve by tumours in the spinal column of abdomen, inflammation of the nerve or damage to it from a poorly executed injection into, or a fall onto, the buttocks. Disc disorders can cause bilateral sciatica (affecting both legs). Radiating abdominal pain may not be due to a constricted nerve, but to muscular pain or pain caused by a hip disorder.

Scleritis. Inflammation of a deep or shallow layer of the sclera, the thick white outer coating which covers most of the eyeball. Not usually viral or bacterial, it is generally the result of an allergic reaction to a disorder elsewhere, such as tuberculosis or certain rheumatic disorders. The cause is also often unknown and the condition is rare, although more common in men than women. The sclera consists largely of connective tissue. If the inflammation is located deep in the tissue, one or more firm swellings occur, but if the seat of infection is shallower, increased blood supply causes red to violet discoloration of the swelling. The swelling is painful, particularly if there is pressure on the eye. If scleritis is seated behind the eye, the eye bulges (exophthalmos), and is painful when moved. A squint may also occur as a result of irritation to the eye muscle.

Scleroderma (persistent systemic sclerosis) Autoimmune disease, principally of older women, and characterized by gradual increase of connective tissue in the skin, followed by hardening (sclerosis). A similar process can also occur in internal organs - in the oesophagus, for example. The condition is related to diseases such as polymyositis and dermatomyositis and can also occur in association with them. All these disorders can be associated with arthritis. There is a benign form, scleroderma, which is restricted to the skin, causing patchy inflammation, hard slippery and pale grey in the centre. In half of cases the disorder spreads further and develops into the severe form, affecting internal organs and causing more serious skin conditions. Changes in pigmentation occur, and calcium is deposited in the skin. Blood vessels are affected, causing circulatory problems in the fingertips which can cause them to die. Constriction of the oesophagus leads to difficulty in swallowing, and when the lungs are also affected there is a danger of respiratory difficulties and pneumonia. The resultant arthritis is similar to chronic rheumatoid arhritisarthsitis Treatment is directed in the first place at the prevention of serious complications. Drugs to dilate blood vessels can help to prevent the death of fingertips and toes; corticosterioids and anti-rheumatic drugs may also be prescribed.

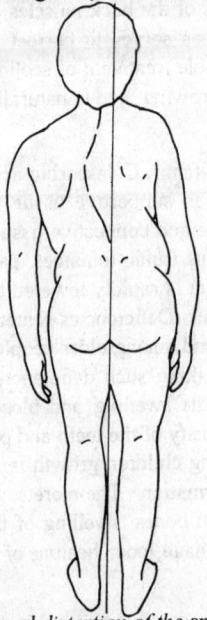

Scoliosis is lateral distortion of the spine which sometimes causes back pain.

Sclerosis. From a Greek word meaning hardening. In *multiple sclerosis* nervous tissue is replaced by connective tissue and appears to harden.

Scoliosis. Lateral crookedness of the spine, often associated with convex crookedness (kyphosis). In cases with one curve it is known as simple scoliosis; if there are more than one, it is termed multiple scoliosis. Usually the vertebrae are also twisted, displacing the ribs on the side of the curvature to form a so-called humpback. Scoliosis can occur at any age, often without recognizable cause; in other cases deformity of the vertebrae is caused by injury, rickets, osteomalacia, osteoporosis or metastasized tumours. Diseases of the spinal column associated with kyphosis can also cause scoliosis. Other causes are disorders or paralysis of the back muscles and pelvic deformities, in which scoliosis serves to correct the position of the lower spine. Reasonable treatment of scoliosis is possible only while the patient is growing, and is naturally dependent on the cause.

Scurvy. Consequence of vitamin C (ascorbic acid) deficiency. The vitamin plays a part in supportive tissue formation, such as dental tissue, cartilage and connective tissue. It is found in all green vegetables, citrus fruits, tomatoes, paprika and red pepper. Vitamin C content is rapidly lowered by cooking, baking and contact with the air. Deficiencies sometimes occur in children on a liquid diet and among older people who neglect their eating. Generally speaking such deficiencies are not severe, with symptoms such as swelling and bleeding of the gums, pain in the joints, porosity of the teeth and possibly subcutaneous bleeding. In young children growth is arrested by disturbances in skeleton formation. The more severe form produces symptoms such as thin bones, swelling of the joints, a strong inclination to haemorrhage, poor healing of wounds and loose teeth.

If the diet contains sufficient virtamin C the above problems should lnot occur, and extra vitamin C is not usually ncessary. If a deficiency clearly exists, however, vitamin C should be taken in the form of tablets or by injection.

Sebaceous cyst. Blockage of the duct of a sebaceous gland in the skin. As the gland continues to secrete sebum (fat), a swollen lump is produced, which can grow several centimetres across.

It is smooth and round, usually light grey in colour and looks like a marble directly beneath the skin. The condition can occur anywhere except on the palms of the hands or the soles of the feet because they have no sebaceous glands. The most frequent complication of sebaceous cysts is that they can become inflamed if their content is contaminated with bacteria. This usually renults in an abscess. The only treatment for sebaceous cysts is to remove them completely. They are loose under the skin and so this is a simple operation, which some family doctors perform themselves.

Sebaceous gland disorders. The two most common sebaceous glands are acne and rhynophyma (strawberry nose).

Sebaceous glands secrete a waxy substance (sebum) associated with hair roots and the small downy hairs that occur all over the skin's surface. Consequently there are sebaceous glands everywhere except on the palms of the hands and on the soles of the feet. With acne, a plug is formed which blocks the duct of the sebaceous gland and the gland swells as a result. This is the blackhead or comedo. If bacteria enter the gland it may become inflamed. In the case of an atheroma cyst, the sebaceous gland duct is completely clogged up and the gland may swell to a diameter of several centimetres. With strawberry nose, the sebaceous glands of the nose become larger than normal without their ducts being blocked. This gives rise to a clinical picture which is also known as whisky nose, although there is no connection with the consumption of alcohol.

Serum sickness. Immune reaction which can occur after the injection of animal serum, formerly used for vaccination. The body identifies proteins in the animal serum as alien, causing an allergic and immune reaction. The disorder occurs if serum protein is present in excessive proportion to the antibodies which the body makes against it. Symptoms can include fever, swollen lymph nodes, skin eruptions or painfully swollen joints. Symptoms occur about 8 days after the injection, sooner and more severely if the patient has previously been in contact

with the serum. Nowadays serum sickness is rare because
most vaccines are purified or prepared synthetically.

Sexual problems. Sexual feelings and their expression are a normal part of human life, but sex is not always without its problems. Many factors can make the sexual aspects of a relationship unsatisfactory. In general, couples are effectively informed
about pregnancy and contraceptives, but knowledge of the various phases and techniques of sexual contact has to be acquired
by experience. It is not unusual for ignorance about anatomical and sexual differences between men and women to be a
source of disappointment. Naturally such ignorance does not
always lead to frustration. A good book about sexuality can
often be illuminating, and when the partners know each other
and are prepared to explain what gives them pleasure most
problems disappear spontaneously. Sexual problems are sometimes caused by physical abnormalities. Phimosis (excessively
tight foreskin), inflammation of the genitals, and so on can
spoil much of the pleasure which sex can give. Sex is not
merely physical, as can be seen from the fact that psychological problems can be a factor in sexual difficulties. Stress and
all sorts of unconscious emotions and fears can stand in the
way of sexual satisfaction. It is important that partners should
be prepared to recognize problems and look for a solution
together. Increased flexibility of social norms and values has
made it possible to obtain help from all sorts of organizations
and individuals, and the fact that many couples take advantage
of such possibilities is clear proof that a healthy sex life is to
many people an important factor in mental and spiritual well-
being.

Shingles. Acute viral infection in a sensory nerve associated with
fever and painful, itchy blisters, occurring particularly in older
people with reduced resistance. It is caused by the chickenpox
virus (*Herpes zoster*), which responds to certain, imperfectly
understood stimuli with renewed activity in one or more sensory nerves and in the skin areas served by those nerves. Thus
the condition affects one side of the body, usually the abdo-

men. The disorder begins with fatigue and fever, followed by
itching in the affected area associated with slight pain which
later becomes stabbing and severe. After 2 to 3 days the affected area becomes blistered; the blistering dries up in 2 weeks.
Shingles in the eye can cause blindness, because the cornea
becomes blistered. The disorder clears up in a few weaks, with
slight loss of feeling or painful oversensitivity of the affected
area. In severe cases neuralgic pain persists in the skin. There
is no specific treatment, but measures can be taken against
itching and pain.

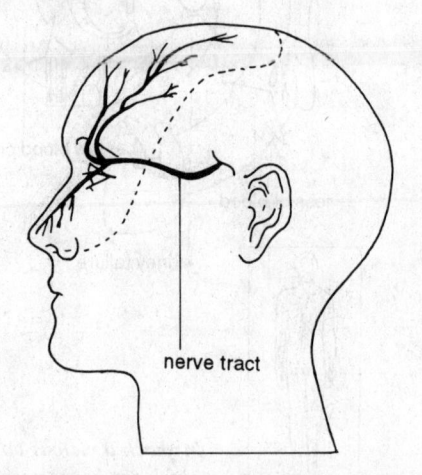

nerve tract

*The skin of the face can be affected by shingles, as can the
cornea.*

Shock. Combination of symptoms resulting from sudden deficiencies
in the circulation of the blood. Shock is characterized by low
blood pressure, rapid heartbeat, cold hands and feet, clammy
skin and changes in mental condition varying from drowsiness
to agitation. The foremost causes of shock are:

  (a) Shortage of blood in the circulatory system;

  (b) Circulatory disorders caused by heart conditions;

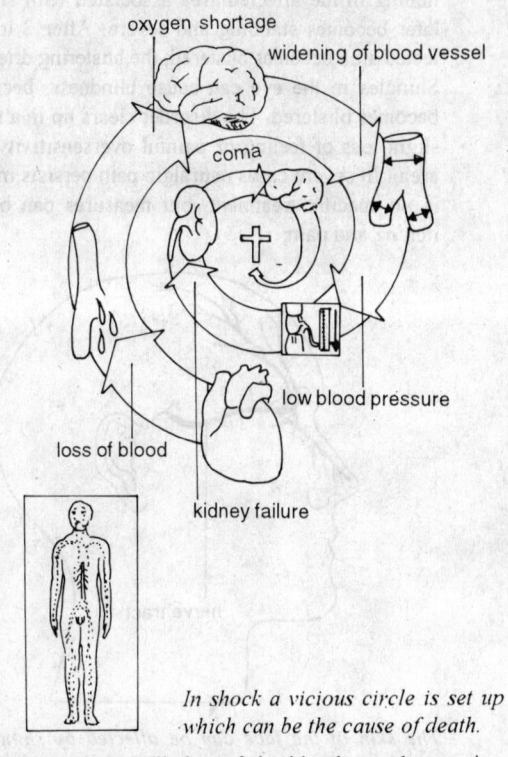

oxygen shortage

widening of blood vessel

coma

low blood pressure

loss of blood

kidney failure

*In shock a vicious circle is set up
which can be the cause of death.*

(c) Sudden severe dilation of the blood vessels, causing
too little blood to flow through the system.

Shock caused by blood shortage is the most common, as a
result of internal or external haemorrhage. Treatment is by
blood transfusion and staunching the haemorrhage, to which
end an emergency operation is almost always necessary

When the heart is the cause it pumps insufficient blood
through the system. This can happen as a result of coronary
infarction, in which part of the heart no longer functions; heart
rhythm disorders can also adversely affect the pumping func-

tion. This form of shock is treated by medication to stimulate the heart and combat rhythmic disorders. If the cause is cardiac infarction the heart often reacts insufficiently to stimulation by drugs, in which case the patient usually dies.

Severe dilation of the blood vessels can result from serious blood poisoning or a violent allergic reaction (anaphylaxis). Treatment consists of fluid replacement by infusion, large doses of antibiotics, and drugs to narrow the blood vessels.

Shoulder, disorders of. Almost always associated with pain and restricted movement, although shoulder pain can also be caused by disorders of the heart, gall bladder or diaphragm. The most important shoulder conditions are fractures of the humerus (upper arm) or clavicle (shoulder blade). The shoulder can also be dislocated by a fall or other accident and injuries to children can cause epiphysiolysis. Arthritis of the shoulder often occurs as a rheumatic disorder; tendon and mucous goblet cell inflammation can be associated with calcium deposits. Shoulder pain also occurs in polymyalgia rheumatica and in neuralgic pain and circulatory disorders caused by a cervical rib. Shoulder conditions can cause frozen shoulder.

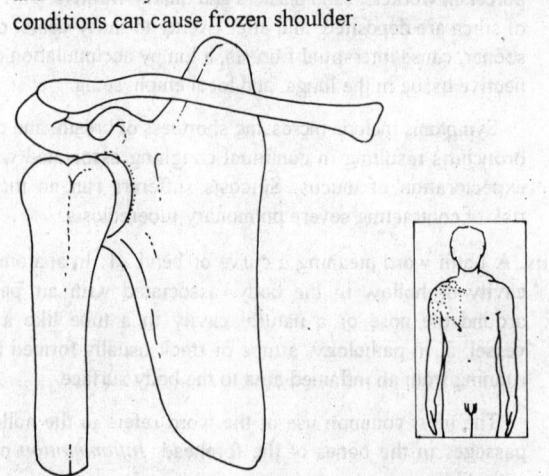

As the shoulder joint is more mobile than the hip it is more likely to be dislocated.

Sickle-cell anaemia. Anaemia caused by increased breakdown of abnormal blood cells. In sickle cell anaemia the red blood cells are not disc-shaped, but look like half moons or sickles. They are not continuously present, but occur when extra demands are made on the body by infection or oxygen deficiency, for example. The condition is congenital, and occurs predominantly in people of African origin. The symptoms are fatigue, pallor, palpitations and vertigo. Sickle cells transport oxygen less efficiently than normal red blood cells, a potential cause of oxygen deficiency, which shows as shortness of breath. The sickle cells are also inclined to clot, causing blockage of the smaller blood vessels, and thus fever, abdominal pain, pain in the arms and legs or lung problems. There is no real treatment for sickle cell amaemia. The best approach is to keep sufferers in good general condition, but generally speaking they do not live to a great age.

Silicosis. Form of pneumoconiosis caused by many years' inhalation of quartz particles (silica). It occurs in miners working in rock, porcelain workers, sand blasters and quarry workers. Tiny grains of silica are deposited, and after twenty to thirty years, or even sooner, cause interstitial fibrosis, a lumpy accumulation of connective tissue in the lungs, and local emphysema.

Symptoms include increasing shortness of breath, and chronic bronchitis resulting in continual coughing associated with the expectoration of mucus. Silicosis sufferers run an increased risk of contracting severe pulmonary tuberculosis.

Sinus. A Latin word meaning a curve or bend. 1. In anatomy, any cavity or hollow in the body, associated with air passages around the nose or a natural cavity in a tube like a blood vessel. 2. In pathology, a tube or track usually formed by *pus* running from an inflamed area to the body surface.

The most common use of the word refers to the hollow air passages in the bones of the forehead. *Inflammation* of their mucous linings causes *sinusitis*.

Sinusitis. Inflammation of one or more of the paranasal sinuses. The sinuses are cavities in the skull connected with the nose, situated in lthe upper jaw, the forehead and behind the eye sockets. Their function is not precisely known. Theory suggests that they form while the skull is growing to prevent it from becoming too heavy. The sinuses have the same mucous membranes as the nose, which also swell if the patient has a cold, and produce a great deal of mucus. The most important cause of sinusitis is a nasal cold spreading to the sinuses, generally more likely if breathing through the nose is restricted. This is also the case if the nasal septum is displaced by a tumour or nasal polyps (protrusions of the mucous membrane). Sinusitis is a regular occurrence in cases of hay fever and chronic bronchitis, which cause swelling of the nasal mucous membrane. This in its turn can close the small opening from the sinuses to the nose, thus trapping any bacteria which may be there, and providing ideal conditions for them to multiply. Therefore, to prevent or cure sinusitis the openings from the sinuses to the nose should be kept as clear as possible.

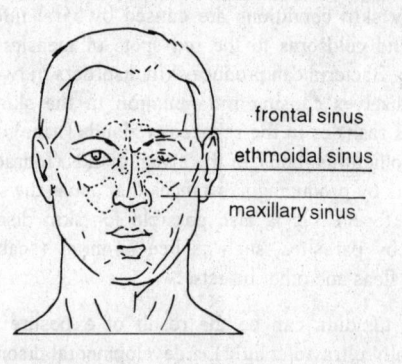

frontal sinus
ethmoidal sinus
maxillary sinus

Sinusitis occurs when a patient has a cold and bacteria enter the nasal sinuses and are unable to get out again because of nasal congestion.

Skin cancer. Collective name for various malignant skin diseases. Most skin tumours are benign, but it is wise to consult a doctor if a birthmark, mole or other protrusion on the skin grows, changes shape or begins to bleed or itch. A birthmark can develop into a melanoma, and basal cell carcinoma can form in skin areas exposed to the sun for long periods (ultraviolet light); this form of skin cancer fortunately does not metastasize, in contrast with a melanoma and spinal cell carcinoma. In the last two cases in particular, early diagnosis is important so that the tumour can be removed by surgery or treated by radiation.

Skin disorders. Disorders of the skin can be divided into a number of categories, both in form and cause.

Eczemas form the largest group. Other large groups are tumours and infections. Other skin conditions are grouped according to certain common features, such as the formation of blisters. Skin conditions have many causes; a number are allergies-contact eczema for example-or skin eruption following the use of certain medicaments.

Many skin conditions are caused by viral infection, from warts and coldsores to the red spots of measles or German measles. Bacteria can produce skin disorders in two ways, first by themselves causing inflammation in the skin (impetigo, barber's rash) or in the sebaceous glands (acne), the hair follicles (folliculitis, boil), or the sweat glands (hidradenitis). The second is by producing substances that cause the skin disorder (scarlet fever). Is is also possible for skin disorders to be caused by parasites, such as lice or mites (scabies, for example), fleas and other insects.

Skin tumours can be the result of exposure to radiation (especially ultraviolet light), a developmental disorder or accumulation of certain substances in the skin (xanthomas). Sometimes absolutely no cause can be found. Skin eruptions can be divided into three categories. The first are on the same level as the skin, and include changes of colour, such as redness, too little or too much pigment, vascular dilation in the skin and discharge of blood in the skin (purpura). The second category are above the level of the skin, including all lumps from less than 1mm (pimples) to larger than 1 cm (tumours) in diameter, and also blisters. Uriticaria (nettlerash) occurs when the skin becomes locally thicker and paler, because of fluid between the skin cells.

The third category includes conditions below the normal level of the skin, retractions of the skin, erosions (abrasion), wounds and ulcers. All skin disorders consist of one or more of these elements, often in combination, such as redness with pimples, or an ulcer with a red edge.

Skin pigmentation, abnormal. May be caused by deficient or excess pigment, but the term also includes localized conditions. There are various diseases with pigment disorders as a symptom, such as hereditary conditions (including albinism and phenylketonuria). Infections such as leprosy can also cause such disorders; here pigment loss is related to nerve failure. Fungal infections such as pityriasis versicolor or overexposure to radiation can also cause a pale patch, possibly a form of skin cancer. A local pigment excess may be a birthmark or naevus. Excess pigment can occur in pregnancy (chloasma) or be caused by a melanoma. Even when the underlying condition is treated, pigmentation may well not return to normal; redistribution of pigment is a lengthy process. If a patch is not too dark it can be disguised with cosmetics.

Skull fractures. There are two main types of fractures: fractures of the cranium, the main dome of the skull, and fractures of the base of the skull. A fractured cranium is often associated with concussion; because various blood vessels run directly beneath the cranium, there is a risk of epidural or subdural haemorrhage. If the bone is pushed inwards (impression fracture) there can be local brain damage with possibly failure symptoms or epilepsy; otherwise few problems are caused.

Diagnosis is by X-rays, and admission to hospital is recommended because of possible complications. Impression fractures are usually reset in the operating theatre.

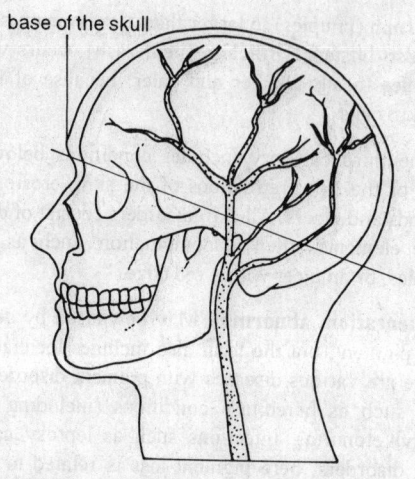

base of the skull

Fracture of the base of the skull can cause tearing of the cerebral blood vessels, causing haemorrhage or infarction.

Sleeping sickness (trypanosomiasis) Infestation with a parasite transmitted by a fly. There are two kinds: *Trypanosoma gambiense* (the West African variety) and *Trypanosoma rhodesiense*, the East African variety); *Trypanosoma cruzi* causes Chagas disease. *Trypanosoma* are protozoal organisms, spoolshaped, with a tail which propels them through the bloodstream and tissue of the host. They pass from a sick person to a healthy one by the tsetse fly. The parasites move through blood and lymph nodes, causing fever, oedema, swollen lymph nodes and temporary skin eruption. After this the parasites can deregulate brain function, causing disturbances in the senses, muscular movement, physical function and sleep regulation (hence the name). If the disease is not treated it is fatal in the long trem, but drug treatment is completely possible.

Sleep-walking (somnambulism) Getting up, walking and performing sometimes quite complicated tasks while asleep, in a state of lowered consciousness, or without being conscious at all. Like nail-biting, bed-wetting and persistent thumb-sucking, sleepwalking is called a 'childhood neurosis symptom', because it generally implies psychological problems. It frequently occurs in children between the ages of 8 and 12, more often than the average in some families. If precautions are taken against potential nocturnal dangers (by locking windows, putting a gate at the top of the stairs, etc.) the condition is not serious, and treatment is not usually necessary. Contrary to general opinion it is not dangerous to wake sleep-walkers or to take them gently back to bed.

Slipped disc. Protrusion of the soft inner core of a vertebral disc, trapping one or more nerves of the spinal column, usually occurring in adults, and often caused by an awkward move when lifting. The condition is also known as a prolapsed or herniated disc. A slipped disc is usually in the lumbar region of the spinal column, and symptoms occur suddenly or in a few days in the form of increasing low back pain (lumbago), and above all pain radiating to buttocks and legs (sciatica), with tingling and possible loss of feeling. A characteristic feature is that pain increases with pressure in the abdominal cavity : with

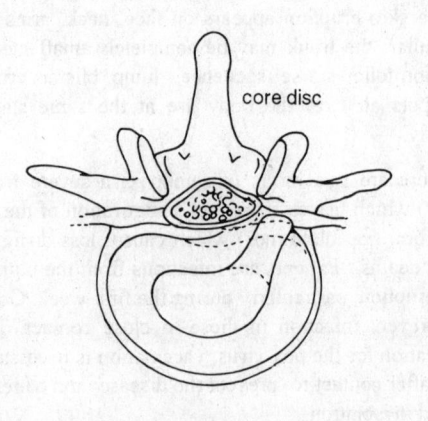

core disc

In slipped disc the soft core of the disc protrudes and may press on the nerves in the spinal cord.

coughing, sneezing or pressure. Discomfort is least acute in the morning; minor reductions in intensity of pain may be noticed, particularly when walking on the toes or heels. Problems with urination or defecation are rare. A slipped cervical disc in the neck is far less common, and causes corresponding pain in one arm. Physical examination shows that pulling or pressing the nerve causes radiating pain. The pain prevents the patient from stretching and raising the affected leg, and often the leg shows reflex disorders; depending on the position of the slipped disc, the knee tendon or Achilles tendon reflex may be weakened. The slipped disc can be made visible by contrast X-ray examination of the spinal column (myelography), and possibly a CAT scan.

Smallpox. Viral infection with the smallpox virus, of which man is the only carrier; this fact has made it possible to eradicate the disease. The virus now exists only in laboratories, and so vaccination is no longer necessary. The pox virus is inhaled, and breeds in the air passages and lymph nodes, from which it moves to the skin and mucous membranes. Roughly 12 days after infection the patient feels sick, and has fever. Four days later a skin eruption appears on face, neck, arms and legs in particular; the trunk may be completely unaffected. The skin eruption follows a set sequence : lump, blister, crust, scar; all the spots all over the body are at the same stage simultaneously.

There are two forms of smallpox: a severe from (variola major) which leaves scars and disfiguration of the face, and a mild form (variola minor) which causes less disfiguration and fewer deaths. Patients are infectious from the outbreak of the skin eruption, particularly during the first week. Good hygiene can prevent infection in those in close contact. There is no medication for the pox virus; vaccination is necessary immediately after contact to prevent the disease, and patients must be treated in isolation.

Soft Sore. Inflammation of the genital organs, caused by the bacterium *Haemophilus ducreyi*. This disease occurs mainly in the tropics and subtropics and is very rarely encountered in Britain. The symptoms of soft sore are soft, painful ulcers or pustules (chancres) on the penis, on or around the labia of the vulva, and around the anus. The pus coming from the ulcers is contagious and the disease is transferred to others through sexual intercourse or manual contact. Following infection, women are less likely to display symptoms than men.

If not treated, the ulceration continues, and swellings occur in the lymph nodes of the groin.

Soft sore resembles syphilis (hard chancre), and various tests must therefore be carried out before treatment can commence. Antibiotics, special rinses and lotions are available for therapy.

Spastic colon. One of the commonest intestinal conditions, affecting an estimated 15 per cent of the population at one time or another. In a large number of patients a link can be shown with psychological factors such as irritability, tension or neuroses. The condition is characterized by periods of spastic contraction of the colon, causing spasmodic pain reduced by defecation or the release of wind. Faeces are often hard, and constipation alternates with slight diarrhoea.

Spasticity. Increased muscular tension as a result of spastic paralysis. The muscles look well-developed, but cannot exert force, flexible movement is impossible. Contractures gradually occur, in which the arms tend to be bent and the legs extended. If spasticity affects one side of the body only, a typical gait results : the leg is thrown outwards at every step, and the arm held upwards with elbow bent, like a wing. Walking is impossible if the condition affects both sides of the body. Life-long physiotherapy is recommended for optimal muscular function.

Speech disorders. Good hearing, control of mouth, tongue and vocal muscles, and normal intelligence are the prerequisites of normal speech; defects can be caused by deafness, spasticity and backwardness. Until a certain age children have difficulty in pronouncing certain sounds such as *r* and *l*. If such difficulties persist after the age of four, they are termed speech defects.

Incorrect pronunciation of consonants or replacing them with other sounds is called dyslasia, and can indicate impaired hearing or motor disturbances; lisping may be caused by dental abnormality, a disturbed relationship with parents or long-term illness. A short tongue or enlarged tonsils do not cause speech defects. Unseparated nasal and oral cavities caused by a congenital cleft palate or by a palate too short to reach the real wall of the nasal cavity cause difficulties in pronouncing, *p, b, t, d, k, s, z, f, v* and *w*. Vowels are distorted, and air escapes from the nose during speech, which normally is not the case. A cleft palate must be operated on as soon as possible to avoid this abnormality. Blockage of the nose causes an inability to pronounce nasals such as *m, n* and *ng*, which sound like *b, d* and *g*. Acquired speech defects can be caused by paralysis of mouth and throat muscles, or by damage to part of the brain-by a stroke, for example. Speech therapy can be effective.

Sperm deficiency. Usually investigated in men from involuntarily childless marriages. The most suitable sperm for such tests is that produced by masturbation; it must be examined under the microscope within an hour. Semen consists of fluid from the prostate gland and seminal vesicles, mixed with spermatozoa from the testicles. On ejaculation prostate fluid is expelled first, then spermatozoa and then fluid from the seminal vesicles. Various abnormalities can occur: too few spermatozoa per ejaculation, no spermatozoa at all, too few active spermatozoa, or only dead or obnormally formed spermatozoa. Fluid from the prostate or seminal vesicles may be inadequate in quantity or of abnormal chemical composition. Such conditions may be congenital, as in Klinefelter's syndrome or in the case of undescended testicles. The testicles can also be damaged by infections such as mumps notoriously. Other conditions which can cause sperm deficiencies are bilateral testicular cysts, variocele, torsion of the testicle, lead poisoning, malnutrition and severe vitamin A and E deficiency. Such abnormalities can often not be treated and result in sterility.

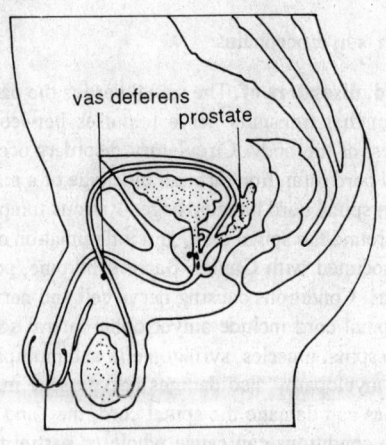

vas deferens

prostate

The presence of blood in the semen is a rare abnormality caused by disorders of the prostate or the vas deferens, but often no cause can be found.

Spider naevus. Skin disorder which looks like a small red spider, caused by severe dilation of a skin capillary; connected blood vessels in the area are also dilated, but to a lesser extent, giving the spider-like appearance. The condition is harmless in itself and affects forehead, neck and arms.

Spina bifida. Congenital condition of the spinal column. It arises in the fourth week of pregnancy because of deficient closure of the nerve tract, leading to incomplete development of one or more spinal arches and incomplete vertebrae. The disorder is serious and not uncommon. A soft swelling is visible at the defective point, usually only covered by spinal membrane (spina bifida aperta). If these membranes tear, the interior of the spinal column is revealed and the fluid exuded is cerebrospinal fluid.

Understandably, normal development of the nervous system is affected, often resulting in paralysis of the legs, with associated incontinence; there may also be foot disorders (club feet) and other congenital abnormalities. Another possible complication is hydrocephalus.

Spinal cord, disorders of. The spinal cord is the part of the nervous
system that transmits nerve impulses between the brain and
the rest of the body. Circulatory disorders occur as a result of
spinal cord infarction through blockage of a major blood vessel
and in spinal cord haemorrhage. Various tumours can occur in
and around the spinal cord, and inflammation of the spinal cord
is associated with Guillan-Barre syndrome, poliomyelitis, and
tetanus. Conditions causing nerve cell and nerve path decay in
the spinal cord include amyotrophic lateral sclerosis, altrophy
of the spinal muscles, syringomelia and multiple sclerosis. Cervical myelopathy also damges nerve tissue in the spinal cord.
Injuries can damage the spinal cord; they and a number of the
above conditions can cause whole or partial transverse lesion
or even breaking of the spinal cord. Disorders of the spinal
cord can cause failure symptoms such as anaesthesia, slack or
spastic paralysis, urinary problems and co-ordination difficulties. Spina bifida is a congenital disorder in which the spinal
cord is not properly covered by the vertebrae.

Spinal cord, tumours of. A distinction is made between tumours
originating in the spinal cord itself (gliomas) or those originating in the spinal mucous membrane (meningiomas and
neurinomas). Other types of tumour can exert pressure on the
spinal column, particularly metastases of cancers of the breast
and lungs to the vertebrae. Malignant growths of the vertebrae
themselves are less common. The symptoms are, depending on
the cause, a slow or accelerating transverse lesion (interruption of the spinal cord) possibly associated with severe radiating pain caused by localized pressure or irritation of the nerves
of the spinal cord. Diagnosis is by X-ray of the vertebrae,
myelography or CAT scan. To remove pressure on the spinal
column, vertebral arches above the condition are removed by
surgery, after which the tumour itself is removed. Gliomas in
the spinal cord are sometimes not removed if this would complete the transvere lesion. Secondary tumours are usually removed unless few failure symptoms have occurred and the

tumours is susceptible to radiation therapy or cytostatic drugs, so that there is a long-term chance of improvement in the patient's condition.

Spinal cord injuries. Damage to the spinal cord can be caused in various ways. A blow to the spine or a fall on the head or buttocks can cause vertebral displacement, resulting in pressure on the spinal cord. This also occurs in a so-called compression fracture, in which a vertebra is pressed inwards, trapping the spinal cord. Patients with arthrosis, chronic rheumatoid arthritis and cervical myelopathy run an increased risk. Concussion of the spinal cord is a short-term function disturbance not involving permanent damage, but causing tingling that may last for minutes or hours and possibly paralysis of the limbs. Contusion of the spinal cord is more serious, and usually occurs in the neck (whiplash injury), sometimes causing smarting pain in the shoulders or arms resembling that caused by a partial transverse lesion, in which case limited or complete recovery is possible. If the transverse lesion completely severs the spinal cord, there is no chance of restoration of function. Damage to the spinal cord is established by X-ray or CAT scan and the exact nature of the injury determined by the symptoms and any reflex abnormalities.

Spinal muscular atrophy. Rare condition involving *decay* of motor anterior horn cells in the spinal cord, causing slack paralysis. There are forms that occur particularly in children and which are probably hereditary; the more severe form rapidly causes invalidity, the more benign form only causes a certain degree of invalidity in later life. Spinal muscular atrophy in adults usually begins between the ages of 40 and 60; the cause is still unkown. The symptoms are increasing slack paralysis, leading to muscular atrophy. Irritation of the motor anterior horn cells causes small muscular contractions (fasciculation). The condition can be a component of amyotrophic internal sclerosis; it can deteriorate gradually and is potentially fatal if respiratory difficulties set in. Diagnosis is by the characteristic clinical picture and electrical tests of muscles. There is no specific treatment.

Spleen. A sponge-like purplish organ about the size of the hand, laying on the left side in the abdomen between the stomach and the left kidney. It functions as a part of the immune defence system and plays a role in the maintenance of the blood, especially the quality of red blood cells. In infants up to age of about five months, the spleen is the source of red blood cells, and even in adults suffering from *anaemia*, it may produce red cells which usually come only from bone marrow. The adult spleen clears the circulation of old red blood cells which it breaks down. People with *malaria* often have much enlarged spleens because the organ collects red cells damaged by the parasites.

Like the thymus and the lymph nodes, the spleen is also a source of lymphocytes. Thus it is likely to enlarge during any infection, but disorders of the white blood cells such as *Hodgkin's disease* and *leukaemia* also have this effect.

However, adult humans are able to survive without a spleen. Its principal functions are shared with the liver and lymphatic system. If a powerful blow to the left side of the abdomen or a broken rib should rupture the spleen, it is usually removed.

Spleen, disorders of. The spleen has a function in the manufacture and breakdown of blood cells, the latter function being the more important. Aging and malformed blood cells are removed from the bloodstream by the spleen and cleared away. In an illness that produces large numbers of malformed blood cells, the spleen becomes overactive. Such disorders include haemolytic anaemia for red blood cells and leukaemia and Hodgkin's disease for white blood cells. Overactivity causes the spleen to swell. The swelling can be clearly felt on physical examination, and also causes abdominal pain by exerting pressure on other organs in the abdomen. The spleen is also able to manufacture blood cells, although generally this facility is not used.

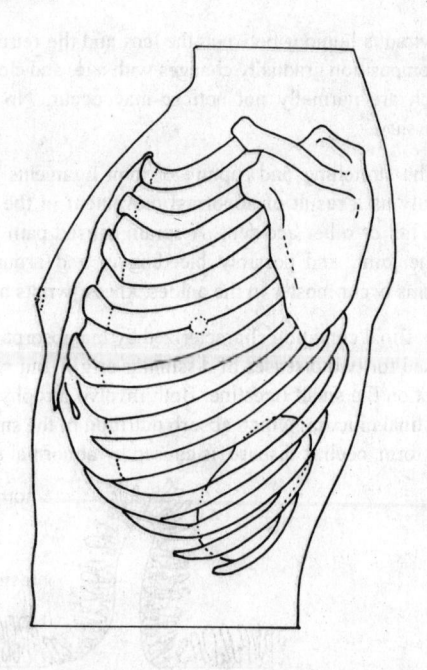

The spleen is in the rear of the upper part of the left-hand abdominal cavity and is protected by the rib cage.

If the bone marrow is no longer able to produce enough blood cells as a result of aplastic anaemia, leukaemia or multiple myeloma, the spleen can produce extra cells, an activity which can again cause it to swell. The spleen always contains large quantities of blood because of its role in blood breakdown; thus if the organ is ruptured, in a car accident for example, there can be massive haemorrhage with risk of shock.

Spots before the eyes (floaters) Small black dots or threads apparently floating before the eyes when looking at a light-coloured surface. They are experienced by almost everybody, although some people are more conscious of it than others and the condition, which is in fact harmless, can be very irksome to them. The floating spots are caused by cloudy points or particles in the vireous humour between the lens and the retina of the eye; its composition gradually changes with age, and cloudy patches-which are normally not noticed-may occur. No treatment is necessary.

Sprain. The stretching and rupture of joint ligaments and capsule, usually as a result of abnormal movement in the joint caused by a fall or other accident. A sprain caused pain and swelling in the joint, and possibly bleeding in and around the joint. Sprains occur mostly in the ankles, knees, wrists and fingers.

Sprue. Intestinal condition characterized by malabsorption. The term is used for two diseases of dissimilar origin, but with the same effect on the small intestine. Both involve atrophy of the small intestinal mucosa, which absorb nutrition in the small intestine. One form, coeliac disease, is caused by abnormal sensitivity of

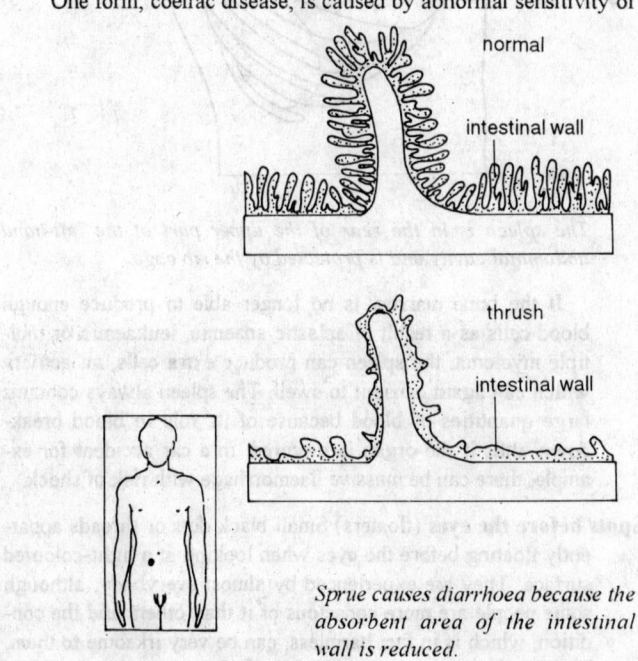

normal

intestinal wall

thrush

intestinal wall

Sprue causes diarrhoea because the absorbent area of the intestinal wall is reduced.

the intestinal mucosa to gluten. The condition can be congenital in children or acquired by adults. In tropical sprue the condition is probably caused by infection. Atrophy leads to digestive difficulties (malabsorption) with symptoms including more frequent defecation, increased faecal fat content, weight loss and symptoms characteristic of vitamin and nutritional deficiency; anaemia is a possibility. It is sometimes difficult to draw a distinction between sprue and other forms of malabsorption. The small intestine can be X-rayed, but biopsy is more likely to lead to correct diagnosis. Coeliac disease should be treated by a gluten-free diet. Tropical sprue can be treated with folic acid and antibiotics.

Squint (strabismus) Condition in which the eyes do not point in the same direction when focused on an object. In order for an object to be seen properly, light reflected by it must be projected at the same time through both eyes on to a certain part of the retina (fovea centralis). If the patient has a squint, then both lines ofsight do not reach this point and thus accurate perception of perspective is not possible. Sometimes one eye deviates inwards, sometimes both. They can also be turned outwards (*strabismus divergens*). Squinting is the most common defect which can reduce sharpness of vision in one eye. It occurs in 5 per cent of the population (25 per cent of children). There are various types. First pseudo-squint: a child can seem to be squinting when this is not in fact the case. It can be caused by an asymmetrical face, broad nose or eyes that are set rather far apart and usually disappears as the face develops. A simple examination reveals whether an abnormality exists.

Stammering. Speech disorder characterized by repetition of the initial sound of a word, entire words or even parts of sentences. There may be strained pauses in speech, followed by sometimes explosive continuation of speech. Symptoms of fear and anxiety also occur when speaking: sweating, palpitation and avoidance symptoms such as saying nothing at all. Stammering begins in childhood as a reaction to problems. It is generally a sign that the child does not feel secure, but there is certainly also a hereditary element, demonstrated by the fact that the problem often occurs more than once in a family and the fact that it is four times more common in boys than girls.

Stein-leventhal syndrome. Complex of symptoms associated with certain functional disturbances of the ovaries. During menstruation it is usual for an ovum to ripen in one of the ovaries (in a follicle, a vesicle filled with fluid). At ovulation the ovum is released, involving hormones from the pituitary gland and hypothalamus. In Stein-Leventhal syndrome this hormonal function is not regulated, and the ovaries are continuously stimulated. The follicles never ripen but are halted at various stages of development, with the result that the ovaries are enlarged

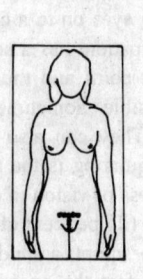

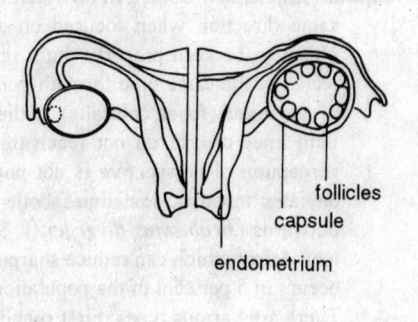

follicles
capsule
endometrium

In Stein-Leventhal syndrome the ovaries are well supplied with follicles, but ovulation often does not occur, thus breaking the normal menstrual cycle.

and surrounded by a rigid capsule; laparoscopy reveals various follicular cysts. Outward symptoms of this syndrome are slight, brief menstruation (oligoménorrhoea) and even complete lack of menstruation (amenorrhoea). First menstruation starts at the usual age. Some women affected complain of heavy, lengthy menstruation; such women are often thickset and have a masculine pattern of hair distribution (hirsutism). Infertility occurs through lack of ovulation.

Sterility. Failure of a wished-for pregnancy to occur for a period of more than a year during which sexual intercourse has occurred during ovulation. The use of the terms sterility and infertility is justified only after an examination from which it is established that abnormalities are present which make it impossible for pregnancy to come about in the normal fashion.

There are many causes of fertility disorders, both in men and in women. The man's production of healthy sperm cells can be disturbed because a testicle has not descended; the higher temperature then hinders good production of sperm. An attack of mumps after puberty can sometimes affect the sperm-producing tissue. Before puberty, the patient recovers from mumps without any harmful consequences where fertility is concerned. The production of sperm can also suffer through poisoning by heavy metals, smoking and exposure to radiation. Abnormalities in the passage from the testicle hinder the transport of sperm cells. Such abnormalities may be congenital or may result from an operation or inflammation.

In women, hoemonal disturbances are often the cause of faulty ovulation. This is usually accompanied by an abnormal menstrual cycle. The number of occasions on which ovulation is possible is thereby much reduced. Stress also influences ovulation. The passage of sperm through the cervix can be rendered difficult by an abnormality in the vaginal mucus. Moreover, congenital abnormalities in the oviduct, or constriction arising from scars formed after inflammation, can impede the fertilized ovum's passage to the uterus. As the above remarks show the causes of reduced fertility can be of many kinds. The investigation of the causes and their possible treatment can take a long time; both the woman and the man should be involved.

Steroid. One of a class of chemical compounds consisting of carbon and hydrogen atoms arranged in four "rings", three haxagons and one pentagon. To this structure, other atoms of carbon, hydrogen and oxygen may be attached in varying patterns which determine the functions of dirrerent steroids.

Steroids are lipids. They include cholesterol and the adreno-
cortical hormones and steroids are the basic material from which
bile salts are formed. The chemical in the skin converted by
sunlight to vitamin D is also a steroid.

Still's disease. Slow disease of the connective tissue in childhood
(juvenile rheumatoid arthritis). The disease is rare. It usually
manifests itself between the ages of two and five. The cause is
still not entirely clear. A distinction is made between the systemic form, showing symptoms of disease elsewhere in the
body, and a form which involves only abnormalities in one or
two joints. Symptoms of the systemic form are varying fever,
loss of appetite, irritability and pains in the joints with swelling, particularly of ankles and wrists. A patchy skin eruption
sometimes occurs as well. The pericardium and lungs may also
be affected.

Stokes-Adams syndrome. Attacks of unconsciousness caused by
the heart suddenly ceasing to pump enough blood to provide
the brain with adequate oxygen: when the supply of oxygen-
rich blood is interrupted for 15 seconds the patient turns

atrial impulse

ventricular impulse

ventricular impulses

pulse

*If the atrium fails, some time elapses before the ventricle takes
over the rhythm: the patient becomes unconscious for this period (Stokes-Adams attack). Ventricular rhythm, and thus the
pulse, are much slower than normal.*

pale and loses consciousness. As soon as the heart starts to
pump enough blood again the brain receives more oxygen and
the patient recovers. Stokes-Adams attacks are the result of
disturbances in cardiac rhythm: total stoppage of the heart,
extremely low heart rate and fibrillation. The latter condition
does no cease spontaneously and can only be corrected by

electric shock. If the heart beats too slowly or not at all it must be stimulated by injection. An effective treatment is the fitting of a pacemaker, to ensure that heart rate remains above a certain minimum.

Stomach, haemorrhage form. Loss of blood from damaged gastric mucous membrane. This can be a complication of conditions such as a stomach ulcer or stomach cancer or can sometimes be caused by severe damage from medicines (aspirin, particularly if used in combination with alcohol). A stomach ulcer is the commonest cause and together with duodenal ulcer is responsible for more than half of all haemorrhage in the upper part of the alimentary canal (oesophagus, stomach,

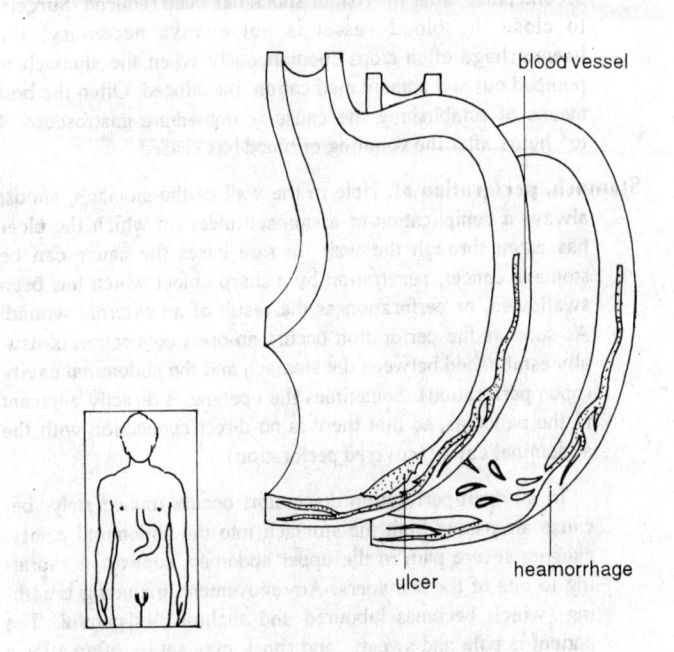

Stomach haemorrhage is caused by an ulcer eating into a blood vessel in the wall of the stomach.

duodenum). Haemorrhage occurs when the ulcer or tumour eats into a blood vessel. Symptoms depend on the extent and rapidity of the haemorrhage. Severe haemorrhage causes vomiting blood (haematemesis), in which the blood is often brownish-black through contact with stomach acid. Such conditions cause nausea and sweating and there is great danger of shock. Smaller haemorrhages cause blackening of the faeces (melaena); in the first instance there are no visible symptoms and laboratory tests have to be carried out on the faeces.

A doctor should be consulted in all cases of stomach haemorrhage. In severe cases immediate treatment including transfusion may be necessary; establishment of the cause takes second place, after the risk of shock has been reduced. Surgery to close the blood vessel is not always necessary; the haemorrhage often stops spontaneously when the stomach is pumped out and antacid medication introduced. Often the best means of establishing the cause is immediate gastroscopy 4 to 5 hours after the vomiting of blood has ceased.

Stomach, perforation of. Hole in the wall of the stomach, almost always a complication of a stomach ulcer, in which the ulcer has eaten through the wall. In rare cases the cause can be stomach cancer, penetration by a sharp object which has been swallowed, or perforation as the result of an external wound. As soon as the perforation occurs an open connection is usually established between the stomach and the abdominal cavity (open perforation). Sometimes the opening is directly adjacent to the pancreas, so that there is no direct connection with the abdominal cavity (covered perforation).

In an open perforation discomfort occurs immediately, because air passes from the stomach into the abdominal cavity, causing severe pain in the upper abdomen, sometimes radiating to one of the shoulders. Any movement, including breathing (which becomes laboured and shallow), is painful. The patient is pale and sweaty, and shock may set in, often after a period in which the pain has decreased. On physical examination the abdomen feels hard and is painful if pressed. The

tension is usually the result of peritonitis. Diagnosis of an open
perforation is confirmed by the presence of air under the diaphragm in an abdominal X-ray; an emergency operation is
necessary to repair the hole. If the perforation is covered, the
symptoms are milder and there is no air in the abdominal
cavity.

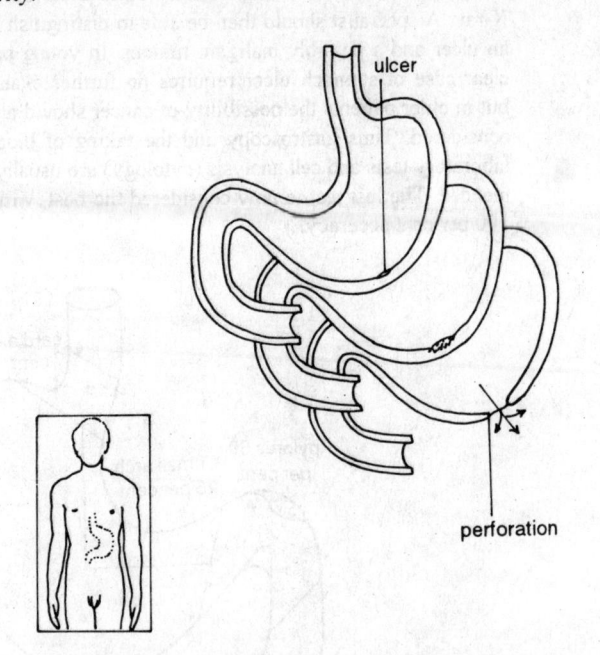

A perforated ulcer eats through the wall of the stomach, releasing gastric juices into the abdominal cavity.

Stomach cancer. Malignant tumour of the mucous membrane of
glandular tissue of the stomach. Together with intestinal cancer this is one of the commonest malignant tumours. It affects
men over the age of 40 in particular. The cause is not clear; a
connection with the eating of salted or smoked fish is sometimes suggested.

Stomach cancer has many symptoms in common with a stomach ulcer: pain a full feeling, nausea, vomiting and loss of appetite and weight. Haemorrhage is a possible complication. An X-ray does not always distinguish between the two conditions either. Tests are made to distinguish between benign and malignant tumours; the simplest method is a barium contrast X-ray. A specialist should then be able to distinguish between an ulcer and a possibly maligant tumour. In young patients a clear case of stomach ulcer requires no further examination, but in older patients the possibility of cancer should always be considered. Thus gastroscopy and the taking of biopsies for laboratory tests and cell analysis (cytology) are usually recommended. The last test is now considered the best, with almost 100 per cent accuracy.

cardia 12.5 per cent

pylorus 50 per cent

small arch 25 per cent

Stomach cancer occurs at various sites within the organ.

Stomach disorders. The stomach is the organ that receives ingested food after it has passed through the oesophagus. It acts as a reservoir, so that large quantities may be eaten at the same time without overloading the intestine. The stomach divides the food into small portions, which are then gradually passed into the small intestine. Digestion begins in the stomach, which produces a strong acid (hydrochloric acid) and a protein-splitting enzyme (pepsin). Stomach acid kills bacteria, thus protecting the alimentary canal against disease. The muscles in the stomach wall ensure good mixing of the food.

Stomach ulcer. Ulcer of the mucous membrane caused by stomach acid, either in the stomach or the duodenum. The conditions is more common in men than women and usually occurs between the ages of 20 and 50. About 80 per cent of such ulcers are duodenal.

Stomatitis. Inflammation of the mucous membrane of the mouth. There are various causes, one of the which is infection from the fungus *Candida albicans,* causing creamy-white patches throughout the mouth, or redness and inflammation of the oral mucous membrane. The condition is also known as oral thrush. The herpes simplex virus, among others, can cause inflammation of the mouth; the virus, which is also responsible for cold sores, causes small blisters throughout the oral cavity. Inflammation of the mouth can be a secondary result of another condition, such as certain blood or serious skin disorders, but also of smoking. *Candida* infection can also be related to other disorders such as diabetes mellitus or cancer. Oral inflammation with the formation of ulcers can occur without a particular cause, in which case it is known as stomatitis aphthosa.

Stretch marks. Subcutaneous marks which form under hormonal influences and during the rapid weight gain of pregnancy. After about the fourth month of pregnancy, marks sometimes appear in the skin of the abdomen, upper legs, buttocks and breasts.

Stroke (cerebrovascular accident) Sudden disturbance of blood supply to the brain, possibly leading to loss of faculties (including loss of feeling and paralysis).

In roughly three-quarters of cases the cause is narrowing of a blood vessel and possibe clot formation, leading to paralysis or aphasia, the inability to speak. These symptoms can be short-lived, if the blood clot dissolves quickly (when it is known as TIA, transient ischemic attack, a temporary disturbance of the blood supply). More serious is a cerebral infarction, after which the symptoms are more likely to persist.

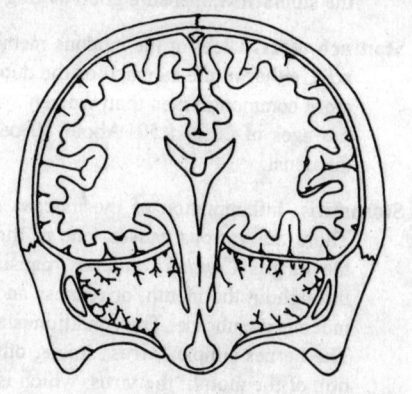

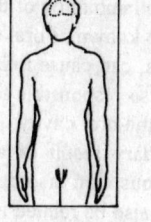

In cerebral infarction the symptoms-such as paralysis-are dependent on the site of the interrupted blood supply.

Strongyloidiasis. Infestation with the *Strongyloides stercoralis* worm, 2 mm long, which occurs frequently in the tropics. About 35 million people are affected. Only the females live in the small intestine where they lay their eggs. The larvae hatch in the body and are excreted with the faeces, then develop into infectious larvae in the ground. These larvae can penetrate into man via the skin, after which they pass through the blood and lungs to the intestine, where they develop into adult worms in 17 days.

Stye. Acute inflammation of a sebaceous gland at the base of an eyelash, causing swelling, redness and pain; an abscess forms around the sebaceous gland, and can break through to the outside. Styes are usually caused by staphylococci; they heal rapidly once the abscess has burst.

Sdden infant death syndrome (cot death) Sudden and unexpected death of an apparently healthy baby, with no explanation being found even after autopsy. Much research into the cause is currently being carried out. A disorder in the rate of breathing and heartbeat during sleep is at present thought to be the most probable cause.

Sudeck's Dystrophy. Dystrophy is wastage of tissue, usually muscles. Sudeck's dystrophy mainly affects wrist or ankles, or another part of the arm or leg. The cause is unknown, but is probably a disorder of the autonomic nervous system. Usually this is a reaction of the nervous system to an (often minor) injury to an arm or leg. For this reason it is sometimes also called reflex dystrophy. First, dilation of the veins causes red and swollen skin. The skin is very sensitive. In the next phase the skin is shiny, and hair begins to fall out, and the veins begin to become constricted. Finally severe venous constriction causes nutritional deficiency in all tissue. Muslces become thinner, bones show osteoporosis, which makes them more brittle. Joint tissue in the affected area also wastes, causing restricted movement.

Suffocation. Oxygen shortage, possibly causing death. Suffocation usually occurs because breathing is obstructed, as in choking. Examples of other causes are drowning, in which water in the lungs prevents breathing, a plastic bag over the head which closes the mouth and nose because it is sucked in and vomiting in unconscious people without the stimulus to cough. A less obvious cause is carbon monoxide inhalation, which drives the oxygen out of the red blood cells and thus prevents the tiusses from being supplied with oxygen. The first symptoms are shortness of breath and fear, followed by unconsciousness; the patient is pale or blue in colour, red in carbon monoxide poisoning.

Breathing stops after a while and, finally, death occurs. The brain cannot continue functioning for more than a few minutes without oxygen and after this it becomes damaged. Help must, therefore, be given quickly. If suffocation seems likely the first step is to free the respiratory tract by removing objects and by wiping vomit from the mouth. If the patient is not breathing, mouth-to-mouth resuscitation must be applied until breathing starts again or help arrives.

Sunburn. Damage to skin caused by excessive exposure to the sun's ultraviolet rays, comparable with a mild first-degree burn.

It usually occurs as a result of sun-bathing.

The skin is normally protected against the rays of the sun by pigment which is formed when the pigment cells are activated by ultraviolet radiation. The skin then becomes tanned.

Sunburn mainly occurs in the spring, when only small amounts of pigment have been laid down. The result is mild sunburn, with redness of the skin and pain.

Second-degree sunburn can occur in serious cases, especially when someone has fallen asleep in the sun. In addition to the redness, blisters also form. Mild sunburn is not a serious condition and heals without leaving any scars. It therefore requires no special treatment. The pain can be relieved by products applied to the skin after it has been exposed to the sun. Suntan oil and suntan lotion are of value only in the prevention of sunburn, not in its treatment. These preparations retard the ultraviolet rays, but do not soothe the pain. Severe sunburn is a serious condition, a form of sunstroke.

Sunstroke. Serious disorder that results from overexposure to heat. It is particularly common in people who do not enjoy perfect health (cardiac and vascular diseases, diabetes or alcoholism). The condition occurs mainly in hot damp weather and is caused by the failure of the heat regulation centres of the brain and the resultant overheating of the body. This may result in certain organs being damaged.

The initial symptoms may be headache, dizziness and nausea. Sometimes there is a fit of epilepsy. Confusion or unconsciousness then sets in and the blood temperature can rise to over 40°C. The liver and kidneys are often damaged by the high temperature. Damage to the heart and brain may also occur. A number of patients die from widespread tissue damage or shock. No time must be lost in treating the condition.

Sweat glands, inflammation of (hidradenitis) Suppurating inflammation of the sweat glands in the armpit or groin. There are special sweat glands at these sites which also produce body odour.

The condition outwardly rather resembles a boil, but a boil is an inflammation of the hair follicles and not the sweat glands. Hidradenitis is caused by the bacterium *Staphylococcus aureus*. It is found on the skin's surface, but causes infection only once it has penetrated deeper. In simple cases, inflammation of the sweat glands can be treated by an ointment which draws out the inflammation. It is sometimes necessary to remove the suppurating contents of the infected glands by making a small incision.

Sweating excessive. Sweating is the body's reaction to an increase in temperature and a means by which it tries to lose heat. The sweat glands are controlled by the central nervous system and consequently someone may also sweat as a result of psychological tension-often known as a cold sweat.

Excessive sweating occurs when the rate of perspiration is higher than normal. It is difficult to define the borderline because there is a good deal of variation over what may be regarded as normal. A person is usually regarded as sweating excessively if problems arise as a result.

Sympathetic nerves. The peripheral nervous system—that is, all nerves except those that make up the central nervous system—is traditionally divided functionally into the voluntary and the autonomic or vegetative nervous systems. The latter is further subdivided into sympathetic and parasympathetic. It is now considered more useful to identify nerve-cells in terms of the transmitters that carry signals between them because drugs, for example, are often designed to block or to mimic these transmitters, but the older functional classification is still used, especially in the study of anatomy.

Although some parasymphathetic and voluntary nerves originate in the brain and the remaining voluntary system begins in the spinal cord, sympathetic nerves originate outside the central nervous system. They begin in ganglia, small nodes or clusters of neurons and nerve-endings lying in a row from top to bottom opposite the spaces between vertebrae on each side of the spinal cord. Each ganglion is connected directly to the spinal cord.

The sympathetic system runs to the skin, eyes, arteries, digestive organs and heart. It regulates sweat glands, body hair follicles, eyelids (also under voluntary control) and pupils, muscles in the arteries and the heart, the amount of air entering the lungs and the rate of digestive activity. Parasympathetic nerves act in the same organs, often with an opposing effect, as well as in the bladder and rectum. The vagus nerve to the heart and stomach is part of the parasympathetic system.

Both parts of the autonomic nervous system depend primarily on the transmitter noradrenaline, though its effect on the behaviour of different neurons differs greatly depending on the cell itself. Some autonomic neurons utilize a different transmitter, serotonin. Some parasympathetic nerves and the entire voluntary system depend on the transmitter, acetylcholine.

Syncytium. A group of cells that have merged, losing their cell walls but retaining their nuclei, so a multinucleate cell within a single corporate membrane. Syncytia occur primarily in heart muscle.

Syphilis (lues, hard chancre) Venereal disease caused by the bacterium *Treponema pallidum*. The disease is very contagious and transmitted by sexual intercourse or oral contact with infected genitalia. It is the 15 to 30 year-old age group that is most at risk of infection.

Infection takes place at the mucous membrane of the genitals and sometimes also via damaged parts of the skin. The mucous membrane of the throat can also become infected.

An average of 3 to 6 weeks after contact with the bacterium, an unlcer, which is not painful but has a hard edge (hard chancre), is formed at the bacterium's point of entry. This ulcer can be on the penis, lips of the vulva, anus lips on the mouth or in the throat. This is first stage syphilis and at this time the patient is extremely contagious. In a few cases the symptoms may pass without being noticed. The ulcer heals without treatment, but the bacterium remains in the bloodstream and quickly passes hard, painless swellings from the lymph glands into the groin. The second stage begins some 6 to 8 weeks after the formation of the ulcer. The symptoms consist of slight fever, headache, loss of appetite, tufts of hair falling out, a red rash on the plams of the hands and soles of the feet, sore throat and sore bones. Sometimes ulcers appear in other parts of the body. These are highly contagious. This stage lasts for a year or longer, and after this the latent stage begins. There are few symptoms at this time, other than occasional inflamed skin lesions. Years later (sometimes 10 to 20 years after infection), the third stage can arise. Skin lesions are characteristic at this point.

Syringomelia. A rare condition, usually of the upper part of the spinal cord. A central cavity forms, surrounded by a kind of scar tissue. The cause is unknown. The condition begins between the ages of 20 and 45 and causes either no serious disability or disability which does not become serious until a late stage. Various nerve fibres can be interrupted as the cavity forms and this leads to reduced sensitivity to pain and temperature in the hands and arms. Later on, lesions in the skin and joints arise because of the interruption of nerves in the autonomic nervous system. Finally, slack paralysis occurs, with atrophy (muscle wastage) in the arms and spastic paralysis with numbness in the legs.

T

Tachycardia. Heart rate of more than 100 beats per minute, usually the result of the heart adjusting to particular circumstances such as physical exertion, fever, infection or anaemia. Sometimes the condition is caused by the production of extra impulses in the wall of the right auricle, giving a heart rate of more than 150 beats per minute, usually for no particular reason, and usually returning to normal within a few minutes to an hour. The heart usually shows no abnormalities, and no treatment is necessary.

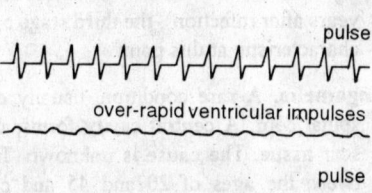

normal ventricular impulses

pulse

over-rapid ventricular impulses

pulse

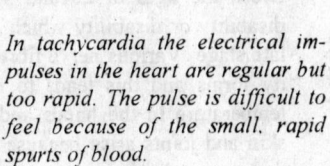

In tachycardia the electrical impulses in the heart are regular but too rapid. The pulse is difficult to feel because of the small, rapid spurts of blood.

Tapeworm (*Taenia*) Infestation with a parasite that lives and grows in the intestine. There are two kinds, the common tapeworm which occurs throughout the world and the armed tapeworm, which occurs in the tropics and subtropics.

Tapeworms live in the small intestine of man, where they feed on liquid food. They can grow to be very long (up to 10 metres) and are long-lived (13 years). Man is usually infested with one or more worms.

The tapeworm has a head with four suckers (scoleces, 1-2 mm long), and the armed tapeworm also has a crown of barbed hooks. A thin neck connects the head to the body, which consists of hundreds (700-1,000) of segments. A fully-grown segment is 2-3 cm long and has male and female reproductive organs (hermaphrodite). When mature a segment contains about 180,000 eggs, and ten such segments are discharged with their eggs each day. The segments remain mobile for several hours, and as they crawl they release their eggs. The eggs are found in faeces, and can be seen moving there, and around the anus. Man, cattle and pigs can be intermediates hosts. The larva emerges from the egg after it has established itself in the intestine of the intermediate host and develops into a bladder worm. Man can be infested by eating raw or under-cooked meat from infested cattle or pigs, and even by handling beef (the eggs of *Taenia saginata* stick to the hands). The outer covering of the bladder worm dissolves in the stomach and the head attaches itself to the small intestine.

Teeth, discoloured. Discolouration of the teeth often occurs through exterior influences, such as colouring matter in food, tobacco or certain medicines. One substance known to have a discolouring effect on the teeth is fluoride. Too much fluoride, as for example in the drinking water during the period when the teeth are growing, can lead to a yellowish-brown, spotty discolouration.

One medicine known for its discolouring effects is tetracycline, the antibiotic. Using it while the teeth are developing can lead to a grey to yellowish-brown discolouration. Tooth discolouration is sometimes the consequence of an injury with dental bleeding, the result being a dark discolouration.

Dental discolouration does not in itself mean that the teeth are any weaker; in fact they sometimes becomes stronger (for example, as a result of too much fluoride). If it is treated, it is mainly for cosmetic reasons.

Teeth, disorders of. Dental caries, also known as tooth decay, is one of the commonest human disorders. Other conditions include periodontitis and gingivitis, disorders of the supporting apparatus (including bone and gums), and abnormalities of tooth position. The first two conditions are firmly related to oral hygiene. Abnormalities of position have a negative effect in two ways; they can have a deleterious effect on dental health, for example because the teeth are difficult to clean, and they can be psychologically troublesome because of their appearance. Common abnormalities are overbite, crowding through lack of space and crooked placing of the teeth associated with faulty alignment of upper and lower jaws (malocclusion).

Teeth, occluded. Poor fitting together of elements in the upper and lower jaw. After dental caries and periodontosis it is the most important dental disorder in older children. The condition occurs in various forms and degrees of severity. In the milk teeth it shows above all in protrusion of the upper jaw: overbite, possibly the result of thumb-sucking. The same overbite can also show in the permanent teeth, but other conditions occur, though less frequently, such as overcrowding of the jaw, causing teeth to grow crookedly. Thumb or finger sucking has already been mentioned; early loss of milk teeth can also cause problems later. The permanent teeth are already starting to develop, and uneven loss of milk teeth, can deleteriously affect their position. It is, therefore, clear that care should be taken to avoid bad sucking habits and to look after the milk teeth and the gums properly. Many problems can be wholly or partly corrected with braces (orthodontics); the prospect of this is not attractive to children in the short-term, but in the long-term they are less likely to suffer from caries.

Telangiectasia. Rare hereditary disorder of small blood vessels, which causes dilation of the capillaries in the skin and in the mucous membrane of nose and mouth. The condition is dominant, that is to say children of a parent with the disease have a 50 per cent chance of inheriting it; telangiectasia occurs equally frequently in men and women. The dilated blood vessels appear on the skin as small red points which disappear if pressed. Because the wall of the small blood vessels is much weaker than normal, bleeding occurs more frequently; patients often have nosebleeds, and sometimes, more seriously, stomach haemorrhage. The inclination to haemorrhage increases with age. Medical help is not needed until the patient is adult, by which time the condition is familiar, as one of the parents is likely to have been treated for it. Although the disorder can cause problems, sufferers' lives are no shorter than average.

Tendon injuries. Injury to the tough connective tissue at the end of a muscle by which it is attached to bone. Tendon injuries limit movement and cause pain at the point of injury. If the tendon is torn completely, the muscle contracts powerfully, with one piece of the tendon attached to it. Tendon injuries can be part of more general damage, such as fractures, or can occur in isolation. They are more likely to occur if the tendon has lost rigidity through inflammation or under-use. Tendon tears the common in sport: in the fingers in handball sports, for example, if the ball is caught incorrectly, possibly causing hammer finger. Footballers may tear the Achilles tendon, usually by being kicked above the heel; normal walking is then impossible because the heel cannot be raised. Tendon tears are often incomplete, and can be treated with splints or plaster; a total tear must be repaired by surgery.

Tennis elbow (epicondylitis) Inflammation of the periosteum and tendons in the bony projections (condyles) of the upper arm on the outside of the elbow. This is the site of the insertions of the muscles that extend the hand and wrist and turn the lower arm. The inflammation arises as a result of irritation of the periosteum. This irritation can result from a blow, but usually it is a matter of the energetic or intensive use of this group of muscles. It may affect tennis players, but equally it can be a consequence of other prolonged activities such as knitting or uising a screwdriver.

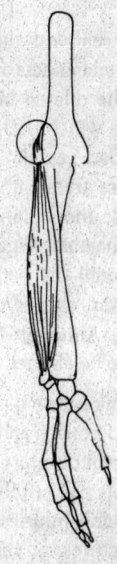

Tennis elbow is caused by chronic irritation and inflammation at the point at which the tendon is attached to the elbow.

Tenosynovitis. Inflammation of the connective tissue sheath surrounding a tendon, resulting from irritation through intensive use. Generally the tendon itself is also inflamed, along with the mucus goblet cells in the area. The wrists are often affected. Symptoms are pain and loss of strength: objects cannot be gripped properly, for example. Fluid may accumulate within the sheath, and precipitated substances in this fluid can cause a grating sound as the tendon moves through the sheath. The condition may also cause ganglion formation, and chronic inflammation can lead to constriction of the sheath, so that the tendon cannot slide smoothly through it, making it impossible to straighten a bent finger, for example, without a sudden movement with an associated click. Tenosynovitis can also be an element of another disease, such as a rheumatic disorder or bacterial infection.

Treatment is by rest of the affected tendon and sheath, if necessary in combination with painkillers and inflammation inhibitors. Serious constriction of the sheath may be corrected by surgery.

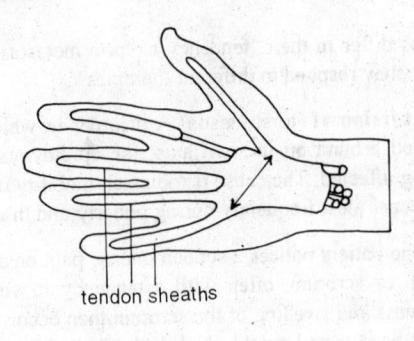

tendon sheaths

The tendon sheaths are joined together, and thus tenosynovitis caused by a small wound can spread through the whole hand.

Testicle, atrophy of. A condition in which the testicles cease to produce sperm and hormones or do so in only limited amounts. The testicles are also usually reduced in size. This condition can occur after orchitis external injuries, torsion of the testicle and undescended testicles.

The testicles of some individuals have a predisposition to atrophy, for example in Klinefelter's syndrome and in testicular feminization.

Atrophy of the testicle frequently leads to infertility.

Testicle, cancer of. The formation of a malignant growth in one of the two testicles, the organs lying in the scrotum which produce sperm. This cancer occurs mainly between the ages 15 and 34.

Initially, an enlargement of the scrotum is often the only symptom of the growth. This is unfortunate, because the patient tends not to go to the doctor unless it is causing pain. By then, however, metastasis has often occurred. An operation is the best means of determining whether a cancer is present. If a growth is disovered, the testicle is removed at once and the tumour is examined under a microscope to determine its cellular composition and whether or not it is malignant. Cellular composition is important, because the various cancers of the testis differ in their tendency to form metastases, and also in how they respond to different therapies.

Testicle, torsion of (torsio testis) A disorder in which a testicle is turned around on its own axis, the epididymis possibly also being affected. The cause is too much mobility in the scrotum. It occurs most frequently during puberty and in young adults.

The patient notices a sudden intense pain on one side of the groin or scrotum, often with a tendency to vomit and faint. Redness and swelling of the scrotum then occur. The condition must be detected quickly and distinguished from, for example, a strangulated inguinal hernia or epididymitis, both of which can give rise to the same symptoms.

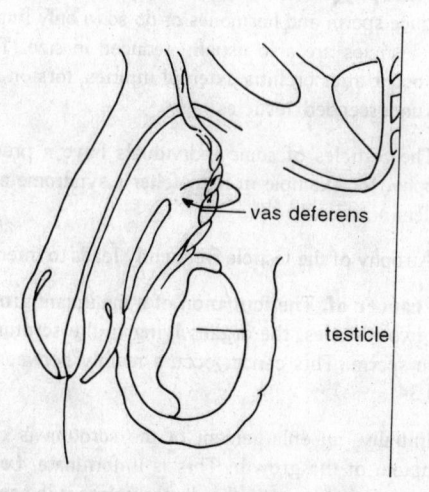

Torsion of the testicle restricts blood supply, with the result that the testicle could die.

The torsion causes a strangulation of the vessels carrying blood to and from the testicle, the testicle is cut off from its oxygen supply, and the tissues may die as a result.

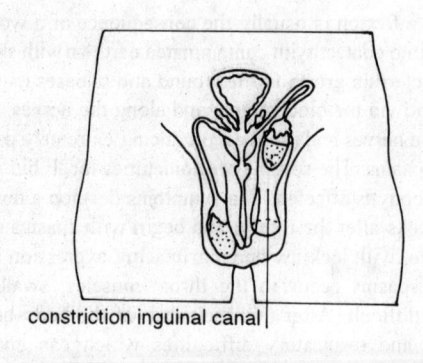

constriction inguinal canal

One or both testicles can be prevented from descending by a constriction in the inguinal canal.

The testicle must be turned back within 4 to 5 hours, otherwise the damage to its tissues is irreparable. This can be done externally by hand, or by an operation. An operation makes it easier to decide whether the testicle can be saved and if it can the surgeon will attach both testicles to the scrotum in order to prevent the condition from recurring.

Testicle, undescended (cryptorchism) Failure of one or both testicles to descend fully into the scrotum via the inguinal canal.

The cause of the testicle's failure to descend is not always clear; hormones may play a part and mechanical obstacles,. such as an inguinal hernia, can retard descent.

If the scrotum is empty, the testicle may lie in the inguinal canal, in the area around the inguinal canal, or in the abdominal cavity. The descent of the testicle into the scrotum is essential for the production of hormones and sperm, because they can be produced only at below normal body temperature and the scrotum's relatively exposed position provided this.

Tetanus (lockjaw) Serious wound infection, caused by the poison (toxin) of the tetanus bacillus (*Clostridium tetani*). This disease is now rare as a result of a vaccination programme.

The infection is usually the consequence of a wound which comes into contact with contaminated earth or with street refuse. The bacterium grows in the wound and releases its toxin. This is spread via the bloodstream and along the nerves, and stimulates the nerves and muscles, producing extremely painful muscular spasms. The spasms are sometimes local, but usually the whole body is affected. The symptoms develop a few days to a few weeks after the injury, and begin with spasms in the jaws and face, with lockjaw and a grimacing expression as a result. When spasms occur in the throat muscles, swallowing becomes difficult. After this the rest   of the body becomes affected, and respiratory difficulties which can endanger the patient's life may arise. When the disease reaches its height, the victim is extremely sensitive towards any stimuli, such as sounds. These can cause a sudden and total spasm. One complication is pneumonia, which may be the consequence of swallowing the wrong way. Sudden spasm can result in the fracture of a dorsal vertebra. The disease is frequently fatal if not treated.

Thalassaemia. A congenital abnormality in which the production of red blood corpuscles is disturbed. The proteins used in the production of red cells are abnormal and as a result the corpuscles are also abnormal. This leads to their rapidly being broken down. Thus, thalassaemia is primarily a disturbance in cell production, combined with a form of haemolytic anaemia.

Persons suffering from thalassaemia sometimes display no symptoms at all and if there are any these are the general symptoms associated with anaemia.

Threadworm (oxyuriasis; pinworm) Oxyuriasis is a disease caused by infestation with the threadworm, common intestinal parasite, and it affects more than 200 million people throughout the world, especially children. The colourless worms live at the junction of the large and small intestine, or sometimes in the caecum, and feed on their contents. The male worms, 3-5 mm in length, remain in the same place, but the females 9-12 mm long, move usually at night, to the skin around the anus as soon as they begin to ovulate and lay their eggs there, after which they die. Threadworms have a life-span of 6 to 8 weeks.

The larvae in the eggs develop very quickly, and can cause infestation within 5 to 6 hours or even sooner. The worms and deposited eggs cause anal itching, Children in particular tend to scratch, and eggs stick to their fingers. If the thumb is sucked, or food is consumed without washing the hands, eggs can get into the mouth. Infection can also result from inhaling air containing eggs from clothes or bedding. From the mouth the eggs reach the intestine, where they develop into larvae and move to the junction of the large and small intestine. They are fully grown within 4 to 7 weeks.

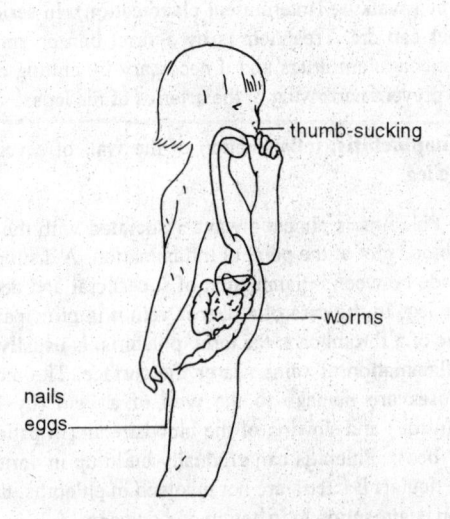

Once threadworm infestation is established, the child often sustains it himself or herself through poor hygiene.

Sometimes eggs are found on or in faeces. A strip of transparent tape can be used to obtain a sample of eggs in order to establish which worm produced them. Infection can be prevented by thorough washing of the skin around the anus with soap and water, regular hand washing, and regular changes of clothes and bedding.

Thromboangiitis obliterans. Inflammation of the walls of large and medium arteries and veins, particularly in the legs.

The cause of this disorder, which occurs partlicularly in young men who are heavy cigarette smokers, is unknown. Inflammation of the walls narrows the blood vessels, and this restricts blood supply to the legs and feet. The symptoms are cold feet and a bluish colouring. When the calf muscles receive too little oxygen-rich blood cramp occurs in the calves when walking (intermittent claudication). In serious cases the toes can die. Treatment is by a strict ban on smoking, use of anticoagulant drugs and if necessary by cutting certain nerves to prevent narrowing of the arteries of the legs.

Thrombophlebitis. Inflammation of the wall of a vein, usually in the leg.

Phlebitis is almost always associated with the formation of a blood clot at the point of inflammation. A distinction must be made between inflammation of superficial and deeper veins of the leg. In the case of a deeper vein it is principally symptomatic of a thrombosis; the term phlebitis is usually reserved for inflammation of veins nearer the surface. The most important causes are damage to the wall of a vein (by injections or infusion) and slowing of the bloodstream (in patients confined to bed). Phlebitis can gradually build up in varicose veins in particular. Bacteria are not involved in phlebitis; the inflammation is a reaction to irritation and damage.

Thrombosis. The presence of a blood clot in a vein or artery.

Although thrombosis can is principle arise in any blood vessel and in any part of the body, it occurs in the veins of the leg in the overwhelming majority of cases. A blood clot can form when the wall of the vein is damaged at some point (due to an inflammation, for example) or when the blood flow is lower than normal (during a prolonged stay in bed, for example). In both cases, blood platelets have the opportinty to attach themselves to the wall of the blood vessel and in this way form a clot. Overweight people, elderly people, and pregnant women run a slightly greater risk of suffering a thrombosis; the combination of taking the contraceptive pill and cigarette smoking also increases the risk.

Thrombosis in a superficial vein in the leg is characterized by pain, redness and swelling of the blocked vein. When a clot forms in one of the deeper leg veins, a thrombotic leg results: there is pain in the calf, with swelling in the leg and shiny skin.

Thrush. Infection of the mucous membrane of the mouth, throat or vagina caused by the fungus *Candida albicans*. The fungus is normally present on the skin and in the mucous membrane and mouth of most people without causing infection. If the host's resistance is lowered by lengthy illness or the use of certain medicines (including cytostatics) the fungus can multiply and cause infection.

If antibiotics are being used normal bacteria are killed and the fungus has the opportunity to grow; oral sprue occurs regularly in patients with blood disorders, tumours or AIDS. Characteristic of the infection are small white patches on the oral mucous membrane which leave a small wound if scratched. The disorder is very painful. Sometimes infection spreads to the oesophagus; in rare cases the small intestine is affected. It can also affect the vagina (candidiasis).

Thymus. A gland in the upper chest behind the sternum and just below and forward of the thyroid gland. During foetal and early infant life, the thymus processes lymphocytes, subsequently called T-cells, which are part of the immune defence system. Chiefly, the thymus provides some physical information by means of which these cells can distinguish between what is foreign to the body and cells that are part of it, between self and not-self in the words of one authority. It may also cause T-cells to differentiate so that they perform different functions in the immune system.

The means by which the thymus accomplishes these tasks are not understood. However, it also secretes a hormone, thymosin, which may extend its task of differentiating new lymphocytes to other parts of the body. In later life, the thymus shrinks and seems to dry up.

Thyroiditis. Inflammation of the thyroid gland, which can be caused by infection; more commonly it is an autoimmune disease involving antibodies against thyroid tissue. A few days or weeks after infection of the air passages (usually by a virus) the thyroid swells increasingly and painfully, and swallowing becomes more difficult. Pain usually radiates to the jaw and ears (de Quervain's thyroiditis). Treatment is by large doses of aspirin and sometimes corticosteroids. Chronic thyroiditis (Hashimoto's disease) is the commonest form; it is an autoimmune condition with no known cause that occurs mainly in women, often associated with little pain, simply enlargement of the thyroid (goitre). After several months most of the normal thyroid tissue is replaced with connective tissue. Treatment with thyroid hormones helps in allowing the gland to return to its normal size. In the early stages of any form of thyroiditis it is possible that excess thyroid hormones will be produced; in the chronic form the gland can sometimes not produce sufficient hormones, in which case continuing hormone treatment is essential.

Thyroid tumour. May be either benign or malignant, and for this reason any lump at the front of the neck should be examined very thoroughly. Lumps in the thyroid occur quite frequently; there may be only one, or the whole gland can be full of them, in the latter case often as a result of persistent goitre. Benign and malignant tumours are more common in women than men.

Tic douloureux. Pain in the face can be caused by various factors. Known syndromes include hemicrania, or migraine, and trigeminal neuralgia.

Hemicrania occurs above all in men and is characterized by regular attacks of disabling throbbing pain around one eye, possibly radiating to the temple and jaw; there are also local disturbances such as streaming eyes, running nose, narrowing of the pupils and drooping eyelid. The attacks occur several times per day for several weeks or months, followed by a long period without attack. The cause is not entirely clear.

Trigeminal neuralgia is also associated with recurrent shooting pain lasting for several seconds in the cheek or jaw, caused by touching a 'trigger spot' such as a nostril or the corner of the mouth. In this condition too there are periods, sometimes lasting for years, which are free of attack.

Tinnitus. Hearing sounds in the ear or head without a source of noise. Buzzing in the ears can be caused by an ear-wax blockage, but it more frequently occurs in an ear that has been damaged in some other way; by loud noise, medication, otitis, surgery, accident or old age. All these are likely to involve slight hearing loss. Tinnitus associated with vertigo is a symptom of Meniere's disease. It can also be caused by high blood pressure, and more rarely by a tumour of the pons.

The cause of tinnitus should always be sought. It is sometimes a genuine noise (a constricted blood vessel or a dragging muscle in the neck), and this may be susceptible to treatment, but in almost half of all cases no apparent cause can be found.

Tonia tonus (Gr. *ton* = stretch) The suffix refers to a disorder of some kind of movement; thus, dystonia is a malfunction in muscle tension or tonus.

Tonsillitis. Inflammation of the tonsils. Tonsillitis occurs predominantly in children and young adults. So-called 'common' tonsillitis is caused by bacteria or viruses. In many cases a viral infection occurs first (while the patient has a cold, for example), which weakens the resistance of the tonsil cells and allows bacteria, almost always haemolytic streptococci, to invade. The symptoms of common tonsillitis are a sore throat, pain when swallowing, a general feeling of malaise, with fever, loss of appetite and headache. The fever can be high, and associated with shivering attacks. Examination of the throat reveals red and swollen tonsils with white spots on the surface, caused by accumulation of pus in the tonsils. Also the lymph nodes in the neck below the ear are enlarged and tender.

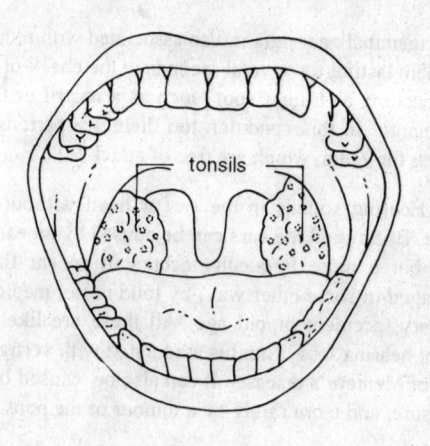

Tonsillitis is usually a bacterial infection of the tonsils: the tonsils are red, enlarged and covered in white spots.

Tonsils, enlargement of. Enlarged tonsils are usually caused by viral or bacterial infection, in the latter case often associated with fever, sore throat and enlarged lymph nodes in the neck. The condition occurs in tonsillitis and, among others, in glandular fever. The tonsils have a protective function against viruses and bacteria, but can lose this, and become a breeding ground for bacteria in particular, and cause infections of the mouth, throat and larynx. Chronically inflamed tonsils are sometimes enlarged, and sometimes associated with a slight sore throat, an unpleasant taste in the mouth and bad breath. The lymph nodes of the neck also swell. A rare cause of swelling of one tonsil is a malignant growth, and this possibility should be borne in mind if one-tonsil grows very quickly.

Tooth Abscess. Inflammation of the part of a tooth where it enters the jawbone. It is often a complication of dental caries (decay). If a tooth is affected by caries, the process can be halted only by completely removing the decayed material and filling the space with a suitable substitute. If this is not done, inflammation arises in the dental pulp-the central part of the tooth, where the nerves and blood vessels run. From there the infection passes down the root canal to the tip of the root. Such inflammation is characterized by intense pain, which is often spasmodic and frequently radiates out into the whole jaw and increases upon contact with heat. If an abscess subsequently forms in the jaw, the symptoms are mainly apparent at the point of infection. They increase when pressure is applied to the abscess. The tooth can come loose at this stage. If the pus can flow away, for instance between the tooth and the gum, the pain is eased; otherwise, it can lead to swelling, pain and even fever and swollen lymph glands.

Inflammation of the root-tip must be treated as quickly as possible by lancing the abscess, allowing the pus to escape. Antibiotics are sometimes prescribed.

Torticollis (wryneck) Characterisitic twisted head position caused at birth by tearing of one of the oblique neck muscles, with resultant haemorrhage and subsequent muscular scarring; the scar tissue shrinks, hence the unusual head position. The condition can also be caused by cutaneous scar tissue shrinkage after severe burns or major inflammation. The skin pulls the head rigidly sideways, and muscle then wastes. Other causes are long-term muscular spasm or paralysis on one side of the neck, and disorders of the vertebrae of the neck such as arthrosis or rheumatic inflammation.

Treatment is by slow stretching of the wasted tissue, possibly combined with cutting of shortened muscles or a skin transplant.

Toxic shock syndrome. A condition mainly seen in young women who use tampons during menstruation, which gave rise to the name 'tampon disease'. However, the phenomenon also occurs without any tampons being used (15 per cent of cases also occur in children).

It is caused by bacterial toxins which may be released in the case of certain infections of the female genital organs. The bacterium can be in a superficial wound, or in a tampon which is left in for too long. In the past, synthetic fibre tampons were available and these absorbed magnesium from the body tissues and weakened their defences, increasing the risk of infection. These tampons have now been withdrawn from sale.

Toxin. A poison produced by plants or animals. Toxins are almost always proteins and act as antigens. Bacteria, for example, may cause disease not by direct destruction of tissue but by means of toxins released into tissues. Antibiotics may control the bacteria, but the toxins must be allowed to clear from the system if they cannot be neutralized with other drugs.

Toxoplasmosis. Infestation by the widespread microorganism *Toxoplasma gondii*. Something like half the world's population has the infestation, usually without displaying any symtoms. Many infected mammals and birds also act as hosts.

The sexual development of the parasite takes place in a cat, the eggs being laid in the cat's intestinal wall and being eliminated from the body along with the stools. After as little as two days development, the egg is capable of infesting a new host when eaten. The development inside the cat is crucial for the dispersal of the parasite, because it is usually only for a short period in cats' lives that they eliminate the eggs along with their stools. The eggs cannot withstand desiccation.

After the egg has been taken in by a man or an animal, the parasites are released in the intestine and enter cells throughout the body. The infestation often passes unnoticed.

Trachoma. A serious, chronic eye disorder which is the most important cause of blindness in the world today. Trachoma is caused by the micro-organism *Chlamydia trachomatis*, and is very infectious. It can readily occur under unhygienic conditions and can be transmitted by flies.

It begins as a lingering conjunctivitis usually in both eyes. Numerous small bumps, bluish-red in colour, appear on the insides of the eyelids. These bumps may reach 5 mm in size. They burst in due course, and scar tisue then forms. Trachoma itself may cause relatively few symptoms. It is the resultant complications (bacterial infections) that may finally lead to blindness. After many years, simple trachoma also leads to scar formation in the cornea and to blindness.

Trachoma is treated by means of antibiotics, specifically tetracyclines. The eye recovers if treated promptly. However, scar tissue is permanent once formed.

Transmitter. A chemical released by a neuron as the end result of the signal that has travelled through the neuron. The transmitter diffuses across the minute gap separating the neuron from the next neuron or from the effector organ and initiates either a signal or a change in the state of the effector. Without transmitters, the nervous system cannot function.

Three transmitters suffice to link together the peripheral nervous system and its many effector organs, but the list of chemicals that operate as transmitters within the central nervous system is much longer and still growing. They include the three peripheral transmitters, noradrenaline, acetylcholine and serotonin, as well as amino acids such as glutamine, which may also become incorporated in proteins, and the recently-discovered opiate-like substances called enkephalins. All of these chemicals are small molecules which can also be easily copied in laboratories. This fact is important because large classes of drugs such as the tranquillizers either mimic or inhibit the actions of transmitters.

In the periphery, transmitters are excitatory; that is, they cause the next neuron to signal or the effector to change state. In the brain and spinal cord, however, some transmitters are inhibitory; that is, they inhibit signalling by the next neuron.

Note that an inhibitory neuron is one which releases an inhibitory transmitter. These opposing functions are thought to be immensely important in the processes of memory and learning, for example.

Transsexualism. A phenomenon in which someone born as a man or a woman is convinced that he or she is of the other sex. The endeavour and desire for the body to be altered to the inward, emotional identity are always present in the transsexual person.

A biologically male transsexual will, by reason of his inner feelings, seek contact with a heterosexually inclined man, and a biologically female transsexual seeks contact with a heterosexual woman. The sexual feelings may also be homosexual, bisexual or asexual in nature. However, transsexuality is not a form of homosexuality. Transsexuals do not regard their relationship as homosexual apart from a few exceptions.

Transverse lesion. Interruption of nerve cells in the spinal canal, resulting in deficient muscle control and lack of feeling from the point of the lesion. It is caused by spinal injury (in an accident, for example) and tumours of the vertebrae (by metastasis) or of the spinal canal. Other causes are inflammation (an abscess), disorders of the blood vessels and in very rare cases a slipped disc.

Cases of total transverse lesion cause persistent paralysis with loss of sensation in parts of the body below the injury. Life-threatening infections can be caused by the inability to urinate and by intestinal paralysis.

Transvestism. The irrepressible need to dress, from time to time, in the manner of the other sex and thereby to experience sexual and emotional satisfaction.

In a wider context, it can also be a part of the desire to assume the role of the other sex (transsexuality), and sometimes it can also be part of the desire of homosexuals to obtain a certain kick from the clothing of the other sex.

However, genuine transvestism occurs mainly in heterosexually inclined men, many of whom are married and have children.

Treatment is very difficult. The most important aim is to remove any guilt feelings and to promote self-acceptance. This occasionally lessens the need for such behaviour.

Tremor. Rhythmic trembling that occurs because of the involuntary contraction of opposing muscles. It occurs mainly when fear, other emotions or cold are being experienced. Some people always have such a slight tremor. These so-called physiological tumours are normal. Senile tremor in old people is an intensification of this normal tremor. Benign family tremor is an intensified physiological tremor which decreases with the use of alcohol and certain medicines. Other members of the family usually also have such a tremor. Another type of tremor occurs in Parkinson's disease. When the cerebellum is affected, a tremor arises, particularly when specifically directed movements are made.

Trench fever. Infection caused by *Rickettsia quintana* and transmitted by lice. *Rickettsiae* have characteristics of both viruses and bacteria, and the various forms cause illnesses with fever and skin rashes as their most important manifestations (including Q fever and typhus). They are transmitted by ticks, lice mites or fleas, which explains the prevalence of the disease at times of war, poverty and undernourishment, and particularly during the two World Wars. Characteristics of the disease are one to two days of high fever, followed by five fever-free days. Skin rashes, mild bleeding, headache and muscular pain can occur. Few patients die of the disease, and it is now rare. Treatment is with antibiotics.

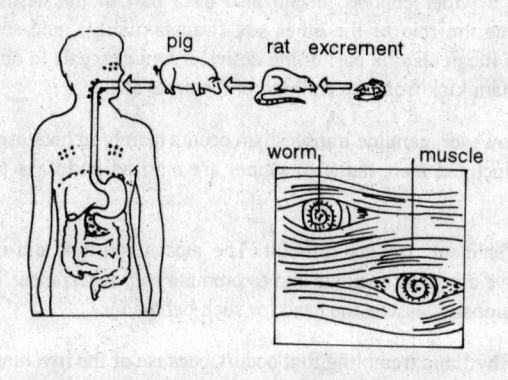

Trichinisis can be caused by eating under cooked pork; the worms infest transverse muscle and cause muscular pain.

Trichiniasis. Infestation with *Trichinella spiralis,* a small thin worm (1.5 to 4 mm long); also called trichinosis. This parasite infests some 28 million people in North America and Eastern Europe. The full-grown worm lives in the wall of the small intestine, where the female gives birth to dozens of live larvae.

These pass through the bloodstream and lodge in muscles, where they can remain encysted for 20 to 30 years. The development of the larvae into full-grown worms in the small intestine can cause diarrhoea and their movements through the body can give rise to fever, muscular pain and oedema, particularly in the eyelids. In serious cases, the brain or heart can be affected by the larvae. Once the larvae have become encysted in the muscles, the symptoms disappear.

Trichomoniasis. Infestation by a flagellate protozoan. This parasite has a world-wide distribution and women aged between 30 and 50 are the group mostly affected.

Three kinds of trichomoniasis occur in humans, but only *Trichomonas vaginalis* can cause symptoms. Most people who are infested are not troubled by the parasite and are carriers. Symptoms arise when the numbers of parasites in the vagina have risen to such an extent that the vaginal wall is damaged.

Inflammation sets in and this forms a good breeding ground for a variety of bacteria. A yellowish-green discharge from the vagina, with itching and pain, are the consequence. These symptoms often recur after every menstruation. Pregnant women are particularly susceptible to trichomoniasis. The symptoms can last for months but their intensity declines with time.

Men are much less frequently affected than women. Inflammation of the urethra and prostate can occur, with resultant pain, itching, problems with urination, and discharge from the penis. The infestation can be transmitted by sexual contact.

Trichuriasis. Infestation with nematode worms of the genus *Trichuris*. They are 3-5 cm long and have a very thin front portion and a fat rear one containing the reproductive organs. They live for roughly eight years. The worms occur throughout the world: approximately 350 million people are infested. At the junction of the large and small intestine the worms probably feed on the contents of the intestine and tissue fluid. They drill their thin section into the intestine wall, while the thick section is free and lays eggs which are then discharged in faeces and develop on the ground.

Tricuspid valve, disosrder of. A condition of the heart valve between the right auricle and the right ventricle. The function of the tricuspid valve is to prevent blood from flowing back from the ventricle to the auricle during the heart contraction of systole. Stricture (stenosis) of the tricuspid valve is rare. Leakage (insufficiency) of the valve can occur as a result of damage caused by endocarditis. The valve can also leak when the blood pressure in the vessels of the lungs, and thus also in the right ventricle, is substantially increased (e.g. in the case of abnormalities of the mitral valve).

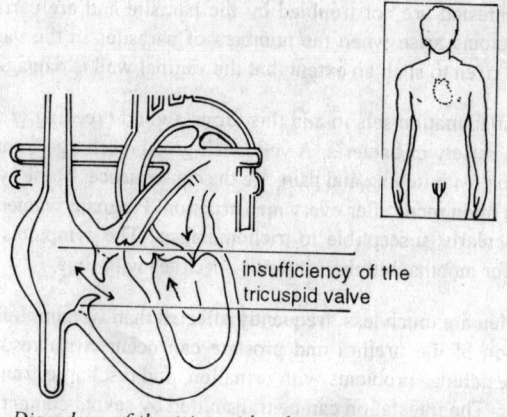

insufficiency of the
tricuspid valve

*Disorders of the tricuspid value are stenosis or leakage of the
valve. If the value leaks, l   d returns to the right atrium each
time the heart beats.*

Trigeminal neuralgia. Facial pain caused by irritation of one or
more branches of the trigeminal nerve. This is the sensory
cranial nerve which innervates the face. Pain in the trigeminal
nerve occurs mainly in older people. It is characterized by
various sharp twinges lasting a few seconds, in the area of one
cheek or jaw. These attacks are often brought on by touching
the nostril, by chewing or by speaking, and may be repeated
constantly. Sometimes there are periods of remission lasting
for years. Before the diagnosis of trigeminal neuralgia can be
made, it is necessary to rule out any other causes of pain in
the face, such as inflammation of the ear, sinuses and jaw. In
addition, eye conditions such as glaucoma and nervous pain
after shingles can also cause pain in the face.

Tuberculosis. An infectious disease caused by the tubercle bacillus
(*Mycobacterium tuberculosis*). This bacterium was discovered by Robert Koch in 1882 and identified as being the
causative agent of TB. Tuberculosis was formerly regarded as
a manifestation of extreme physical decline as a result of malnutrition, poor hygiene and poverty, and it was known as (gal-

loping) consumption or phthisis because of the considerable emaciation it caused. The name tuberculosis arose in the nineteenth century after the characteristic inflammatory tubercles, which were found in the organs of deceased patients. Hereditary factors, physical condition, diet, race and age are factors contributing to a person's susceptibility to the disease and the course taken by it. Most patients are between 18 and 30 years old.

Tubular necrosis, acute. Sudden loss of kidney tubules, with resultant kidney failure. Acute tubule necrosis can be caused by a reduction in the supply of blood and oxygen to the kidneys, and also by poisonous substances such as mercury, carbon tetrachloride and some antibiotics. The excretion of large quantities of haemoglobin in the urine, such as after the failure of a blood transfusion, can also be a cause, as can the elimination of the muscle protein myoglobin in crush syndrome.

Anuria or oliguria initially develops lasting for 1 to 3 weeks, and there are symptoms of uraemia. Treatment on a dialysis machine may be necessary at this stage. Depending on the cause, kidney function may be gradually restored.

Turner's syndrome. A congenital abnormality in which a sex chromosome is missing. The woman has only one X-chromosome instead of two (or one chromosome and part of the second X-chromosome). This abnormality occurs during or frequently after, the fertilization of the ovum.

Women suffering from this syndrome are frequently short, have a short and wide neck, and the lower arm is at an angle to the upper arm. The development of the breasts is retarded. The ovaries consist only of slivers of tissue, without any ova. There is therefore also no ovulation or menstruation, with resultant infertility. The vagina and uterus are however present. The syndrome is usually recognized at an early age by the outward appearance of the girl. It can be confirmed by scraping cells from the mucous membrane of the cheeks and sending them for karyotype analysis. The treatment consists of administering the sex hormones which are normally produced by the ovary, and possibly also in giving anabolic steroids to stimulate an increase in height.

Typhoid fever. A serious infection caused by the bacterium *Salmonella typhi*. A similar clinical picture can be caused by the agent responsible for a form of paratyphoid. Infection can be transmitted by unboiled milk, water or by food infected by carrier.

The disease begins after an incubation period of about 7 to 14 days, with headaches, swollen abdomen and abdominal pain, nausea, and diarrhoea, sometimes preceded by constipation. The body temperature gradually rises in the course of the first week to over 40°C. A skin rash and red spots (roseola) sometimes appear in the second week. In some cases, typhoid can cause an inflammation of the cerebral membrane or pneumonia. Serious complications are possible, such as intestinal bleeding or intestinal perforation.

U

Ulcer. Deep defect in the skin or mucous membrane, formed by the death of tissue.

An ulcer shows little tendency to recover, in contrast to a wound which heals much more easily. Skin ulcers occur regularly, and have very varied causes. Bacteria, parasites, fungi etc. can cause ulcers. Examples are leprosy, yaws, leishmaniasis and syphilis. Disorders in the blood supply to a particular part of the skin lead to the death of tissue, with an ulcer resulting (as for example with bedsores). Abnormalities in the nerves can give rise to numbness. As a result, sharp objects are not felt and can easily cause wounds (in diabetes, for example). An ulcer forms a good culture medium for bacteria and gangrene can result. Gastric and duodenal ulcers are regular occurrences. These ulcers arise through the effect of the gastric juices upon the mucous membrane. The resistance of the mucous membrane has usually already been reduce. Tension (stress), operating through the nervous or hormones, may disturb the balance between the resistance of the mucous membrane and the corrosiveness of the gastric acid, with ulcers possibly forming as a result.

Ulcerative colitis. Chronic inflammation and ulceration of the large intestine, without specific cause such as a bacterium or virus, often occurring in older children and young adults, but sometimes in later life. Ulcerative colitis is probably an autoimmune disease: the body produces defences against its own tissue. Psychological factors may also be involved, but this is doubted nowadays. The most important symptom is diarrhoea containing blood and mucus, passed up to 40 times per day according to the seriousness of the condition. Sometimes only blood and mucus are passed. Other symptoms are a diminished sense of urgency, fever, loss of weight, convulsive abdominal pain and general malaise, all changing with the severity of the disorder, which tends to flare up and then subside for a time. Serious forms can lead to anaemia and protein deficiency. Complications are perforated stomach ulcers or abscesses and fistulas in the intestine, also inflammation of the eyes and joints and a skin condition (erythema nodosum). The risk of intestinal cancer is increased. If the condition is suspected, rectoscopy provides an adequate diagnosis; this examination is necessary to eliminate other intestinal disorders such as enteritis, malignant tumours or other causes of inflammation of the large intestine, such as dysentery.

Umbilicus, infection of. Usually occurring within the first six days after birth. The severed umbilical cord is an open wound liable to infection. The cause is usually a staphylococcus, whose source must be sought in the immediate surroundings. Tetanus infection can also occur, probably as a result of poor hygiene. If infection sets in, the skin around the navel becomes red and swollen, and the navel itself discharges fluid containing pus. The principal danger is contamination via the large blood vessels behind the navel, which can lead to blood poisoning (sepsis). Umbilical infection can be avoided by binding the remaining section of the umbilical cord with sterile gauze and handling the baby in as hygienic a manner as possible. If infection nevertheless occurs, it can be treated with antibiotics.

Umbilicus, prolapsed. The umbilical cord can become trapped between the baby's head and the birth canal during labour. The condition cannot be diagnosed with certainty except by internal examination during labour. The condition is caused by occipito posterior presentation, transverse presentation or head presentation in which the size of the head is not in proportion with the size of the birth canal, as is the case with the small head or a premature baby or a constricted pelvic aperture. Because a prolapsed umbilical cord can be badly crushed during labour it is potentially dangerous to the child, causing oxygen shortage and therefore possibly brain damage. To lessen the risk, the child should be delivered by Caesarean section.

Uraemia. Complex of symptoms causes by accumulation of waste products in the blood normally excreted with the urine, usually the result of kidney failure, or disturbances in the body's salt or water content. Accumulated waste products are stored in the body or try to leave it by other means, thus causing disorders of the alimentary canal such as nausea, vomiting and diarrhoea, a smell of ammonia on the breath and yellowish grey, severely itching skin. General symptoms such as listlessness and fatigue are caused by reduced intake of nutrition and anaemia. There may also be thirst, muscular contractor and complaints caused by high blood pressure such as headache and oedema. Severe uraemia can result in coma, epileptic convulsions and blindness, and can be fatal.

Treatment is directed at removing the cause of the reduced kidney function. The production of waste products can be limited by a reduced protein diet. If the cause cannot be treated or the condition is severe, an artificial kidney (dialysis) may be used; persistent severe impairment of kidney function may require a kidney transplant.

Urethra, stricture of. A condition which can seriously restrict the flow of urine from the bladder. It occurs in various forms, congenitally most frequently in boys. Another form is caused by urethritis or damage to the urethra by the passage of small kidney stones or by foreign bodies such as hairpins, which children may insert in play. In men over the age of 40 the condition is usually caused by an enlarged prostate. Urination is difficult, which may result in urinary retention, in which some urine remains in the bladder, increasing the likelihood of cystitis and bladder stones. Treatment is by stretching the urethra; if the prostate is enlarged the section causing the obstruction can be removed by an operation via the urethra.

Urethritis. Inflammation of the urethra, the tube that carries urine from the bladder. A distinction is usually made between inflammation caused by gonorrhoea and the normal form, which is more common; in 25 per cent of such cases no cause can be found (non-specific urethritis, NSU). Almost all forms can be

transmitted by sexual intercourse. The condiition is often associated with cystitis, and causes smarting during urination and
an increased desire to do so. The urine often contains blood or
pus, and urethral discharge may occur; any discharge should
be examined to establish the cause of the inflammation and to
ascertain which antibiotics to prescibe. At the same time information should be sought about sexual contacts, both to establish a possible source and to prevent passing on the infection.
Any sexual partners should be treated at the same time.

Urinary disorders. Abnormalities in the quantity and or composition of the urine. Normally, 1 to 2 litres of urine are produced
daily. When less than 100 ml are produced, the condition is
known as anuria. Low urination can also be the consequence
of urine retention. Frequent urination is usually the result of
cystitis. Abnormally high urine production occurs in diabetes,
chromic kidney failure, the recovery phase of tubule necrosis,
and in other conditions.

Urination, difficult. Inability to urinate normally. Difficulty in
emptying the bladder may arise from sclerosis of the neck of
the bladder, a congenital stricture in the urethra, or narrowing
of the urethra, such as often occurs in elderly men with an
enlarged prostate. Urine is passed in a thin, weak stream and
this requires much time and effort, often with subsequent
dribbling. Apart from narrowing of the urethra, another cause
can be external pressure on the urethra. In women, this often
results for prolapse of the bladder or pregnancy. A swollen
pelvis or bladder can also be the cause. In a number of spinal
cord disorders, the nerve paths to the bladder are imparted, and
in consequence it can be difficult or impossible to empty the
bladder. When there is difficulty in passing urine, some urine
frequently remains in the bladder (urine retention). A bladder
stone can suddenly close the neck of the bladder during
urination, and this is accompanied by considerable pain.

Urticaria (nettlerash) Itchy skin condition consisting of pink raised
patches (urticae), which can occur suddenly; they disappear
within a few days. Some people get nettlerash after eating

certain foods, notoriously strawberries and chocolate, and some medicines can cause it.

The condition can also accompany certain infections, both bacterial and viral, or worm infestation. There are also numerous other causes, some of them unknown.

Treatment in the first place is by avoiding contact with the substance that causes the condition. Because this is not always possible, and because the cause is sometimes unknown, the doctor often has to resort to treating the symptoms with anti-histamine tablets, to block the effect of histamine, which causes the symptoms. Soothing ointments may also be prescribed.

Urticaria is also used to describe the condition for which scrofula is the usual medical term. This is also an itchy skin condition, occurring predominantly in children. The skin of arms and legs is covered with tiny pimples, often with a little blister on top.

The cause is usually an allergic reaction to insect bites, particularly those of dog or cat fleas. The condition occurs above all in the late summer and autumn. The child tends to scratch the itchy spots and the wounds thus caused are prone to bacteria infection and thus also to impetigo.

Treatment is aimed at preventing infection by controlling fleas from pets.

Uterine myoma. Benign tumour of muscle fibres in the wall of the womb. Uterine myomas usually occur in the muscular wall of the uterus itself (intramural), but they may also be located below the layer of mucous membrane (submucous) or below the capsule on the outside edge (subserous). The muyoma grows in the direction of least resistance and is effectively encapsulated by surrounding tissue. The size of the tumour can vary between a few milimetres and the dimensions of a small football. Sometimes more than one myoma occurs at one. Myomas grow under the influence of oestrogens, therefore do not occur before puberty. A uterine myoma usually becomes smaller after the menopause, and no new myomas then arise. They can increase in size during the first half of pregnancy. Uterine myomas may cause discomfort, but need not necessarily do so; this depends on size and location. Uterine myomas are often discovered by chance. When the myoma is below the layer of mucous membrane, lengthy and copious menstruation can occur because the uterus can no longer contract so well. Anaemia can then

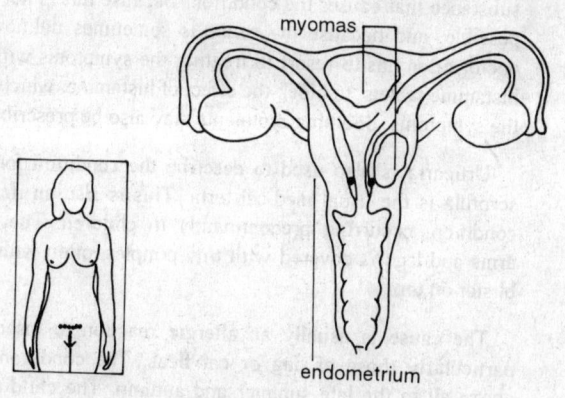

Myomas can cause irregular growth of the endometrium and menstrual difficulties.

arise. A uterine myoma does not in itself cause pain, but if the uterus attempts to expel a myoma from the cavity, this can lead to intense cramp. Complications are unusual, and malignant degeneration is extremely uncommon. A uterine myoma can sometimes die if it grows quickly and there is an insufficient supply of blood (during pregnancy or when it turns on its own axis). A large uterine myoma can also lead to complications of presentation: the foetus may enter an abnormal position because of the lack of space. On internal examination the presence of a uterine myoma is detected as a lumpy mass. It is sometimes necessary to perform a laparoscopy in order to be certain.

Uterine Polyp. Benign protrusion of mucous membrane inside the womb, sometimes large enough to protrude through the cervix.

Polyps cause a watery discharge containing blood, sometimes bleeding during intercourse (so-called contact bleeding), also excessive menstrual flow and painful menstruation, because the womb tries to eject the polyp. Polyps protruding from the neck of the womb can be 'twisted off in hospital. A polyp that has been removed is usually sent for microscopic examination. Uterine polyps are generally removed under anaesthetic by a gynaecologist. In young girls a particular form of cancer resembling a polyp can occur, and a careful distinction must be made between the two conditions.

Uterus, disorders of. The uterus (womb) can be affected by many disorders, not all of which cause discomfort. A congenital deformity of the womb causes difficulty only if it prevents pregnancy or makes it difficult to fit an intra-uterine device (coil). The same is true of uterine myoma or polyp, which cause pain, pressure or excessive menstrual flow only if they become very

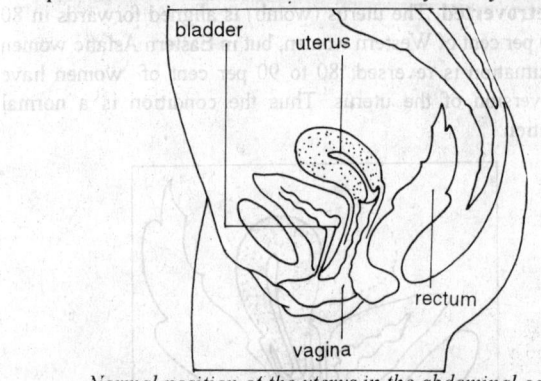

Normal position of the uterus in the abdominal cavity.

large. Prolapse of the uterus can cause discomfort, but many women suppress the fact and delay consulting a doctor. They may complain of fatigue and dizziness, then find these to be symptoms of anaemia caused by excessive menstrual flow resulting from a disorder of the womb. Itching or vaginal discharge can also be the reason for consulting the doctor; they are symptoms of a uterine polyp and infection. Cancer of the endometrium (womb lining) and cervical cancer start to cause discomfort at a late stage. All this suggests that women should undergo regular check-ups, particularly smear tests. Some uterine conditions can be treated by the family doctor; others are the province of a gynaecologist or team of specialists.

Uterus, prolapsed. Condition in which the uterus (womb) hangs too low in the vagina, or sometimes protrudes from it, particularly after the menopause, and often connected with an earlier difficult childbirth. The prolapsed womb can also pull on the bladder, causing bladder, complaints. Prolapse gives a heavy feeling in the lower abdomen, and risk of bladder infection is increased. It is caused by stretching of the ligaments which support the womb and stackening of the pelvic muscles. It can be prevented by care during childbirth, post-natal muscular exercise and avoiding excessive weight.

Uterus, retroverted. The uterus (womb) is aligned forwards in 80 to 90 per cent of Western women, but in Eastern Asiatic women the situation is reversed; 80 to 90 per cent of women have retroversion of the uterus. Thus the condition is a normal variation.

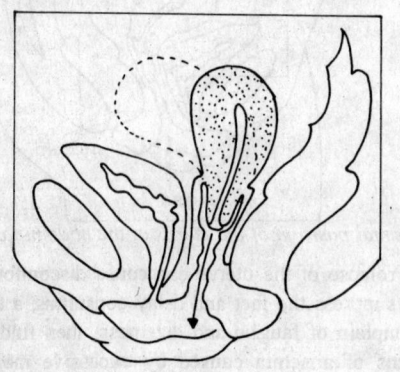

Slack muscles and ligaments allow the uterus to protrude into the vagina in uterine prolapse

V

Vaccination. The word derives from L vacca=cow, and was introduced by the English physician, Edward Jenner, who discovered and publicized the technique for preventing smallpox by vaccination with a less virulent strain of the same virus which he knew as cowpox. The cowpox virus antigens caused appropriate cells in the immune defence system to form antibodies and to prepare themselves by increasing their number so that if the smallpox virus itself should appear, it could be attacked and destroyed.

When the French chemist, Louis Pasteur, developed a protection against rabies three-quarters of a century later, he suggested that it be called a vaccination in honour of Jenner although it had nothing to do with cowpox or cows. Properly, Pasteur's inoculum of dead rabies bacteria should have been called an inoculation. Similarly, all the shots now available to protect us against *cholera, diphtheria, German measles, measles, poliomyelitis, tetanus, typhoid fever, whooping cough, yellow fever* and other diseases work with the same organic machinery as does vaccination. These inoculations are now almost universally known as vaccinations, moreover.

Vagina, Atrophy of. Shrinkage of the mucous membrane lining of the vagina. After the menopause the oestrogen production of the ovaries decreases. All the internal sexual organs become smaller and the layer of mucous membrane in the vagina becomes thinner. If the ovaries are removed or irradiated, the same occurs because no oestrogens are produced. The reduced layer of mucous membrane can cause smarting and lead to pain during sexual intercourse. The membrane bleeds easily and likelihood of infection is increased. Discharge, itching and sometimes loss of blood occur if infection sets in. An internal examination should be carried out in such cases, because these are also symptoms of cancer of the uterus or cervix. Atrophy of the tissue around the neck of the bladder can result in the symptoms of cystitis. Vaginal atrophy after the menopause is treated by applying oestrogen cream to the vaginal mucous membrane. Oestrogen tablets may also be prescribed. In addition to the usual side-effects of oestrogens, menstruation begins again if the womb has not been removed. If irradiation or removal of both ovaries is the cause of vaginal atrophy, the sudden shortage of oestrogens is compensated for with oestrogen tablets. These are often combined with progesterone, the other hormone normally produced by the ovaries.

Vagina, disorders of. In rare cases the vagina is missing altogether; this condition is usually accompanied by various congenital disorders. Congenital cysts occur regularly in the wall of the vagina and are harmless. A septum can also occur in the vagina. Sometimes the hymen is rigid and has no opening, preventing the passage of menstrual blood. Such disorders do not usually come to light until puberty. Some of them can be remedied by surgery. Abnormalities within the vagina usually occur later. The commonest is vaginitis, usually accompanied by vaginal discharge and itching of the vulva. After the menopause, the mucous membrane can become thin and dry (vaginal atrophy) causing discomfort. Benign vaginal tumours occur rarely, and cancer of the vagina more rarely still. When the vaginal wall becomes too weak, the bladder and rectum can protrude into the vagina (cystocele and enterocele). This mainly occurs after several difficult childbirths. Prolapse of the womb can also occur because the pelvic floor muscles have slackened. It is then difficult to retain the urine. This condition may be remedied by means of a pessary, but sometimes an operation is necessary.

Vagina, tumour of. Vaginal tumours are rare, and usually benign, as in Gartner's cysts, small cavities full of liquid in the wall of the vagina. There is often more than one such cavity and only rarely do they cause discomfort. Others cysts can be formed by sebum and sweat glands in the lower end of the vagina. Sometimes a cyst forms as a result of endometriosis. Such cysts are painful during menstruation because blood accumulates in the cavity. They often occur in scar tissue, and are removed if they cause discomfort. Warts (condylomata accuminata) are the consequence of viral infection and can arise in the event of protrcted discharge. They disappear after treatment with podophyllin or silver nitrate; they can also be frozen off. Fibroids are small benign tumours in the vagina which should be submitted to laboratory tests after removal. Malignant tumours in the vagina occur only very rarely. The initial symptoms are painless loss of blood, or an odorous discharge, with pain at a later stage. Cancer of the vagina requires extensive surgery. Women whose mothers used diethylstilbestrol (DES) during pregnancy are more prone to benign, and sometimes also malignant, disorders of the gland tissue of vagina and cervix, and should undergo regular checks.

Vaginal discharge. The sexually mature vagina is kept moist by a discharge that originates from the vaginal wall and the cervix; its quantity and thickness vary with the menstrual cycle. A large quantity of clear mucus is produced during ovulation and discharge also increases before menstruation. In the vagina there are bacteria which form lactic acid and ensure that the vaginal fluid is acidic, a means of protection against vaginal infections. The discharge increases when blood supply to the vagina increases during sexual excitement and pregnancy. The quantity and acidity of the discharge both decrease after the menopause. Any unusual conditions in the vagina can alter the nature of the discharge. Soap, vaginal douches and the like may irritate the vagina and kill off acid-forming bacteria, which increases the likelihood of infection. An ill-fitting pessary or forgotten tampon can also lead to an abnormal discharge. Young girls may insert foreign bodies into the vagina when playing. The most common reason for abnormal discharge is vaginal infection. Infections of the cervix (gonorrhoea and genital herpes) also cause abnormal discharge. Erosion of the cervix, or a polyp, results in reduced discharge without demonstrable infection. A complete examination should be carried out if the discharge is protracted, especially if blood is also being lost. A smear test is most useful. Treatment of the discharge depends on the cause.

Vaginismus. Involuntary contraction of the muscles around the opening of the vagina which prevent penetration by the penis during intercourse, often leading to frustrations and loss of libido.

Some women are able to find satisfaction in other sexual activities and attain orgasm. There are various causes, such as fear of sexual intercourse because of an unpleasant occurrence in the past (such as rape), an upbringing in which sex is regarded as sinful, or a physical abnormality in which vatomos,is occurs in order to prevent pain.

Vaginitis. Infection of the vaginal mucous membrane. One of the first symptoms is increased secretion and a white discharge, together with itching and smarting. The nature of the secretion, the colour, the smell if any, and the density, help to determine the cause of the inflammation. Diagnosis is by vaginal examination with a speculum and microscopic examination of the secretion. The most frequent causes of vaginal inflammation are infections such as candidiasis, chlamydia or trichomonas. Infection with the fungus *Candida albicans* leads to a thick, creamy, whitish-yellow secretion with itching. The labia are frequently red and swollen. Fungus infection can occur during pregnancy, when the patient is on the pill, in diabetes and when antibiotics are used. Treatment is by means of fungicides in vaginal tablets, creams or tampons. The application of yoghurt-soaked tampons can also help. The sexual partner must usually be treated as well. A condom should be used in sexual intercourse for some time. A greenish, foamy secretion with a fish-like odour is an indication of a trichmonas infection. The infection is usually transmitted by sexual intercourse, but this need not necessarily be so. Treatment is usually by means of an antibiotic drug. The partner is treated at the same time, and condoms should be used in sexual intercourse to avoid the disease passing to and fro between the partners. Vaginal inflammation is not caused only by infections. Vaginal atrophy or washing the genitals with soap can cause reddening and smarting of the vaginal wall as well as vaginal secretion.

Varicocele. Abnormality of the blood vessels which drain the testis, a kind of varicose vein, nearly always occurring on the left side. The cause is increased pressure in the veins below the testicle, particularly when the patient is standing up. The patient often does not notice the variocele but sometimes suffers from a heavy feeling in the affected half of the scrotum, and a certain amount of pain.

Varicose veins. Abnormally dilated and tortuous veins, usually occurring in the legs. A vein can dilate if blood pressure increases, for example because the valves in the vein are not functioning properly, or because flow of blood out of the vein is restricted. The original condition is also important : some people have leg veins with naturally less rigid walls. Varicose veins are more likely to occur in pregnancy if the patient has a job involving standing or is overweight. Varicose veins of the leg look like twisted blue cables under the skin. The legs feel tired and heavy, to a lesser extent when they are moved. There is often no clear link between the severity of the condition and the extent of the varicose veins. Three principal treatments are possible. Elastic support stockings close the veins by pressure and reduce discomfort, a simple but effective method particularly recommended in mild cases or during pregnancy. Treatment by injection involves the introduction of an irritant into the veins, causing the wall to become inflamed and the varicose vein to shrivel and close. Alternatively the veins may be completely removed by surgery.

Venereal diseases. Contagious diseases transmitted by sexual contact, also known as sexually transmitted diseases. Most involve inflammation of the skin and mucous membranes. Besides well-known disorders such as syphillis and gonorrhoea there are many others now known to fall into this category, such as genital herpes, or conditions like lymphogranuloma venereum and granuloma inguinale. Disorders such as AIDS and hepatitis B can also be transmitted sexually, but are not usually classified as venereal diseases. Veneral diseases are not only transmitted by penis-vagina contact, but also by anal intercourse, contact of mouth with genitals or anus, mouth-to-mouth kissing or contact of mouth or genitals with infected skin. Symptoms of venereal disease are not always restricted to the genital organs. Treatment should begin as soon as possible to prevent further spread through the body. The likelihood of catching a venereal disease is greatest between the ages of 15 and 30, because people in this group have the most varied contacts. Venereal disease cannot be prevented by innoculation or similar methods. Wearing a condom gives some protection. The only other thing that can be done is to pay careful attention to possible symptoms in oneself and one's partner, such as discharge, ulcers, cuts or swellings. A doctor should be consulted if there is the slighest doubt. Women are more likely to suffer from venereal disease without being aware of it, and thus women with many sexual contacts are advised to undergo regular ckecks. Treatment, often also of the sexual partner(s), is usually with antibiotics. Sexual intercourse should be avoided until recovery is complete.

Ventricular septal defect. Hole in the septum between the heart's ventricles. Ventricular septum defect is a congenital heart disorder; only in exceptional cases does it occur spontaneously, for example after a heart attack in which part of the septum dies. The consequence of a congenital ventricular septum defect is that blood flows from the left ventricle (where blood pressure is high) to the right ventricle (where the pressure is much lower). This causes pressure to rise in the right ventricle, and thus also in the blood vessels of the lungs. The seriousness of the symptoms depends on the size of the defect: a small hole causes little or no discomfort but a large one may be accompanied by retarded growth, shortness of breath rapid tiring and pneumonia. In a number of cases, minor defects heal of their own accord after a few years, so that treatment is not necessary. A heart operation to close the opening is carried out if the defect does not appear to be healing spontaneously or if the hole is large. In the latter case, it is preferable to carry out the operation within a few months of birth.

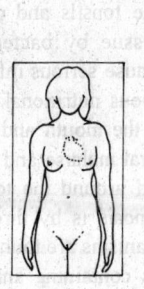
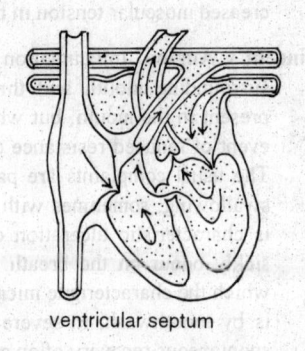

ventricular septum

A hole in the ventricular septum causes mixing of oxygen-rich and carbon dioxide-rich blood in the right ventricle because pressure is higher on the left than the right.

Vertebral disc disorders. Conditions relating to the elastic discs of cartilage between the spinal vertebrae. The spinal column derives its flexibility from these discs. These disorders are frequently accompanied by vertebral conditions. They usually lead to a restriction in the mobility of the spinal column and are often combined with pain. The best-known vertebral disc condition is dorsal hernia (slipped disc). In this condition, the softer core of the disc protrudes into the spinal canal, and as a result pressure is applied to the nerves. This leads to pain, and loss of function can arise. Hernia occurs mainly between the lowest lumbar vertebrae and is usually caused by placing an undue load on the spinal column, specifically the vertebral discs. Surgery is often required.

Vertigo. Collective name for a number of sensations of movement, dizziness or a feeling of lightheadedness. The sensation can be of spinning or falling away, and is caused by disorders of the inner ear, of the eighth cranial nerve (which carries stimuli from the auditory organs and the organs of balance), the brain

stem or the cerebellum. The condition can also be caused by
the use of certain medicines, disturbing one's centre of balance; lightness of the head is also associated with headaches,
concussion, dyplopia, low blood pressure and anaemia. Increased muscular tension in the neck may be a direct cause.

Vincent's Angina. Inflammation of the tonsils and often also of
surrounding mouth and throat tissue by bacteria normally
present in the mouth, but which cause serious infection in the
event of reduced resistance or serious nutritional deficiencies.
The usual complaints are pain in the mouth and difficulty in
swallowing, sometimes with general malaise and fever. There
is characteristic ulceration on and around the tonsils, and a
sickly odour on the breath. Diagnosis is by throat swab on
which the characteristic micro-organisms are found. Treatment
is by mouthwash, in severe cases containing antibiotics, but
spontaneous recovery often occurs.

Virilism. Appearance of male external sexual characteristics in a
girl or woman. This   takes place under the influence of male
sex   hormones (androgens).   The clitoris becomes enlarged,
and hair distribution resembles a man's (hirsutism), with hair
on the chest and face. The voice deepens, the breasts either do
not develop or become smaller, and menstruation does not occur.
A female baby with excess androgens can look just like a boy
at birth. The clitoris looks like a penis and the labia may have
shrunk. This may happen if the mother is taking medication
containing androgens or if the baby girl has a disorder of the
adrenal cortex. The production of androgens in the adrenal
cortex is then increased because of the absence of an enzyme
(congenital adrenogenital syndrome). When the disorder is
contracted at a later date it is known as the acquired
adrenogenital syndrome. The cause is then usually an androgen-
producing tumour in the adrenal cortex. In an enzyme disorder
treatment consists of hormone therapy. Any tumour (benign or
malignant) is removed. Treatment causes most signs of virilism
to disappear, although male hair distribution and an enlarged
clitoris often remain. Cosmetic removal of the hair, and

correction of clitoris size by plastic surgery, are both possible.

Virus. An organism consisting of genetic material in the form of either DNA, like most plants and animals, or RNA (see chromosome, gene), usually wrapped in a rigid coat of protein and possibly other chemicals. Viruses are the smallest known infectious agents, passing through the pores of filters which will trap bacteria. However, all known viruses contain a substance, usually a protein, either in the coat or associated with the genetic material which acts as an antigen.

Viruses cannot reproduce themselves and in that sense, are not living. In order to reproduce themselves, they must invade a cell. Once inside, the viral coat dissolves, the genetic material takes over the cell's reproductive machinery and reproduces copies of the virus. When they leave the cell, it is destroyed, causing the most common symptoms of any viral disease. However, some viruses, for example the A.I.D.S. virus and herpes, also deposit their genetic material inside the genetic material of the cell. It remains within the healthy cell for some indeterminate period of time, whereupon it emerges from the cell's nucleus and acts like any other reproducing virus.

Vitamin. A nutrient like protein, carbohydrate or fat, but required only in minute quantities. In the absence of vitamins, however, the body develops severe symptoms and eventually dies. We cannot synthesize vitamins but vitamin D can be made by skin cells in sunlight.

Vitamins A, D, E and K cannot be dissolved in water but are fat-soluble. It is possible to take in too much of these vitamins because they are stored in fat cells within the body. Excesses of vitamins A and D can be poisonous; for example, an excess of vitamin D causes *anorexia, hypertension, kidney failure, nausea* and *vomiting*.

Vitaminsa B and C are water-soluble. Amounts excess to requirements are removed in the urine.

The great majority of people eating Western diets obtain

adequate supplies of vitamins from their food. During pregnancy and early growth and after wasting illnesses, supplements may be recommended by the doctor, but self-dosage with vitamins is at best a waste of money and in the case of the fat-soluble vitamins, a threat to health.

Vitamin deficiency. Because vitamins do not form a coherent group, this term includes a number of different conditions with different causes. Vitamin deficiency is by no means always the consequence of inadequate nutrition. Two principal groups should be distinguished: vitamins soluble in fat (A, D, E and K) and those soluble in water (the rest). The following is a brief list of some important vitamins, the food source, and the cause and consequences of a possible shortage.

Vitamin A occurs in animal products (cod liver oil, milk, butter) but mainly in vegetable matter (greens, root vegetables, tomatoes) in the form of a pro-vitamin, carotene, which the body can convert. Shortage occur through poor diet. Symptoms in mild cases are night blindness and dry skin. Severe cases cause serious eye conditions (conjunctival dehydration) and skin conditions (dehydration and callus formation).

Vitamin B consists of 4 groups (vitamin B complex): vitamins B_1 B_2 B_6 and B_{12}. Vitamin B_1 (thiamine) occurs in liver, kidneys, wholemeal grain products, pulses and lean meat. Shortage causes beriberi, with characteristic nerve inflammation and heart weakness. Vitamin B_2 is contained in among other things milk and other dairy produce, green vegetables and liver. Deficiency causes cracks in the corner of the mouth, ophthalmia, excessive sensitivity to light (photophobia), sometimes oedema and difficulties in swallowing.

Shortage of vitamin B_6 causes no distinct symptoms, but anaemia can occur in certain cases. Vitamin B_{12} is found in meat, milk and liver. Deficiency usually occurs through shortage of 'intrinsic factor' in the gastrointestinal tract, which means that the vitamin cannot be absorbed. This condition, known as pernicious anaemia, often occurs after stomach resection, because the vitamin is produced there. Treatment is by injection; oral treatment is effective only in association with intrinsic factor. Vitamin C occurs in fresh vegetables, citrus fruits, tomatoes and paprika. Deficiency is almost always the result of an inadequate diet. Symptoms include bleeding of the gums and poor healing of wounds. Severe cases lead to scurvy.

Vitamin D is contained in liver; egg yolks and butter. At the same time it can be formed in the skin by the effect of UV light. The vitamin is needed for calcium metabolism, and is thus involved in bone formation. Vitamin D deficiency causes poor calcification of growing bones in children, and thus rickets, with thickening at the growth discs and crooked bones, especially at the end of the calf bones. In adults decalcification sets in, and thus weakening of the bones (osteomalacia), with additional muscular weakness and listlessness. Treatment is by considerable quantities of the vitamin. There is much propaganda for giving children vitamin D in the winter, but the usefulness of this procedure is still in some doubt.

Vitamin E is found in green vegetables and wheat germ. It seems to be a material essential in the body's mebabolic system, but the symptoms typical of a shortage are not known; anaemia in children is a possible one. Vitamin K occurs in many natural products, and is also produced by bacterial synthesis in the gastrointestinal tract. Deficiency caused by poor diet is rare, but damage to the gastrointestinal tract, by antibiotics, for example, can cause a shortage. Vitamin K is involved in the coagulation of blood, and shortage can lead to difficulties in coagulation. Treatment is by the administration of vitamin K.

Vitiligo. Disorder in the pigmentation of the skin. Pale patches occur as a result of the disappearance of pigment, mainly on the backs of the hands, the face and around the anus. They can form over a period of a few days. The spots are usually only noticed when they are already some centimetres in size or very numerous. The condition can spread over the whole body. There is no pigment at all in the affected areas, so the skin looks snow-white, which is particularly striking in dark-skinned people. Vitiligo is caused by the disappearance of all the pigment cells in the affected areas, most commonly as a result of the formation of antibodies against pigment cells in an autoimmune disease. There is no effective treatment. Spontaneous recovery of the affected patches has been observed in a minority of cases, but the process takes a long time. If the condition does not heal spontaneously or does not heal quickly enough, the only possible solution is to camouflage the most serious patches by using a skin-coloured masking cream.

Volvulus. Twisting of an intestinal loop around its own axis, possible because practically all the small intestine and a small section of the large intestine (sigmoid colon) are attached to the abdominal wall only by a single membrane containing the intestinal blood vessels. Volvulus is a very rare condition, usually congenital in children; volvulus of the sigmoid usually occurs in older patients as a result of constipation. It is common among some tropical peoples.

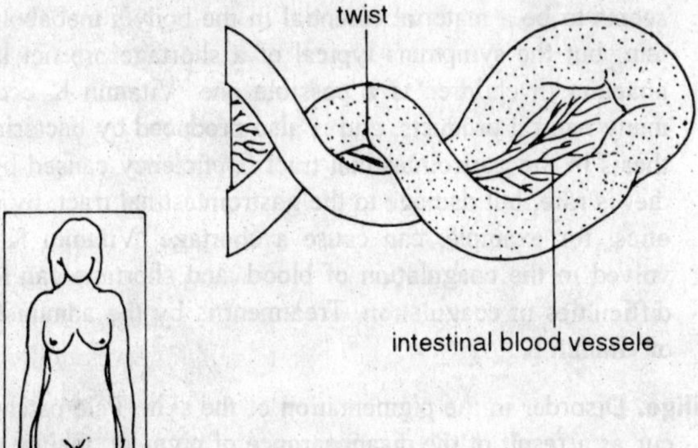

twist

intestinal blood vessele

In volvulus the intestine twists on its axis around the membrane containing the blood vessels, which are trapped, thus threatening tissue death.

The clinical picture is the same as that of acute intestinal obstruction (ileus), causing eventual death of the affected section.

On examination, it is not essential to distinguish between this and other causes of obstruction: possible obstruction is grounds enough to institute surgery, because of the risk of intestinal perforation and shock. If the affected section is dead it must be removed; in other cases it is sufficient to twist the volvulus back and secure it, so that the condition cannot recur.

Vomiting. Forcible regurgitation of the contents of the stomach. Vomiting has various causes, which may lie in the abdomen, the stomach and intestine itself, the brain, or other disorders that stimulate the brain. Psychological causes should not be ruled out. Brain conditions can cause vomiting by stimulating the vomiting centres in the brain, and this can also occur as a result of pressure on the brain, brain tumours, migraine, meningitis and disorders of the organs of balance. Psychological causes are reaction to stress, a disgusting sight or smell, or conditions such as anorexia nervosa or bulimia. Associated factors and symptoms must be examined to establish the cause.

Von recklinghausen's disease. Hereditary disorder involving characteristic skin patches and tumours of the skin and nerve tissue. In the nerves of spinal cord and brain, neurinomas and neurofibromas usually occur; they are normally both benign tumours. They can be very close to the spinal cord or brain, and cause discomfort by pressure. On rare occasions neurofibromas can become malignant. Tumours can also occur in or on the skin at the extremities of nerves that run into the skin. The resulting patches are coffee-coloured, and there can be massive local connective tissue formation with resultant enlargement of parts of the body. Bone tumours and crookedness of the spinal column (scoliosis) may also occur.

W

Walking difficulties. There can be various causes because walking involves a complex interplay of many muscles and joints-not only the leg muscles, but the muscles of the buttocks, back, trunk and arms. Disorders occur in diseases of the central nervous system and disorders of the nerves serving the hips and legs in particular. Abnormalities also occur as a result of muscle, tendon and joint conditions, and malformation of the legs and feet. The scissor walk, in which the legs cross, occurs in spasticity. Paralysis of the calf nerve, which is responsible for pulling the foot forward, causes the foot to point down when the knee is raised; thus people with this condition have to raise the knee particularly high in order to be able to walk. If the shin nerve fails, the calf muscle is not stimulated, and the foot points upwards, so that the front of the foot does not touch the ground. If the calf muscle and Achilles tendon waste, the rear of the sole of the foot is raised and the toes bend beneath it; the foot is aligned with the lower leg and the patient has to walk on his toes.

Wart (verruca) Benign swelling of the skin that results from a virus infection.

Warts measure anything from a few millimetres to a few centimetres in diameter and can occur anywhere on the skin. A wart begins as a small excrescence of the upper layers of the skin. This swelling expands into a small growth typically resembling a miniature cauliflower. The wart is then covered with a thick horny layer so that it has a greyish-brown colour and feels hard. Warts occur mainly on the fingers and backs of the hands of schoolchildren. They also occur on the soles of the feet. Warts in the region of the beard or near the sex organs can look quite different. Warts usually disappear of their own accord after a few years, and treatment is therefore not really necessary. For cosmetic reasons or to avoid contagion, they can be treated by being frozen with liquid nitrogen or by being cut out. Another method is to dissolve the horny layer with a special solvent or an oinment.

Weak contractions. Contractions which are not powerful enough during childbirth to dilate the womb and bring labour to completion. Contractions can be weak from the outset, but they can also become weaker after an initially good start.

Factors that may lead to weak contractions are: a uterus which has been overstretched as a sesult of a multiple pregnancy or hydramnios, abnormal presentation and a full bladder. The contraction often becomes stronger after emptying the bladder.

If the uterus is not being dilated, the contractions may weaken because of physical and psychological exchaustion. In this situation it is important to know whether there are any specific labour problems. If this is so it is usually necessary to bring about delivery by artificial means, such as a Caesarean section.

Weight loss. Persistent decrease in body weight, in medical terms including only abnormal cases, not justifiable or desired weight loss. Weight loss can have many causes, by no means all of them dependent on conditions of the digestive organs. The conditions which may be responsible can be divided into two principal groups: malabsorption (difficulties in absorbing food and disorders of the intestinal mucous membrane) and malignant tumours of the intestines. Weight loss is characteristic of both groups, and in a number of cases the first symptom. Very occasionally conditions such as tapeworm can cause weight loss, as can metabolic disorders such as diabetes mellitus and hyperthyroidism, and malignant tumours in other organs can also be responsible. Psychological causes (anorexia nervosa) are also possible.

Well's disease (leptospirosis) Disease caused by the bacterium *Leptospira icterohaemorrhagiae*, which usually infects rodents living in the wild. This disease occurs the world over. The animals, mainly brown rats, excrete the bacterium along with their urine. The bacteria survive better in fresh water and the chances of humans becoming infected are greatest in a damp area where there is mud and puddles. The number of cases of Weil's disease has been decreasing over the last few years; because the bacteria cannot survive the increasing levels of pollution being found in water. The disorder occurs mainly in people who swim or fall into infected water, and among sewerage workers and farm labourers.

Welder's eye. Acute inflammation of the cornea as a result of exposure of the eye to ultraviolet radiation, as from arc welding and UV lamps ; a form of ophthalmia. It causes damage to the cornea which becomes evident 6 to 12 hours after exposure to the UV light. The eye can also be exposed to excessive quantities of UV light in winter sports, causing a similar condition.

Welder's eye is extremely painful. The eye is red, weeps and is excessively sensitive to light; small pinpoint damaged spots can be seen on the cornea. The condition is easily prevented by wearing protective goggles. No special treatment is needed other than painkillers; the cornea should have recovered within 24 hours.

Wernicke's disease. Serious disorder caused by a deficiency of vitamin B_1. It leads to haemorrhages in the brain stem and certain low-lying parts of the brain. The chief cause is failure to eat properly because of alcoholism.

The symptoms include diplopia (double vision) caused by paralysis of the eye muscles and by pressure on the eyeballs. Other characteristic features are trembling hands and disorders in co-ordination, with resultant difficulty in walking and other actions of all kinds. Vitamin B_1 deficiency also often causes widespread neuropathy, and Korsakoff's syndrome with amnesia occurs. There are usually disturbances of consciousness. Serious B_1 deficiency can endanger life in the long term.

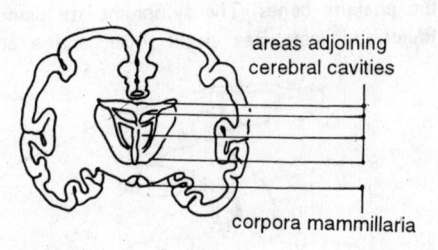

areas adjoining
cerebral cavities

corpora mammillaria

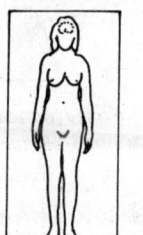

In Wernicke's disease tiny haemorrhages in certain parts of the brain cause loss of memory and difficulties in walking.

Other disturbances can alo arise from alcohol abuse, such as cirrhosis of the liver, anaemia and epilepsy. The diagnosis is made on the basis of the characteristic clinical picture, and the blood is also examined (with the vitamins being determined as well). Treatment consists of remaining in bed, stopping drinking alcohol, and a diet rich in calories and vitamins with injections of vitamin B_1 in large doses. The visual problems and the disturbances in co-ordination usually disappear within a few days under treatment. Neuropathy and Korsakoff's syndrome may continue for many months.

Whiplash injury. Damage to the spine in the nape of the neck, caused when it is suddenly jerked forwards and backwards. It happens usually when the rear of a car in which the victim is travelling is hit in a collision. Injury to the spinal cord occurs in a few cases, with mild symptoms of concussion or contusion of the spinal cord. Concussion of the brain may also occur.

Whitlow. Inflammation of the subcutaneous tissue of the fingers which has spread to the bone of the phalanx. The condition is caused by bacteria (usually in association with an inadequately disinfected cut) which establish themselves in the marrow of the phalanx bones. The symptoms are pain in the affected finger and sometimes slight fever, and a complete cure is

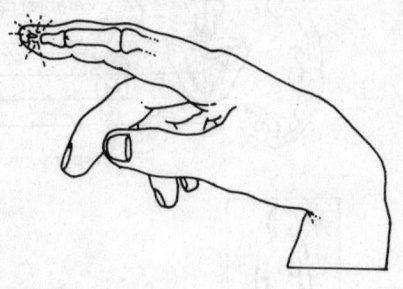

Whitlows are caused by a deep, infected wound of the periosteum; this inflammation of the terminal phalanx of the finger can cause its loss.

usually possible with antibiotics. It is advisable to rest the hand by searing a sling during treatment. The symptoms disappear within days, but the treatment should be continued at length to avoid recurrence of the inflammation. If treatment is not effective, for example because the becteria are resistant to the prescribed antibiotic, complications may occur; this is also the case if the condition remains completely untreated. The most important complications are destruction of the affected phalanx or the formation of a fistula. In the latter case pus from the inflamed phalanx can reach the surface of the skin, reducing pressure on the finger; inflammation becomes chronic. If the phalanx is destroyed, the finger usually stiffens, as the other bones grow together.

Whooping Cough (pertussis) Bacterial infection of the air passages that occurs in childhood. The incubation period lasts for one to two weeks, and the condition is highly contagious, particularly in the early stages. There is no danger of infection after the sixth week, even though the cough may persist. Infection is possible only by direct contact. The symptoms follow three stages: inflammation of the upper air passages (catarrhal stage) in the form of a cold in the nose, sneezing, coughing and a slight fever. The child is listless and irritable. The symptoms worsen after a few days to a week, and the cough takes on the typical whooping cough character (convulsive stage). The coughing comes in fits of short coughs followed by a shrieking inhalation and expectoration of mucus. The tongue protrudes, and the face becomes red or purplish-blue; this is the first real indication of whooping cough. Infants often do not have the shrieking inhalation, but they are very constricted, and the cough is often associated with vomiting. The child does not seem particularly ill between the attacks, although their frequency can be wearing and in very young babies it is the exhaustion caused by the coughing that makes the disease dangerous. The recovery stage begins after four to six weeks, when the attacks diminish in frequency and violence. Diagnosis is usually certain from the characteristic cough; in less obvious cases it can be confirmed by blood tests and saliva cultures.

Wilm's tumour. A highly malignant tumour of the kidney, occurring mainly in children under the age of five.

There is usually a marked swelling of the abdomen. No specific symptoms may occur until late stage, apart from reduction in appetite and loss of weight. Complaints arising at a later stage are stomach ache and the presence of blood in the urine (haematuria). The tumours are usually not detected unless there are metastases, which most often occur in the lungs or the bones.

Wilson's disease. Inherited condition of the body's copper metabolism. This mineral accumulates in the liver, the brain and elsewhere.

The disease usually manifests itself between the 10th and 30th year of life as a result of an enlarged and functionally disturbed liver, and abnormalities in the central nervous system. In the latter case, paralysis or psychiatric disorders may be the consequence. The characteristic feature is the formation of a greyish-green ring (consisting of copper granules) around the iris of the eyes. Treatment with a substance that assists the elimination of copper from the body (penicillamin) can prevent damage to the liver or the nervous system. This treatment must be continued for the rest of the patient's life.

Withdrawal symptoms. Symptoms that occur in giving up a substance (such as alcohol or drugs) to which the patient is addicted. In the case of morphine-type addiction withdrawal symptoms are particularly severe. Sweating, low blood pressure, abdominal cramps, diarrhoea, anxiety, tension, trembling and epileptic symptoms occur. Withdrawal symptoms from other addictions are usually less severe, and restricted to a feeling of tension, restlessness and irritability. A specific symptom is delirium tremens in chronic alcoholism. Withdrawal symptoms fro cocaine and amphetamines include drowsiness, fatigue hunger and depression. If the addiction occurred because of psychological problems, these recur with renewed vigour when the habitis kicked, thus causing a physical and psychological vicious circle.

Worms. Millions of people are infested by parasitic worms, although in Europe parasitic infestations are mainly introduced by tourists and foreign employees.

There are three major groups of worms: roundworms, flukes and tapeworms. Males and females occur only in round worms; the other worms are hermaphroditic, having both male and female sex organs.

The part of the world where a particular worm occurs depends on the conditions the eggs need in order to develop into larvae. Some require a damp, warm soil in order to be able to develop into a larva which can enter a new host (examples are hookworm and strongyloids). These worms are often encountered in the tropics. The flagellate worm and the eel-worm are not so demanding; they occur the world over. The commonest worm in Britain is the threadworm.

Some larvae can develop only inside another animal species (such as mosquitoes and snails). This species then functions as an intermediate host (vector), while the human is the main host in which the full-grown worms live. This applies for example to thread-worms and schistosomes.

Humans are infested by the larvae or eggs which either penetrate the skin or are eaten with food. In some types of worms, infection occurs through the bite of a mosquito.

Not all infested people fall ill; they become carriers of the worms. The question of whether they fall ill is determined by, among other factors, the number of worms, their size and the resistance of the person infested. Infestation can be detected from the eggs or larvae in the stools.

The clinical pictures which arise are very varied and depend on the type of worm. Treatment is usually by medication.

X

Xerophthalmia. Abnormality in which the secretion of tears is reduced, so that the cornea and conjunctiva of the eye are not sufficiently moist.

The symptoms consist of irritation, pain and redness. The absence of lachrymal fluid may cause damage to the cornea. In one form of xerophthalmia, Shigren's syndrome, the secretion of fluid by all the mucous membranes of the eye, nose and mouth is also disturbed. Apart from dry eyes, the mouth and nose are therefore also dry. This is an autoimmune disease. A less common cause is a paralysis of the facial nerve or vitamin A deficiency.

Xerophthalmia is detected by examining the eye and measuring lachrymal secretion (Schirmer test). Filter papers are used to measure the quantity of lachrymal fluid formed over a set period. With Shigren's syndrome, therapy consists of administering eye drops in order to moisten the eye; vitamin B complex is sometimes useful. The syndrome cannot be cured. If a deficiency of vitamin A is the cause, this vitamin can be administered.

Y

Yellow fever. Viral infection prevalent in Central and South America and Africa, which occurs in Western Europe in travellers from these areas. The virus multiplies in the Aedes mosquito, and for the rest of its life span the insect can transmit the virus to man.

There are two kinds of yellow fever, the urban variety, in which human beings carry the virus, and the jungle type in which a mosquito transmits the virus to man from infected monkeys.

The virus causes damage to the liver and the kidneys and the onset of the disease is marked by high fever (40°C), severe headaches, back and muscular pain. The mucous membranes of the mouth, nose and throat swell and become painful; the patient complains of pains in the stomach, nausea and vomiting. Jaundice sets in after a few days, with slight skin, stomach and intestinal bleeding, and the kidneys are also affected. In mild cases the conditions begins to improve after a few days, in serious ones a second period of fever begins, after an initial improvement. At this stage organ failure and death are not uncommon.

In cases of suspected yellow fever the patient must be admitted to hospital. There is no specific therapy, all the doctor can do is ease the symptoms. Travellers to areas where yellow fever is endemic must be vaccinated, and such immunization will provide one or two years' protection against the disease.

Z

Zinc undecenoate (Zinc undecylenate) An antifungal with uses similar to those of undecenoic acid.

Zollinger-Ellison syndrome. A rare disorder in which there is excessive secretion of gastric juice due to high levels of circulating gastrin, which is produced by a pancreatic tumour (benign or malignant) or an enlarged pancreas. The high levels of stomach acid cause peptic ulcers, which may be multiple, in unusual sites (e.g. jejunum), or which quickly recur after vagotomy or partial gastrectomy. Treatment with a histamine-blocking drug, by removal of the tumour (if benign), or by total gastrectomy is usually effective.

Zona pellucida. The thick membrane that develops around the mammalian oocyte within the ovarian follicle. It is penetrated by at least one spermatozoon at fertilization and persists around the blastocyst until it reaches the womb.

Zonulolysis. The dissolution of the suspensory ligament of the lens of the eye (the zonule of Zinn), which facilitates removal of the lens in cases of cataract. A small quantity of a solution of an enzyme that dissolves the zonule without damaging other parts of the eye is injected behind the iris a minute or two before the lens is removed.

Zoonosis. An infectious disease of animals that can be transmitted to man. See anthrax, brucellosis, catscratch fever, cowpox, glanders, Q fever, Rift Valley fever, rabies, ratbite fever, toxoplasmosis, tularaemia, typhus.

Zoophilism. The sexual attraction to animals, which may be menifest in stroking and fondling or in sexual intercourse (*bestiality*).

Zymotic disease. An old name for a contagious disease, which was formerly thought to develop within the body following infection in a process similar to the fermentation and growth of yeast.